FUNDAMENTALS OF
Cardiovascular Pharmacology

G. D. JOHNSTON
Department of Therapeutics and Pharmacology
The Queen's University of Belfast
Northern Ireland

JOHN WILEY & SONS, LTD
Chichester · New York · Weinheim · Brisbane · Singapore · Toronto

Other Wiley Editorial Offices

John Wiley & Sons, Inc., 605 Third Avenue,
New York, NY 10158-0012, USA

VCH Verlagsgesellschaft mbH, Pappelallee 3,
D-69469 Weinheim, Germany

Jacaranda Wiley Ltd, 33 Park Road, Milton,
Queensland 4064, Australia

John Wiley & Sons (Asia) Pte Ltd, 2 Clementi Loop #02-01,
Jin Xing Distripark, Singapore 129809

John Wiley & Sons (Canada) Ltd, 22 Worcester Road,
Rexdale, Ontario M9W 1L1, Canada

Library of Congress Cataloging-in-Publication Data

Johnston. G. D.
    Fundamentals of cardiovascular pharmacology/G. D. Johnston.
        p.   cm.
    Includes bibliographical references and index.
    ISBN 0-471-97013-1 (alk. paper)
    ISBN 0-471-85471-9 (pbk)
    1. Cardiovascular agents.   2. Cardiovascular system–Diseases–
Chemotherapy.   I. Title.
    [DNLM: 1. Cardiovascular Agents–pharmacology.   2. Cardiovascular
Diseases–drug therapy.   3. Cardiovascular System–drug effects.
WG 166 J72f 1999]
RM345.J64 1999
615'.71–dc21
DNLM/DLC   99-14219
for Library of Congress   CIP

British Library Cataloguing in Publication Data

A catalogue record for this book is available from the British Library

ISBN 0 471 97013 1 (cloth)
ISBN 0 471 85471 9 (pbk)

Typeset in 10/12pt Palatino by Dobbie Typesetting Ltd, Tavistock, Devon
Printed and bound in Great Britain by Biddles Ltd, Guildford, Surrey
This book is printed on acid-free paper responsibly manufactured from sustainable forestry, for
which at least two trees are planted for each one used for paper production.

Dedication

This book is dedicated to:

Barbara

Gail   David

Kate   Peggy

Contents

Preface

Most authors of moderate-sized textbooks on drug therapy either confine themselves to a discussion of basic pharmacology and say little about drug selection and clinical use, or concentrate on practical therapeutics and largely ignore the pharmacological background. In this book I have attempted to combine practical clinical utility with information on the principles of cardiovascular pharmacology on which clinical practice rests. This book therefore is primarily aimed at young postgraduate students who require information on pharmacology and drug therapeutics. It is also suitable for undergraduates who require extra information on cardiovascular drug therapy.

Few areas of medical practice have developed more in the last 30 years than has the drug treatment of cardiovascular disease, and few areas of therapeutic practice can claim to have a healthier evidence-base than the subject of cardiovascular pharmacology. However, in view of the rapid mushrooming of medical knowledge, it has become increasingly difficult for doctors, including specialists, to keep up-to-date with the changes in drug therapy. This volume represents a distillation of what I perceive to be important pharmacological principles and current information on the use of drugs in cardiovascular medicine. The opinions expressed may not always include all the available evidence and some areas may be omitted altogether. I can certainly claim to have more than a passing knowledge of the drug treatment of most cardiovascular diseases but have more limited knowledge on the topics of cardiovascular physiology and receptor pharmacology outlined in the first two chapters. These cannot be considered comprehensive reviews of the topics under discussion but they hopefully provide a useful background for the understanding of drug action covered in the later sections of the book.

I would like to thank a number of people who have assisted me in the preparation of this book. I am particularly grateful to my secretary Doris Howe for her dedication, industry and tolerance during the preparation of this manuscript, and without whose help the volume would never have been completed. I am also greatly indebted to Adrienne Ruddock, who transformed my sketches into useful and well constructed diagrams, and to Briegeen Girvin, for her assistance with literature searches and the provision of source material. I also greatly appreciated the help and support of Janie Curtis and Monica Twine of John Wiley & Sons during the various stages of the book's development. Finally, I would like to thank all members of the Department of Therapeutics and Pharmacology for their help in preparing the manuscript, and my family for their perseverance during the many hours I spent at home writing the book.

This is my first attempt to produce a single-author textbook and any errors in the text are entirely my responsibility. Any corrections and criticisms by the reader would be much appreciated. Unlike Professor Brian Leonard, who produced the first volume in this series, *Fundamentals of Psychopharmacology*, I did not have the privilege of researching and writing the text in the tranquillity of the Radcliffe Science Library in Magdalen College, Oxford. I hope the text has not suffered too much as a result.

G. D. Johnston

Introduction

Effective drugs to treat heart disease have been available for over two thousand years. The first account of the value of the digitalis leaf was by the Roman historian Tacitus (59–120 AD) who related the fate of the king of Parthia an independent kingdom in northern Iran flourishing between 250 BC and 224 AD. The son attempted to kill his father, who was at death's door with dropsy, by administering a mixture containing leaves of the purple foxglove. To his great annoyance his father recovered and appeared as though he would live for a long time. The son eventually had him strangled. Digitalis, usually in the purified form of digoxin or digitoxin, remains an effective drug for the treatment of heart failure accompanied by fast atrial fibrillation. There has been considerable debate since the turn of the century, however, as to whether digitalis is effective when heart failure is accompanied by regular sinus rhythm. This question was finally resolved 2 years ago with the publication of the DIG (Digitalis Investigation Group) study which demonstrated a reduction in the number of hospital admissions due to heart failure, no overall effect on mortality, and a tendency to increase sudden death probably due to arrhythmias.

Not only have a number of important drugs withstood the test of time—notably organic nitrates to treat angina pectoris, narcotic analgesics to relieve the pain of acute myocardial infarction, and digitalis to treat heart failure—a number of older drugs have been used for new indications and their modes of action have been elucidated. The discovery of the important regulatory properties of prostaglandins and the metabolic pathway involved in their biosynthesis shed considerable light on the antiplatelet effects of aspirin, and the identification of endothelium-derived relaxing factor as nitric oxide provided a clearer explanation of the cellular mode of action of the organic nitrates.

An important watershed occurred with the development of the beta adrenoceptor antagonists by Sir James Black in the 1960s. For the first time in the treatment of cardiovascular disease it was possible to design specific molecules based on the chemical structures of endogenous hormones which would interact with receptors and alter important physiological processes. These techniques have been refined and developed further to produce a variety of new and important cardiovascular drugs which act as receptor antagonists (angiotensin II and endothelin antagonists), enzyme inhibitors (angiotensin converting enzyme and HMG co-enzyme A reductase inhibitors) and ion channel modulators (sodium channel blockers and potassium channel activators).

The purpose of this book is to provide medical undergraduates, postgraduate students, practising physicians and cardiologists with an overview of the principles and practice underlying the subject of cardiovascular pharmacology. Chapter 1 provides a short introduction to some of the concepts used to describe aspects of cardiovascular function which are important for the understanding of drug action on the heart and vasculature. Chapter 2 summarises the cellular modes of action of the principal cardiovascular drugs, and Chapter 3 documents the factors which influence the concentration of drugs at their sites of action and the intensity of their effects as a function of time. The remaining chapters deal with the drug treatment of individual diseases. In each chapter the author discusses the pathophysiology of the condition, the evidence for drug treatment, and the clinical pharmacology of the agents used to treat the disease. By using this book I hope that the reader will gain some insight into the subject of cardiovascular drug therapy, and will develop a growing interest in this exciting and expanding area of drug therapy.

1 Principles of Cardiovascular Function

Blood flow and capillary diffusion

The cardiovascular system represents a network for moving a variety of chemicals from one location within the body to another. Its design and organisation permit the use of a very small volume of circulating fluid to control the chemical composition of the total internal environment. The processes of flow and diffusion and the physical principles governing these processes are fundamental to the understanding of cardiovascular function.

Factors influencing blood flow

Figure 1.1 represents a segment of a blood vessel within the body with a length (L) an internal radius (R) through which blood flows (Q). Fluid flows along the vessel when the pressures P_1 and P_0 are unequal, i.e. when there is a pressure difference (ΔP) between the ends of the blood vessel. Vascular resistance is a measure of how difficult it is to make fluid flow through the vessel or how much pressure difference is required to permit fluid to flow. The relationship between flow, pressure and resistance is described in the basic flow equation:

$$\text{Flow} = \frac{\text{pressure difference}}{\text{resistance}}$$

or

$$Q = \Delta P / R$$

where Q is the flow rate (volume/time), ΔP the pressure difference (mmHg) and R the resistance to flow (mmHg×time/volume). The basic flow equation can be applied to a single tube or to networks of tubes such as the vascular bed of an organ or the entire vascular system. Although pressure is best expressed as units of force per unit area, it is customary to express pressures in millimetres of mercury. For example, mean arterial

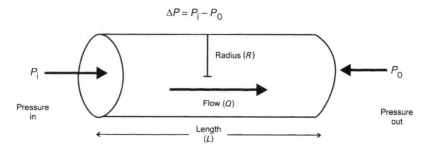

Figure 1.1.   Factors influencing flow through a blood vessel.

blood pressure is said to be 100 mmHg because it is the same as the pressure at the bottom of a mercury column 100 mm high. All cardiovascular pressures are expressed relative to atmospheric pressure which is approximately 760 mmHg at ground level.

From the work of the French physician, Poiseuille, who performed experiments on fluid flow through small glass capillary tubes, the following equation was derived incorporating the radius and length of the tube and the viscosity of the fluid flowing through it.

$$R = \frac{8L\eta}{\pi r^4}$$

where r is the internal radius of the tube, L the length of the tube and η the viscosity of the fluid. The clinical importance of this relationship in cardiovascular physiology and pharmacology is that resistance to flow is inversely proportional to the fourth power of internal radius of the tube. For example, halving the radius will increase the resistance by sixteenfold. It is not surprising, therefore, that most effective antihypertensive drugs dilate peripheral blood vessels to lower blood pressure. Poiseuille's equation ideally applies to uniform flow with a homogeneous fluid in a rigid tube. Although all these conditions do not apply to blood vessels within the body, the approximation is close enough to permit useful conclusions to be drawn from the relationship.

The concept of bulk transport

The movement of substances between organs within the cardiovascular system can be described by the concept of bulk transport. The rate at which a substance (X) is transported by this process depends solely on the concentration of the substance in the blood and the blood flow to that organ.

$$\text{Transport rate} = \text{flow} \times \text{concentration}$$

$$\dot{X} = \dot{Q}[X]$$

where $\dot{X}$ is the rate of transport of X, Q the blood flow and $[X]$ the concentration of X in the blood. This principle can be extended to determine the rate at which a tissue utilises a substance by considering the transport rate to and from a tissue. This relationship is known as the Fick principle and can be formally stated as follows:

$$\dot{X}_{TC} = \dot{Q}[(X)_a - (X)_b]$$

where X_{TC} is the transcapillary efflux rate of X, Q the blood flow, $(X)_a$ the arterial concentration and $(X)_b$ the venous concentration. This relationship is commonly used to determine cardiac output and organ blood flow.

Solute diffusion across capillaries

Diffusion across capillaries depends on four principal factors: the concentration difference, the surface area for the exchange, the diffusion distance and the permeability of the capillary wall to the diffusing substance. Capillary beds permit large quantities of materials to enter and leave the blood because of their large surface area and the presence of very narrow capillary walls. Each capillary consists of a single layer of endothelial cells joined to form a tube. The ease with which a particular solute crosses the capillary wall is known as the capillary permeability. Lipid soluble substances such as oxygen and carbon dioxide cross the capillary wall easily while small polar compounds move through water-filled channels or pores (Figure 1.2) at variable rates.

The permeability varies substantially from organ to organ so that brain capillaries have few pores while renal capillaries and those in fluid-producing glands are more leaky.

Fluid movement across capillaries

The movement of fluid between the capillary and interstitial compartments is important in a variety of physiological and pathophysiological situations, including the maintenance of circulating blood volume, saliva, sweat, urine production and tissue oedema formation. The movement of fluid out of the capillaries is known as filtration while the movement into capillaries is referred to as reabsorption. Fluid flows through transcapillary channels in response to pressure differences between the interstitial and intracapillary

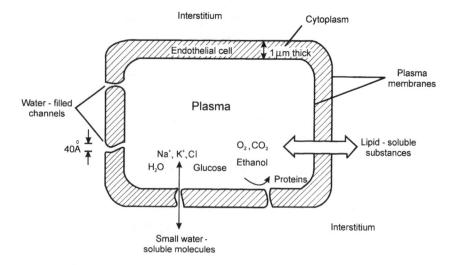

Figure 1.2.   Transcapillary solute diffusion pathways.

fluids, although hydrostatic and osmotic pressures also play important roles (Figure 1.3).

The hydrostatic pressure inside capillaries, which is about 25 mmHg, is the driving force which permits blood to return to the right side of the heart from the capillary bed. This pressure is also responsible for the flow of fluid through the transcapillary pores into the interstitium where the hydrostatic pressure is close to zero. This is counterbalanced by the osmotic pressure which results from the fact that the protein content of plasma is higher than in interstitial fluid. Fluid is therefore drawn into the capillaries. Oedema (increased amounts of interstitial fluid) can therefore result from increased hydrostatic pressure (congestive cardiac failure and gravity-dependent oedema) or reduced osmotic pressure (reduced plasma proteins seen in chronic liver and renal disease).

Cardiac muscle—electrical and mechanical properties

Electrical properties of cardiac cells

Skeletal and cardiac muscle contraction is initiated by rapid changes in voltage which occur on the cell membrane. These changes are known as the action potential. Cardiac muscle cells, however, differ from skeletal muscle cells in three important ways which promote synchronous rhythmic excitation of the heart: the action potentials can be self-generating, they can be conducted from cell to cell, and are usually of long duration.

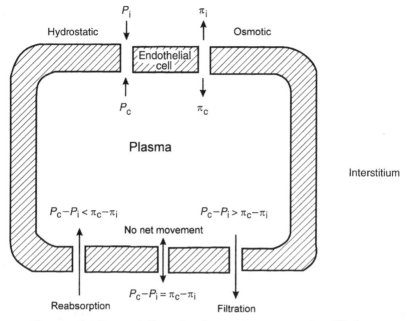

Figure 1.3.   Factors influencing the movement across capillaries.

All cells have an electrical potential across their membranes because the ionic concentrations of the cytoplasm are different from those of the interstitium, and ions diffusing down concentration gradients across semipermeable membranes produce electrical gradients. The ions principally involved are sodium, potassium and calcium. Sodium and calcium concentrations are greater in the interstitial fluid than inside the cell while potassium ions have greater intracellular concentrations. The diffusion of ions across the cell membrane occurs through channels which are composed of protein molecules which span the membrane and are specific for individual ions. Channels exist in various configurations that are either open, closed or inactivated. The permeability of the membrane to a specific ion is directly related to the number of channels that are open for that ion at a given instant.

Figure 1.4 represents a cell in which the concentration of potassium is greater inside the cell than outside and the membrane is only permeable to potassium. As a result of the concentration difference, K^+ ions will diffuse out of the cell. Negative charges such as protein anions are unable to leave the cell. As K^+ ions move out of the cell, the inside of the cell becomes more electrically negative and the interstitium more electrically positive. This creates an electrical potential across the membrane which attracts the K^+

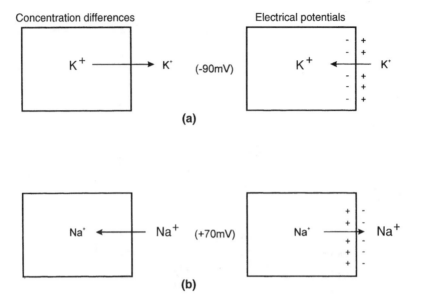

Figure 1.4. The electrochemical basis of membrane potentials. (a) Cells which are permeable to potassium only; (b) cells which are permeable to sodium only.

back into the cell. When the electrical forces tending to pull K^+ into the cell exactly balance the concentration forces tending to drive it out, the resulting potential is known as the potassium equilibrium potential. Assuming an intracellular concentration of 145 mmol/l and an extracellular concentration of 4 mmol/l this potential is approximately −90 mV.

Using the same reasoning for Na^+ which has higher concentrations outside the cell than inside, the sodium equilibrium potential is approximately +70 mV with an extracellular concentration of 140 mmol/l and an intracellular concentration of 10 mmol/l. Cell membranes, however, are not permeable to one ion only, and when the membrane is permeable to sodium and potassium the membrane potential lies between the equilibrium potential of the two ions. By the same reasoning, if the membrane is more permeable to K^+ than Na^+, the closer the membrane potential will be to −90 mV and if the membrane is more permeable to Na^+, the closer the membrane potential will be to +70 mV. Calcium ions also participate in the cardiac action potential. Like Na^+, Ca^{2+} has a higher concentration outside cells than inside. The equilibrium potential for Ca^{2+} is approximately 100 mV and the cell membrane tends to become more positive on the inside when the membrane becomes more permeable to Ca^{2+}. Under resting conditions, most heart muscle cells have membrane potentials close to the potassium equilibrium potential. Electrical and concentration gradients favour Na$^+$ entry into the resting cell. However, sodium entry under resting conditions is maintained by low permeability to sodium and an active sodium pump which exudes Na$^+$ from the cell.

The generation of cardiac cell action potentials

The action potentials of cells from different regions of the heart have different characteristics. Some cells within the specialised conducting system spontaneously initiate action potentials while standard myocardial cells do not, except under special conditions. Cardiac pacemaker-type cells demonstrate fast response action potentials while ordinary cardiac muscle cells have slow response action potentials (Figure 1.5). Fast response action potentials have a rapid depolarisation period (phase 0), with a significant overshoot, a rapid reversal of the overshoot potential (phase 1), a long plateau (phase 2) and a repolarisation (phase 3) to a stable and large negative resting membrane potential (phase 4). In contrast, the slow response action potentials have a slower initial depolarisation phase, a smaller amplitude overshoot, a shorter and less stable plateau phase and a repolarisation to a relatively unstable resting potential (Figure 1.5).

The membrane potential of any cell at a particular instant depends on the relative permeability of the cell membrane to specific ions. Cardiac action potentials occur as a result of transient changes in the ionic permeability of the cell membrane which are triggered by an initial depolarisation. Phase 0

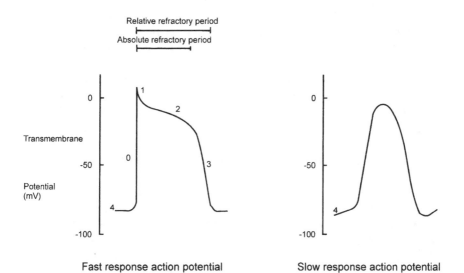

Figure 1.5. The time course of membrane potentials during 'fast' and 'slow' response action potentials.

of the cardiac action potential occurs as a result of a sudden increase in the permeability to sodium ions. This is known as the fast inward sodium current and rapidly moves the membrane potential towards the sodium equilibrium potential. This short-lived period is followed by slower phase characterised by an increase in the membrane's permeability to calcium and a decrease in the permeability to potassium accompanied by a slow increase in sodium permeability (see Figure 8.3). These slow inward currents prolong the depolarised state of the membrane and produce the plateau or phase 2 of the cardiac action potential. The initial fast inward sodium current is small in cells which have slow response action potential and the slow rise is principally due to an inward movement of calcium ions. In both types of cell, the membrane is repolarised (phase 3) to its original resting potential as the permeability to potassium increases and the permeabilities to sodium and calcium return to their resting values. These changes are referred to as the delayed outward currents.

The role of ion channels in controlling membrane potential

The graded changes in membrane permeability which occur with each action potential are brought about by altered permeability of ion channels located on the cell membrane. These channels are either fully open or closed and there are no graded states of partial opening. The factor which is graded, however, is the percentage of time during which the channel is open, i.e. its probability of being open. Certain types of channel are referred to as voltage-gated channels or voltage-operated channels since their probability of being open depends on the membrane potential. Other types of channels known as ligand-gated channels or receptor-operated channels are activated by certain neurotransmitters and other specific signal molecules. Some of the voltage-gated channels respond to sudden changes, but not to slow changes in membrane potential. To explain this, it has been postulated that these channels have two independently operating gates—an activation gate and an inactivation gate, both of which must be open for the channel as a whole to open. Each gate responds to different voltages and time courses. In the resting state with a membrane potential of about $-80\,\mathrm{mV}$, the m (activation) gate of the fast Na^+ channel is closed but its h (inactivation) gate is open (see Figure 8.2). As the membrane is rapidly depolarised, the sodium channels become strongly activated to facilitate the rapid flux of sodium ions. This is because the m gate opens more quickly than the h gate closes. Phase 0 is therefore the period when the m gates rapidly open but the h gates have not had time to close. Phase 1 represents the period when the h gates start to close. The initial membrane depolarisation also activates the (d) gate of the Ca^{2+} channel to open after a brief delay permitting the slow inward current of Ca^{2+} ions which assist in maintaining the depolarisation during the plateau phase of the action potential. Eventually repolarisation occurs by a delayed inactivation of the Ca^{2+} channel (closure of the f gates) and an opening of K^+ channels. The h gate remains closed during the remaining period of the action potential. This effectively inactivates the Na^+ channel and contributes to the long refractory period which lasts until the end of phase 3. With repolarisation complete both gates of the sodium channel return to their original position and the channels are now ready to be reactivated by the next depolarisation.

In the slow response action potential which is seen in non-specialised cardiac muscle cells, the strong activation of the fast Na^+ channel is not observed. Slow depolarisation allows the h gates to close as the activating m gates are opening. The depolarisation beyond the threshold is slow and is principally due to the influx of Ca^{2+} through the slow calcium channels (Figure 1.6).

While certain areas of the heart have a predominance of cells with fast-type action potentials and some areas have a predominance of slow-type action potentials, all cardiac cells can exhibit both types depending on how rapidly they depolarise to the threshold potential.

Rapid depolarisation to the threshold potential is frequently forced on a cell by the occurrence of an action potential in an adjacent cell. Persistent depolarisation of the resting membrane, which can occur with high extracellular potassium concentrations, can inactivate the fast channels by closing the h gates without affecting the calcium channels. In these circumstances all cardiac cell action potentials exhibit slow-type action potentials.

Propagation of cardiac action potentials

Action potentials are propagated from cell to cell because adjacent heart muscle cells have regions called gap junctions through which internal electrical current passes easily. The speed at which an action potential travels through a region of cardiac tissue is called the conduction velocity. This varies considerably in different areas of the heart and is directly related to the diameter of the muscle fibre. In the atrioventricular node the cells have a small diameter and conduction is much slower than in the large-diameter cells in the Purkinje rapid conduction system. Conduction velocity is also related to the intensity of the local depolarising currents which are in turn directly determined by the rate of rise of the action potential. In general, rapid depolarisation favours rapid conduction. Other factors which alter conduction velocity in different areas of the heart are variations in the electrical properties of the gap junctions, cytoplasm and cell membranes.

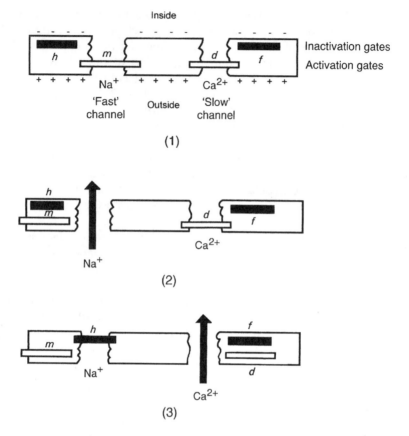

Figure 1.6. (1) Resting cell membrane; (2) sodium entry during fast response action potential; (3) calcium entry during fast and slow response action potential.

The action potential initiated by the sino-atrial node cell initially spreads progressively through the atrial wall (Figure 1.7). As demonstrated in Figure 1.7, the action potentials in the atrioventricular node are similar in shape to those of the sino-atrial node and both types of cell have faster spontaneous resting depolarisation than any other cardiac cells in the conducting system. As a result of the small size of the nodal cells and the slow rate of rise of their action potentials, the cardiac impulse travels very slowly through the atrioventricular nodal tissue. This delays the transfer of the cardiac impulse from the atria to the ventricles and, therefore, the ventricles contract slightly after the atria in each cardiac cycle. Conduction is most rapid in the Purkinje system because of sharply rising action potentials and the large diameter of the cardiac cells. Cardiac impulses,

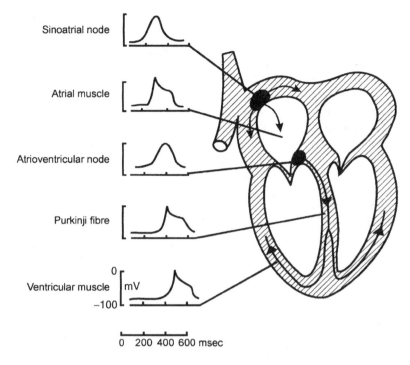

Figure 1.7. Single-cell voltage recordings at different sites along the cardiac conduction system.

therefore, arrive almost spontaneously to cells throughout the left and right ventricles.

Control of heart rate

If there were no external influences on the sino-atrial node, the heart rate would be about 100 beats/minute. This is known as the intrinsic heart rate. Outside factors do, however, have a major effect on heart rate. The two most important mechanisms are the sympathetic and parasympathetic divisions of the autonomic nervous system and the fibres from both systems terminate in the sino-atrial node. Stimulation of parasympathetic fibres which travel to the heart through the vagus nerve release acetylcholine at the sino-atrial node. Acetylcholine increases the permeability of the resting membrane to K^+ and decreases the diastolic permeability to Na^+. This has two principal effects on the resting potential of cardiac pacemaker cells; the resting membrane potential moves closer to the K^+ equilibrium potential and slows the rate of spontaneous depolarisation of the resting membrane. Overall, the time required for the resting membrane to depolarise to the threshold level is prolonged and the heart rate slows. Since there is continuous activity of cardiac parasympathetic nerves at rest, the resting heart rate of a healthy adult is usually between 60 and 70 beats/minute. Sympathetic nerves release noradrenaline which increases the inward currents carried by Na^+ and Ca^{2+} during the period of diastole. These changes increase heart rate by increasing the rate of diastolic depolarisation. There are a number of other factors which can alter heart rate. These include temperature, atrial wall stretch and variations in ion concentration and circulating hormones. Factors that increase heart rate are said to have positive chronotropic effects and those that decrease heart rate have negative chronotropic effects. The autonomic nervous system can also influence the conduction velocity. Increased sympathetic activity increases conduction velocity (a positive chronotropic effect) and increased para-sympathetic activity decreases conduction velocity (a negative chronotropic effect). These effects are most marked at the atrioventricular node.

Excitation–contraction coupling

Muscle action potentials trigger mechanical contraction by a process known as excitation–contraction coupling. The principal effect of the process is a dramatic rise in the intracellular free Ca^{2+}. The intracellular free Ca^{2+} concentration before contraction is less than $0.1\,\mu M$, but after activation of the contractile apparatus reaches almost $100\,\mu M$. As the wave of depolarisation spreads over the muscle membrane and down the T tubules (Figure 1.8), Ca^{2+} is released from the sarcoplasmic reticulum into the intracellular fluid. The main trigger for this release appears to be the entry of calcium into the cell via the L-type calcium channels and an increase in Ca^{2+} concentration just under the sarcolemma on the surface of the cell and throughout the T-tubule system. Although the amount of Ca^{2+} that enters the cell during a single action potential is small, it is essential for triggering calcium release from the sarcoplasmic reticulum and for maintaining adequate Ca^{2+} levels in the intracellular stores. When the intracellular Ca^{2+} level is high, links called cross-bridges form between two types of filaments with the muscle cells. Sarcomere units (Figure 1.8) are jointed end to end at Z lines to form myofibrils which are present along the length of the muscle cell. Thick and thin filaments slide past each other to reduce the size of each sarcomere during contraction. Bridges form when regularly spaced myosin heads from thick filaments attach to regularly spaced sites on the action molecules in the thin filaments. In the resting state the interaction of actin and myosin is inhibited by troponin and tropomyosin. Calcium interacts

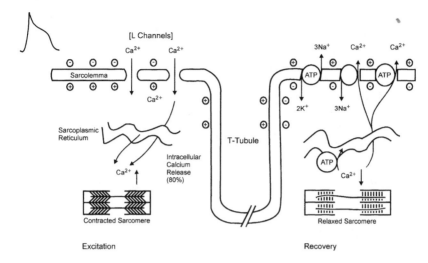

Figure 1.8. Sarcomere shortening and excitation–contraction coupling.

with troponin C to induce a change in configuration which removes the inhibition of the actin sites on the thin filament. A variety of processes participate in the reduction of intracellular Ca^{2+} to terminate the contraction. Most is actively taken up by the sarcoplasmic reticulum by the action of Ca^{2+} ATPase pumps. The remainder is extruded from the cell by the Na^+–Ca^{2+} exchanger and Ca^{2+} ATPase pumps located in the sarcolemma (Figure 1.8). Unlike excitation–contraction coupling in skeletal muscle, different intensities of actin–myosin interaction and hence contraction can result from a single action potential initiated in cardiac muscle. This seems to be dependent on variations in the amount of Ca^{2+} reaching the myofilaments and hence the number of cross-bridges activated during the muscle contraction. The duration of the cardiac muscle cell contraction is almost the same as that of the action potential. Therefore, the electrical refractory period of a cardiac muscle cell is not complete until the mechanical response is over. As a result heart muscle cells cannot be activated rapidly enough to produce tetany or prolonged muscle contraction. This is important for an organ whose function as a pump depends on intermittent contraction and relaxation.

Cardiac output and the control of stroke volume

Cardiac output is defined as the number of litres of blood pumped by the ventricles every minute and this volume is continually adjusted to meet the body's varying transport needs. Cardiac output is, therefore, the heart rate in beats per minute multiplied by the stroke volume (the amount of blood ejected from each ventricle with each beat). Rapid changes in cardiac output are mostly brought about by changes in the autonomic nervous system which can affect heart rate and stroke volume.

Control of stroke volume

Three important functional factors influence the relationship between the volume of blood within the ventricle and the volume expelled during one cardiac cycle. An increase in the ventricular volume produces an increase in the ventricular circumference and hence a lengthening of cardiac muscle cells. An increase in intraventricular pressure at a given volume results in an increase in the tension of individual cardiac muscle cells. Finally, as the ventricular volume increases, a larger force is required from each muscle cell to produce a given intraventricular pressure. This last relationship refers to the law of Laplace which states that there is a relationship between the forces within the walls of any curved fluid container and the pressure of its contents.

During diastole the progressive increases in ventricular pressure and volume combine to increase muscle tension which passively stretches the resting cardiac muscle to greater lengths along its resting length–tension curve (Figure 1.9). End diastolic pressure is referred to as ventricular preload because it sets the resting tension of the cardiac muscle fibres at the end of diastole. At the beginning of systole the ventricular muscle cell develops tension isometrically (at constant length) and intraventricular pressure rises (Figure 1.9). After the intraventricular pressure rises sufficiently to open the aortic or pulmonary valve, ventricular ejection begins as a consequence of ventricular muscle shortening. Systemic arterial pressure is often referred to as the ventricular afterload because it determines the tension that must be developed by cardiac muscle fibres before they can shorten. During systole, cardiac muscle simultaneously generates active tension and shortening. The changes in ventricular volume during ejection are determined by the degree of shortening of muscle fibres during contraction which in turn depends on the length tension–relationship of the muscle cells and the load against which they are shortening. After the aortic and pulmonary valve close the cardiac muscle cells relax isometrically. Ventricular wall tension and intraventricular pressure decrease in parallel during isovolumetric relaxation because the ventricular radius is constant throughout the final period of systole.

Preload and the Frank–Starling relationship

The Frank–Starling law, based on experimental observations, states that the heart contracts more forcefully during systole when it is filled to a greater degree during diastole. Assuming all other factors remain the same, stroke

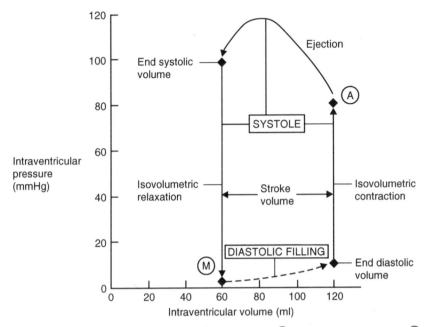

Figure 1.9. The ventricular pressure–volume cycle. (A)—Aortic valve opens. (M)— Mitral valve opens. Reproduced from Sunagawa, K., Sagawa, K., Maughan, M. L. Ventricular interaction with the vascular system in terms of pressure–volume relationships. In Yin, F. C. P., Ed. *Ventricular/Vascular Coupling*. New York: Springer Verlag GmbH & Co. KG, 1987: 210–39. Reproduced with permission.

volume will increase as cardiac filling increases. The same relationship exists for each muscle fibre within the ventricular wall (Figure 1.10). Increases in preload produce increases in stroke volume because longer initial fibre lengths greatly enhance muscle shortening. This occurs without significantly changing the final length to which the muscle shortens against a constant total load (Figure 1.10). This is not accompanied by a significant increase in the end systolic volume since the enhanced force of contraction, resulting from the larger end diastolic volume through the Frank–Starling relationship, ensures that the extra blood entering during diastole is ejected during systole.

Afterload and stroke volume

Increased afterload has a negative effect on cardiac muscle shortening provided the preload is maintained constant. This is because cardiac muscle cannot shorten beyond the length at which its peak isometric tension-generating potential is equal to the total load imposed upon it. Normally

16

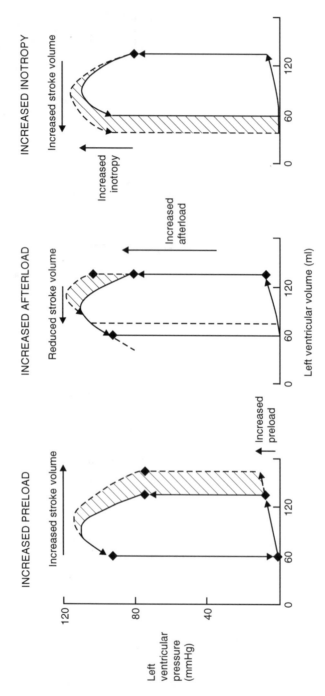

Figure 1.10. Effects of increase preload, afterload and inotropy on the ventricular pressure–volume cycle.

afterload is kept constant because arterial blood pressure is maintained within a narrow range. In conditions such as hypertension and mechanical obstruction to the outflow of the ventricle, stroke volume tends to be reduced by the changes in the pressure–volume loop (Figure 1.10). The cardiac muscle cells have reduced ability to shorten against the afterload created by these conditions. In these circumstances the end systolic volume is decreased.

Myocardial contractility and stroke volume

Inotropic agents such as noradrenaline produce an upward shift of the peak isometric length tension curve (Figure 1.10). This will result in an increase in the shortening of a muscle contracting with constant preload and afterload. Stroke volume will increase by decreasing the end systolic volume without directly influencing the end diastolic volume.

Cardiac function curves

One of the most useful ways to represent the Starling relationship is to plot cardiac output against cardiac filling pressure (Figure 1.11). Each curve demonstrates how cardiac output is changed by changes in preload if inotropic activity and heart rate are held at a constant level. The main influence on inotropic function is the activity of the sympathetic nervous system. Cardiac output increases because heart rate and inotropic activity increase. The relationship observed in patients with impaired ventricular function is also illustrated. The importance of this in patients with heart failure will be discussed later.

Factors influencing myocardial oxygen consumption

Since the heart obtains its energy requirements entirely from aerobic metabolism, myocardial oxygen consumption is directly related to myocardial energy use and hence the splitting of ATP. Basal metabolism accounts for about 25% of myocardial oxygen consumption and muscle contraction for the remaining 75%. The energy expended during the isovolumetric contraction phase of the cardiac cycle accounts for almost 50% of the total, although the heart does not perform any external work during this period. The energy required for isovolumetric contraction depends largely on the intraventricular pressure or cardiac afterload. Cardiac afterload is therefore the principal determinant of myocardial oxygen consumption, and vasodilator drugs which decrease afterload are widely used to reduce oxygen requirements in angina pectoris and congestive cardiac failure. Energy utilisation during isovolumetric contraction is directly related to wall tension and hence to preload.

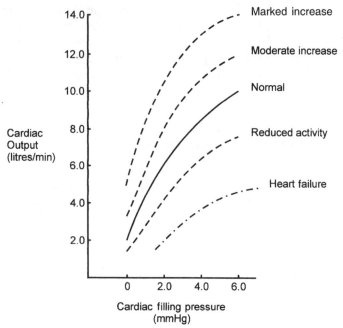

Figure 1.11. Relationship between cardiac sympathetic activity and cardiac function curves. Reproduced from *Mechanisms of contraction of normal and failing heart*. Braunwald, E., Ross, J. Sonnenblick. New England Journal of Medicine Medical Progress series. 1967, Copyright Little, Brown and Co., Published in G.B. by J. A. Churchill Ltd, London, reproduced with permission.

Reductions in preload also tend to reduce energy requirements for isovolumetric contraction.

Increasing myocardial contractility has important consequences for basal metabolism, isovolumic wall tension generation and external activity. Heart muscle uses more energy by rapidly developing a given tension and shortening by a given amount than in performing the same manœuvre more slowly. The net result is described as the energy wasting effect of increased contractility. This may help to explain why drugs which increase myocardial contractility are associated with increased mortality in patients with heart failure. Heart rate is also clearly an important determinant of myocardial oxygen consumption since the energy consumption is the product of energy cost per beat and the number of beats. In general, improving the efficiency of each cardiac contraction results in lower oxygen requirements than increasing heart rate. Drugs which increase heart rate in patients with angina pectoris tend to worsen the symptoms while greatest benefit in this condition is seen with drugs which reduce resting and exercise heart rate such as verapamil and beta adrenoceptor antagonists.

Pressure–volume relationships in the peripheral vasculature

Peripheral blood volumes

About 60% of the total circulating blood volume is contained within the veins of the body organs. This large reservoir is usually referred to as the peripheral venous pool. A second but smaller reservoir of venous blood is called the central venous pool and is contained within the large veins of the thorax and right atrium. About 20% is contained in the pulmonary system and heart chambers and the remaining 20% in the arteries (12%), arterioles (3%) and capillaries (5%). When peripheral veins constrict, blood is displaced from the peripheral venous pool and enters the central pool. An increase in the central venous volume and thus pressure increases cardiac filling. This in turn augments stroke volume through the Frank–Starling relationship.

Peripheral blood pressures

Blood pressure decreases in the consecutive parts of the arterial system as illustrated in Figure 1.12. The mean arterial pressure decreases by a small amount within the larger arteries. A substantial decrease occurs in the arterioles and the pulsation is almost completely dampened within these vessels. The mean capillary pressure is approximately 25 mmHg and continues to decrease in the venules and larger veins as blood returns to the right side of the heart. The central venous pressure is normally slightly greater than 0 mmHg.

Peripheral vascular resistance

We have previously identified the relationship between flow, pressure difference and resistance with the equation $Q = \Delta P/R$. The large decrease in pressure which occurs as blood flows through the arterioles provides the greatest resistance. This resistance is mainly affected by adjustments in the internal diameter brought about by contraction and relaxation of vascular smooth muscle. The overall resistance to flow through the entire vasculative system is called the total peripheral resistance. Since flow in the different organs is usually arranged in parallel, the vascular resistance of each organ contributes to the total peripheral resistance in the same way as an electrical circuit.

$$\frac{1}{R_{\text{total}}} = \frac{1}{R_1} + \frac{1}{R_2} \cdots + \frac{1}{R_n}$$

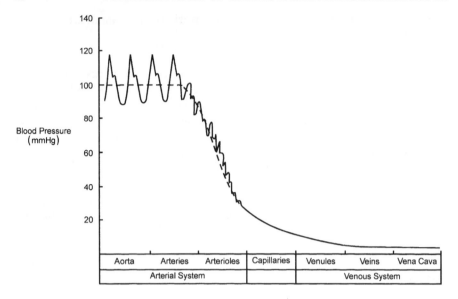

Figure 1.12. Changes in blood pressure at different sites within the circulation. Reproduced from Rowell, L. B. (1986). *Human Circulation Regulation During Physical Stress*. Oxford University Press, New York.

Vascular compliance

Although the large arteries and veins provide a small portion of the overall resistance to flow, their elastic behaviour is very important to overall cardiovascular function since they behave as reservoirs and large amounts of blood can be stored within them. The elastic properties of vessels are usually described by the term 'compliance' which describes how much the volume changes (ΔV) in response to a given change in transmural pressure (ΔP):

$$C = \frac{\Delta V}{\Delta P}$$

The elastic properties of veins are very important for the control of the venous system as a blood reservoir. Veins are much more compliant than arteries so that small changes in venous pressure cause a significant amount of blood to move in or out of the peripheral venous pool. For example, the venous pooling which occurs on assuming the upright position is counteracted by venoconstriction and reduced venous compliance. Vasodilator drugs, particularly organic nitrates, increase venous compliance and impair this response to changes in posture.

The elastic properties of arteries permit them to function as a reservoir on a beat-to-beat basis. This property of arteries has an important role in converting pulsatile flow from the heart into a steady flow through the vascular beds of systemic organs. During the early rapid phase of cardiac ejection, the arterial volume increases because blood enters the aorta more rapidly than it passes into the systemic arterioles. Therefore, part of the work done by the heart in ejecting blood is used up in stretching the elastic walls of arteries. During the latter part of the cardiac cycle, arterial volume decreases because flow out of the arteries exceeds flow into the aorta. During this time the previously stretched arterial walls recoil to shorter lengths and give up their stored energy. This energy projects the blood through the peripheral vascular beds during diastole. Decreases in arterial compliance which occur with age, hypertension, diabetes and other conditions predisposing to atherosclerosis, produce characteristic changes in the arterial pressure wave (Figure 1.13). The pulse pressure and mean arterial pressure tend to increase, the systolic upstroke is steeper and the diastolic waveform shows a reduced gradient with dampened oscillations.

Mean arterial pressure

This is one of the most commonly measured variables in cardiovascular physiology and pathology. It is the mean effective pressure that drives blood through the systemic vasculature and is described by one of the most fundamental equations in cardiovascular medicine.

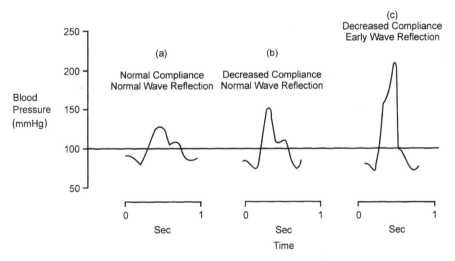

Figure 1.13. Changes in the arterial wave form associated with increases in arterial compliance.

$$BP = CO \times TPR$$

where BP is systemic blood pressure, CO is cardiac output and TPR is total peripheral resistance. Changes in mean arterial pressure can therefore only result from changes in cardiac output or total peripheral resistance. Calculating the true mean arterial pressure depends on determining the mean pressure at which the area above the pressure line is equal to the area below the pressure line (Figure 1.14). In practice usually only the systolic and diastolic pressure are known and therefore a commonly used approximation is the diastolic pressure added to one-third of the pulse pressure. This is relatively accurate for pressures within the normal range, but is less accurate in patients with higher systolic and diastolic blood pressures.

$$P_M = P_D + \tfrac{1}{3}(P_S - P_D)$$

where P_M is the mean blood pressure, P_D the diastolic blood pressure and P_S the systolic blood pressure.

Hormonal influences

Under normal circumstances hormones exert a relatively minor role in controlling vascular tone when compared with local and neural influences.

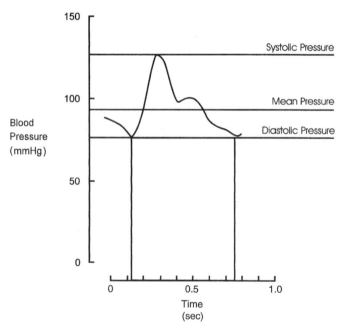

Figure 1.14. Diastolic, systolic and mean blood pressure.

During activation of the sympathetic nervous system the adrenal medulla releases adrenaline and noradrenaline into the circulation. Under normal circumstances the circulating levels of these hormones are probably too low to exert a significant effect on vascular smooth muscle. High circulating levels have important effects, however, when there is activation of the sympathetic nervous system, and in general the cardiovascular effects of high levels of circulating catecholamines parallel the direct effects of the sympathetic system. In addition to the alpha receptors which mediate vasoconstriction, arterioles in many organs have beta adrenoceptors which mediate vasodilatation. Vascular beta receptors are more sensitive to adrenaline than alpha receptors. Low levels of circulating adrenaline cause vasodilatation while higher levels produce alpha receptor mediated vasoconstriction. Vascular beta receptors are not innervated and are therefore unaffected by noradrenaline released from the sympathetic vasoconstrictor nerves.

The polypeptide hormone, anti-diuretic hormone, has vasoconstrictor properties in addition to its effects on water balance. Direct vasoconstriction occurs at very high levels of this hormone and probably only has a role in maintaining blood pressure in hypovolumic and haemorrhagic shock. The same is true of the octapeptide angiotensin II, although this hormone has an important role in regulating salt and water balance and vascular control within the kidney. It is also probably involved in the pathophysiology of essential and renal hypertension.

Vasodilator and vasoconstrictor prostaglandins, derived from arachidonic acid by the action of cyclooxygenase, are important vasoactive substances in ischaemic and inflammatory situations, but probably have a relatively minor role in the maintenance of blood flow in the normal coronary and peripheral circulation. Histamine, synthesised and stored in the secretory granules of mast cells and circulating basophils, also has a potent vasodilator effect. More important, however, is its effect on vascular permeability. This is achieved by causing separation of the junctions between endothelial cells, outward movement of tissue fluid and the formation of local oedema. Histamine is very important in a variety of pathological conditions, but like the prostaglandins has a minor role in normal cardiovascular regulation. Bradykinin and other kinins have similar actions to histamine and are about 10 times more active as vasodilators on a weight for weight basis. These agents and flow-related shear stress increase intracellular calcium levels, nitric oxide synthase production and hence the levels of nitric oxide. This small molecule diffuses into adjacent smooth muscle cells and relaxes vascular smooth muscle. Flow-related endothelial production of nitric oxide is an important factor in increasing blood supply to exercising muscle. The vascular endothelium also produces another important vasodilator substance, endothelium derived hyperpolarising factor (EDHF), and several constrictor factors, particularly endothelin 1.

Neural influences

Sympathetic vasoconstrictor fibres innervate arterioles in all systemic organs and represent the most important reflex control of the vascular system. Release of noradrenaline from the nerve endings increases vascular tone by interacting with alpha receptors on the smooth muscle cells. Most blood vessels do not receive innervation from the parasympathetic nervous system. However, nerve fibres which release acetylcholine are present in the vessels of the brain and heart, but they appear to have a minor role in the control of blood vessel tone.

Arterial pulse pressure

The arterial pulse pressure is defined as the systolic blood pressure minus the diastolic blood pressure. The two main factors defining pulse pressure are the stroke volume and arterial compliance. The pulse pressure is approximately equal to the stroke volume divided by arterial compliance:

$$P_P = \frac{SV}{C_A}$$

where P_P is the pulse pressure, SV the stroke volume and C_A the arterial compliance. Since arterial compliance decreases with age, pulse pressure increases and usually to a greater degree than mean arterial pressure. However, acute increases in pulse pressure are largely due to increases in stroke volume. Changes in total peripheral resistance have little impact on pulse pressure. Recent evidence suggests that increased pulse pressure is a more important risk factor for stroke and ischaemic heart disease than mean arterial pressure in older patients.

Coronary blood flow

Coronary blood flow is mainly regulated by local metabolic mechanisms and therefore responds rapidly and accurately to changes in myocardial oxygen consumption. The relative importance of the various factors is unclear, but adenosine released from myocardial muscle cells would appear to be a likely candidate.

During systole the forces on the outside of the coronary arteries cause them to collapse and vascular resistance increases. As a result, for a large area of the myocardium coronary flow is lower during systole than during diastole despite the fact that coronary perfusion pressure is greatest during this period (Figure 1.15). This is most marked in the left coronary artery since systolic compression is much less in the muscle of the right ventricle.

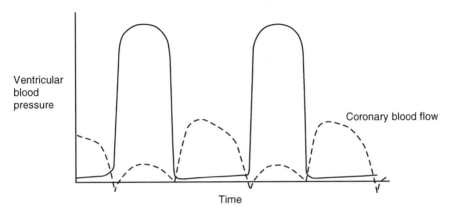

Figure 1.15. Relationship between ventricular blood pressure and coronary blood flow in the left coronary artery. Reprinted from Berne, R. M., Levy, M. P. *Cardiovascular Physiology* 5th edn. 1986: 200. St Louis by permission of the publisher CV Mosby.

Systolic compressional forces are greater in the endocardial layers of the ventricular wall than in the epicardial layers. Normally these regions can make up for reduced flow during systole by increased flow in diastole. However, when coronary blood flow is reduced, for example in coronary artery disease, the endocardial layers of the left ventricle are usually the first regions of the heart to have difficulty maintaining a flow sufficient for their metabolic needs. For this reason myocardial infarctions most frequently involve the endocardium of the left ventricle. Coronary arteries are well supplied with sympathetic nerves which normally cause vasoconstriction. However, when the activity of the sympathetic system increases, coronary blood flow tends to increase. This occurs because increased sympathetic activity increases myocardial oxygen consumption and the local metabolic vasodilator influences overwhelm the sympathetic vasoconstrictor effects.

2 Cellular Mechanisms of Cardiovascular Drug Action

Introduction

Most drugs achieve their pharmacological effect by interacting with cellular macromolecules. This interaction alters the function of the cell component and initiates a series of biochemical and physiological changes which are characteristic of the drug's action. The term "receptor" is used to describe these macromolecules, and this concept of drug action implies that most drugs do not create effects but modify existing physiological systems. Proteins form the majority of drug receptors. Important examples in cardiovascular pharmacology include receptors for catecholamines and angiotensin II, enzymes involved in metabolic and regulatory pathways such as angiotensin converting enzyme (ACE) and phosphodiesterase, and surface proteins which act as gates controlling the entry of sodium, potassium and calcium ions into cells. Cardiovascular drugs acting on receptors for endogenous regulatory ligands such as noradrenaline, angiotensin II and endothelin, are often very specific because these receptors are designed to recognise and respond selectively to individual signalling molecules. Drugs which bind to physiological receptors and produce the effects of endogenous regulatory ligands are termed agonists. For example, isoprenaline is a beta agonist which like endogenous catecholamines, increases the rate and force of cardiac contraction. Other drugs bind to receptors and prevent activity of the endogenous ligand. These compounds are known as antagonists. Propranolol, a beta adrenoceptor antagonist, blocks the action of catecholamines at the beta receptor and so reduces heart rate, inotropic function and peripheral blood flow. Some other agents are less effective than the full agonists and are referred to as partial agonists. Under certain circumstances these drugs can act as antagonists depending on the activity of the endogenous ligands. For example xamoterol, a $beta_1$ partial agonist increases inotropic activity at rest when sympathetic activity is low, but acts as a beta antagonist following exercise when sympathetic activity is high.

Structure–activity relationships and the implications for drug design

The chemical structure of a drug determines its intrinsic activity and affinity for the receptor. The relationships between drugs and receptors are usually very precise, and small modifications of the molecular configuration can result in major changes in the pharmacological properties. For example the (+) enantiomer of sotalol has class III antiarrhythmic activity and no beta adrenoceptor blocking effect, while the (−) enantiomer has beta adrenoceptor antagonist activity and no additional antiarrhythmic properties. A large number of clinically useful agonists and antagonists have been developed by altering the structure of physiological agonists. Using this approach it has been possible to produce drugs which have a more favourable ratio of therapeutic to toxic effects, are more selective for certain tissues, or which have additional beneficial properties. However, selective localisation of drug action within the body does not always depend on selective distribution. If a drug acts on a receptor that serves functions common to several cells, then its effects will be widespread. Digoxin is an important inhibitor of $Na^+/K^+ATPase$, an enzyme which is essential for most cells throughout the body. At therapeutic concentrations digoxin exerts a positive inotropic effect on myocardial cells and delays conduction in nodal tissue. At high concentrations digoxin causes generalised inhibition of ion transport processes which results in widespread toxicity involving the gut, heart and central nervous system. The effect of digoxin is therefore non-selective, but at appropriate concentrations the drug exerts a selective cardiac effect. On the other hand, if a drug interacts with receptors which only occur in a small selection of tissues, the drug action will be more specific. In clinical pharmacology such a drug is usually less toxic and has a wider margin of safety. However, if the differential effect is a vital one, the drug could be potentially very dangerous. The effect of botulinus toxin on the motor end plate is one such example.

The structure and function of receptors

Receptors have two distinct functions: to facilitate the binding of a ligand and to convey a signal to the target cell to produce a physiological effect. The presence of these two apparently distinct functions has led to the concept of two functional domains within the receptor; a ligand-binding domain and an effector domain. The presence of different receptors for several ligands which act by similar biochemical mechanisms and of multiple receptors for a single ligand which act by unrelated mechanisms supports this dual concept. The actions at a receptor can be exerted directly on the effector proteins or indirectly by intermediary cellular molecules known as transducers. The receptor, the cellular target and these intermediary molecules are referred to as the receptor–effector system or signal transduction pathway. The effector protein is often not the final step in the pathway and may synthesise or release another signalling molecule, the second messenger.

Receptors can now be conveniently grouped into several functional families whose members share a common mode of action, and for the large majority, a common structure. For each receptor family there is at least a basic understanding of the ligand binding, the effector domains and how agonist-binding influences the receptor activity. Figure 2.1 illustrates the main receptor families, and Figure 2.2 two important second messengers, calcium and cyclic AMP (adenosine monophosphate).

A large number of receptors involved in cardiovascular physiology and pharmacology belong to the group of receptors known as the G protein-coupled receptors. These are a group of membrane receptors which regulate distinct effector proteins through the mediation of a group of GTP-binding proteins known as G proteins. Receptors for catecholamines, eicosanoids and several peptide hormones employ G protein-coupled receptors. These receptors act by facilitating the binding of GTP to specific G proteins. GTP binding activates the G protein which in turn regulates the activity of specific effectors (Figure 2.3). Important effectors include adenylcyclase, phospholipases and ion channels for calcium, potassium or sodium. A single cell can express several G proteins, each of which may respond to several different receptors and regulate a number of effectors with characteristic patterns of selectivity.

G proteins are bound to the inner surface of the plasma membrane. They are described as heterotrimeric molecules with α, β and γ subunits and are classified according to the structure of the alpha subunit. These polypeptides have very homologous guanidine nucleotide binding domains and characteristic domains which interact with receptors and effectors. When the system is inactive, GDP is bound to the alpha subunit (Figure 2.4). This is facilitated by the formation of an antagonist–receptor complex which promotes the dissociation of the bound GDP. Binding of GTP activates the α subunit which then probably dissociates from the $\beta\gamma$ subunits to interact with a membrane-bound effector (Figure 2.4). The final events in signal transmission involve hydrolysis of GTP to GDP by a GTPase intrinsic to the α subunit and the subsequent reassociation of the α and $\beta\gamma$. The G proteins, therefore, appear to act as molecular switches which produce different signals by acting through their α and $\beta\gamma$ subunit effects. Several receptors in an individual cell can activate a single G protein. For example, several agonists stimulate adenylcyclase using a single G protein known as G_s. Agonists and antagonists of these systems are widely used in cardio-vascular pharmacology. In contrast, in other regulatory systems a single

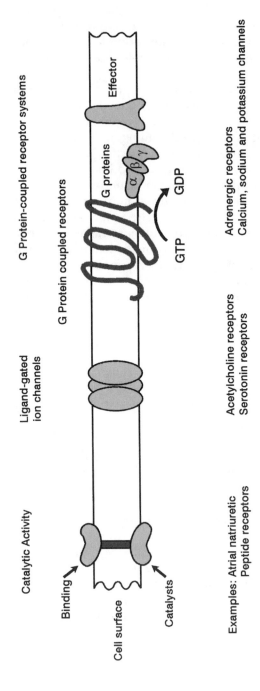

Figure 2.1. Types of receptors for endogenous agonists involved in cardiovascular pharmacology.

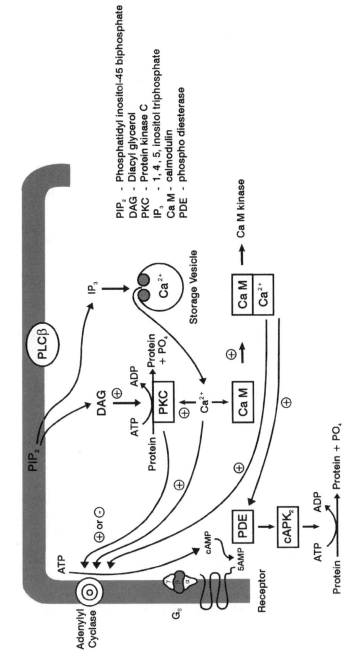

Figure 2.2. Interactions between the second messengers, calcium and cyclic AMP.

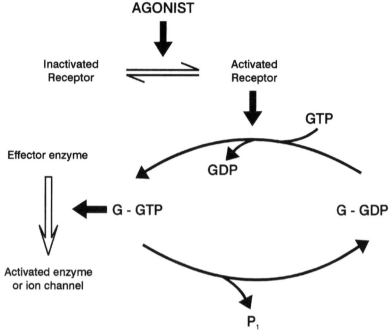

Figure 2.3. Guanine nucleotide-dependent activation–inactivation cycle of G proteins. The agonist activates the receptor which promotes the release of GDP from the G protein (G) allowing the entry of GTP into the nucleotide binding site. In this bound state the G protein regulates the activity of the enzyme or ion channel.

receptor can control more than one G protein and a single G protein can regulate several different effectors.

Second messengers in the cytoplasm

Physiological signals are integrated within the cell by a series of interactions between second messenger pathways. Second messengers influence each other directly by altering the others metabolism and indirectly by sharing intracellular targets. These interactions allow the cell to respond to different agonists singly or in combination, producing an integrated series of second messengers and responses.

Cyclic AMP is one of the most important second messengers involved in cardiovascular physiology and drug action (Figure 2.2). It is synthesised by adenylcyclase in response to activation of a number of different receptors. Stimulation is mediated by G_s and inhibition by one or more G proteins known as G_i. There are at least 10 tissue-specific adenylcyclase isoenzymes,

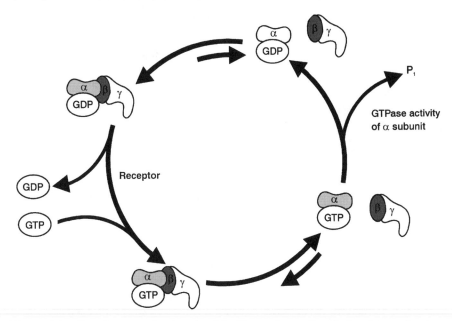

Figure 2.4. Regulatory cycles involved in G protein-mediated signal transduction.

each with its own pattern of responses. Some are inhibited by the $\beta\gamma$ subunits of the G protein which allows activation of the G proteins other than G_s to inhibit adenylcyclase activity. Some isoenzymes are stimulated by $\beta\gamma$ subunits and others by calcium–calmodulin complexes.

The hydrolysis of cyclic AMP is catalysed by a number of phospho-diesterases and the extrusion of cyclic AMP from the cell is achieved by a number of regulated active transport systems. In most situations cyclic AMP activates cyclic AMP dependent protein kinases which regulate several intracellular proteins by catalysing their phosphorylation. A variety of phosphodiesterase inhibitors have been developed for the short-term management of heart failure. They are relatively selective inhibitors of type III phosphodiesterase (Table 2.1). As a result they produce peripheral vasodilatation and increase the force of contraction and the velocity of relaxation of cardiac muscle. On the other hand, inhibition of cyclic nucleotide phosphodiesterase is one of the important mechanisms of the antiplatelet effects of dipyridamole (Table 2.1).

Another important second messenger is the cytoplasmic concentration of calcium which is controlled by the regulation of several different calcium specific channels in the plasma membrane and by its release from intracellular storage sites (Figure 2.2). Drugs which alter vascular tone, the contraction of myocardial cells and myocardial conduction will

Table 2.1. Selective inhibitors of cyclic nucleotide phosphodiesterase isoenzymes

Isoenzyme family	Cellular activity	Examples of selective inhibitors	Cardiovascular effects
I	Ca^{2+}, calmodulin – regulated with different Km values for cGMP and cAMP hydrolysis	Vinpocetine	Vasodilatation
II	cGMP-stimulated cGMP hydrolysis with high Km for cAMP	None available	—
III	cGMP inhibited cAMP hydrolysis low Km for cAMP and cGMP	Milrinone Amrinone Enoximone Vesnarinone	Positive inotropic activity Inhibition of platelet aggregation Vasodilatation
IV	Low Km for cAMP hydrolysis	Rolipram	—
V	High and low Km isoforms for cGMP specific hydrolysis	Dipyridamole Sildenafril	Inhibition of platelet aggregation Vasodilatation with organic nitrates

cAMP – cyclic adenosine 3',5'-monophosphate.
cGMP – cyclic guanosine monophosphate.
Km – Michaelis–Menten constant.

influence the concentration of intracellular calcium. Calcium channels can be opened by electrical depolarisation, by phosphorylation involving a cyclic AMP-dependent protein kinase, or by G$_s$, K$^+$ and Ca^{2+} itself. Opening can be inhibited by other G proteins (G$_1$ and G$_0$) and one channel responds to several cellular influences.

Increased concentrations of cytosolic Ca^{2+} potentiate the contraction of cardiac and vascular smooth muscle cells. The entry of extracellular calcium is more important in initiating the contraction of myocardial cells, while the release of calcium from intracellular storage sites is as important as extracellular entry in the contraction of vascular smooth muscle. In addition, the entry of extracellular calcium can trigger the release of additional calcium from intracellular stores. The cardiac glycosides which increase the force of cardiac contraction and constrict vascular smooth muscle increase the levels of intracellular calcium in inhibiting the ion membrane pump K$^+$/Na$^+$ATPase (see Figure 6.2). On the other hand, decreased intracellular concentrations can be achieved by calcium channel antagonists which reduce calcium entry into the cell and by other vasodilator drugs such as minoxidil and nicorandil which activate the potassium channels on the cell membrane (see Figure 4.6). Beta$_1$ adrenoceptor agonists and phosphodiesterase inhibitors increase intracellular calcium indirectly from intracellular storage sites and phosphodiesterase inhibitors may sensitise the cardiac contractile proteins to the effect of calcium ions. The negative inotropic effects of beta$_1$ adrenoceptor antagonists are related to reduced concentrations of calcium ions available for myocardial contraction.

Calcium regulates cellular activity by interacting with several protein mediators, in particular protein kinase C and calmodulin. Protein kinase C has several substrates which are involved in other signalling systems. Calmodulin also has a wide range of regulatory activities.

Receptor regulation

Receptors do not only initiate regulation of cellular function but they are subject to a variety of homeostatic and regulatory controls. For example, continued stimulation of receptors with agonists can result in a state of desensitisation or down-regulation. When this occurs the same concentration of an agonist results in a diminished physiological response. Several mechanisms are responsible. In some situations only the signal from the stimulated receptor is attenuated in a process known as homologous desensitisation. This can involve covalent modification, destruction of the receptor or its relocation within the cell. Receptor synthesis is also subject to feedback regulation. In other situations, receptors for different agonists which act on a single signalling pathway can demonstrate reduced effect when only one is continuously stimulated. This process is known as heterologous desensitisation and can occur either as a result of modification of each receptor by a common feedback mechanism or from involvement of the effector pathway distal to the receptor. One of the best examples in cardiovascular pharmacology is provided by the changes which occur when adrenergic receptors are continually stimulated by beta adrenergic agonists. Exposure of catecholamine-sensitive cells and tissues to adrenergic agonists causes a well-described progressive decrease in their capacity to respond to these hormones. The desensitisation occurs at several points in the signalling pathway. It can occur at the receptor, G proteins, adenylcyclase and cyclic nucleotide phosphodiesterase. The pattern of receptor tolerance varies according to the degree to which these different components are modified. Desensitisation may be limited to the receptor (homologous) or by diminished responsiveness to a variety of receptor-mediated stimulators of cyclic AMP synthesis (heterologous). Stimulation of receptor phosphorylation frequently leads to decreased sensitivity to further catecholamine stimulation. The receptors are phosphorylated by several different protein kinases. All cases of desensitisation, however, result in deceased coupling to G_s and decreased stimulation of adenyl-cyclase.

On the other hand, supersensitivity to endogenous agonists can occur after withdrawal of receptor antagonists. The sudden withdrawal of beta adrenoceptor antagonists can result in increased heart rate, blood pressure, angina pectoris and a greater risk of developing an acute myocardial infarction. In some of these situations increased receptor sensitivity may be due to the synthesis of additional receptors.

Tolerance to organic nitrates in angina and heart failure is a common clinical problem. Nitrates, after entering the vessel wall, are eventually converted to nitric oxide which is thought to stimulate guanylate cyclase to produce cyclic GMP. The cyclic nucleotide thus formed produces vasodilatation as the level of intracellular calcium ions decreases. Sulphydryl groups are required for the formation of nitric oxide and the stimulation of guanylate cyclase. Vascular tolerance occurs when the sulphydryl groups are oxidised by excess nitrate exposure.

Classification of cardiovascular receptors and cardiac drug effects

Traditionally, drug receptors have been classified primarily on the basis of the effect and relative potency of selective agonists and antagonists. By applying mathematical principles to dose–response relationships it is possible to estimate dissociation constants for the interaction between receptors and individual agonists and antagonists. It is also possible to measure the specific binding of radioactively labelled drugs to receptor sites in tissue and to calculate the density of receptors per cell. For example, it has been calculated that each myocardial cell in the dog contains about 85 000 beta adrenoceptors.

Receptors on the autonomic effector cells

Two chemicals have been identified as neurotransmitters in the peripheral nervous system. These are acetylcholine and noradrenaline. Both are synthesised principally in the nerve endings of the nerve terminals and are stored in the synaptic vesicles until released by nerve impulses (Figure 2.4).

Neurotransmission in the peripheral nervous system occurs at four main sites. Acetylcholine is released at the pre-ganglionic synapses in the sympathetic and parasympathetic ganglia, parasympathetic post-ganglionic neuroeffector junctions and all motor end plates in skeletal muscle. Neurones that release acetylcholine are called cholinergic neurones. Noradrenaline is the transmitter released at most sympathetic post-ganglionic neuroeffector junctions and these neurones are called adrenergic or more strictly, noradrenergic (Figure 2.5).

The receptors for acetylcholine and related compounds (cholinoreceptors) and for noradrenaline and related chemicals are clearly different. Acetylcholine will not interact with receptors for noradrenaline and noradrenaline will not interact with cholinoreceptors. This is equally true for adrenoceptor and cholinoreceptor antagonists.

Cholinoreceptors

It was recognised by pharmacologists at the turn of the century that the action of acetylcholine on effector systems innervated by parasympathetic post-ganglionic neurones (smooth muscle cells, cardiac muscle cells and exocrine gland cells) resembled the action of a naturally occurring plant alkaloid called muscarine. Furthermore, these effects could be antagonised by atropine, another plant alkaloid. Acetylcholine also produced effects similar to those of the tobacco alkaloid nicotine on autonomic ganglia and the adrenal medulla. It remains popular to refer to the effects of acetylcholine on visceral effectors as muscarinic effects and to the effects on autonomic ganglia and adrenal medulla as nicotinic effects. The receptors are known as muscarinic and nicotinic cholinoreceptors respectively. At the skeletal muscle end plate, the action of acetylcholine also resembles that produced by nicotine although the receptors are structurally different to those occurring in the autonomic ganglia. Atropine, a muscarinic blocking drug is sometimes used to increase heart rate in patients with bradycardia and hypotension after an acute myocardial infarction and in patients with carotid sinus syncope.

Adrenoceptors

Noradrenaline is the neurotransmitter released at the adrenergic nerve terminals (Figure 2.5). The adrenoceptors on the innervated tissues not only interact with noradrenaline but also with adrenaline from the adrenal gland and a variety of synthetic compounds such as isoprenaline and phenylephrine. The responses produced by these agonists differ quantitatively and qualitatively from one another. A variety of antagonists have been developed which are remarkably selective in blocking the various effects

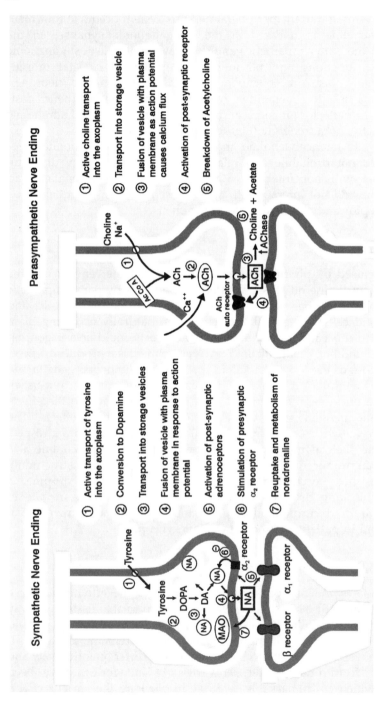

Figure 2.5. Comparison of the stages involved in neurotransmitter synthesis and metabolism at the sympathetic and parasympathetic nerve endings.

of noradrenaline and adrenaline. On the basis of the observed selectivity of these agonists and antagonists, Ahlquist proposed the existence of two types of adrenoceptors, alpha and beta. It subsequently became necessary to further divide the alpha receptors into α_1 and α_2 and beta receptors into β_1 and β_2.

The alpha$_1$ adrenoceptors are located at post-synaptic sites on tissues innervated by adrenergic neurones. The alpha$_2$ adrenoceptors are mostly located pre-synaptically and are involved in the feedback inhibition of noradrenaline release from the nerve terminal. Alpha$_2$ adrenoceptors also occur post-synaptically. The beta$_1$ adrenoceptors are found mainly in the heart and adipose tissue, while beta$_2$ adrenoceptors are located in a number of sites including the bronchial smooth muscle and the blood vessels supplying skeletal muscle. Activation of the alpha adrenoceptors in vascular smooth muscle produces vasoconstriction, while stimulation of the beta$_2$ adrenoceptors in blood vessels of skeletal muscle produces vasodilatation. Activation of beta$_1$ adrenoceptors in cardiac tissue increases heart rate and contractile force. Noradrenaline and adrenaline are potent alpha adrenoceptor agonists, while isoprenaline has little alpha receptor activity at therapeutic concentrations. Adrenaline and noradrenaline are, therefore, potent vasoconstrictors in those vessels containing alpha receptors. On the other hand, isoprenaline and adrenaline are potent beta$_2$ adrenoceptor agonists and produce vasodilatation in skeletal muscle.

Adrenoceptor antagonists

Adrenoceptor antagonists reduce the effectiveness of sympathetic nerve activity by preventing the naturally occurring agonists from interacting with their receptors.

Alpha adrenoceptor antagonists

A large number of compounds possess alpha adrenoceptor blocking activity including the neuroleptic agents, chlorpromazine and haloperidol. However, there are only a few agents whose main therapeutic effect is due to alpha blockade. These clinically important drugs fall into three chemical groups; the haloalkylamines such as phenoxybenzamine, the imidazolines such as phenothalamine and the quinazoline derivatives, prazosin and doxazosin. The haloalkylamines produce an irreversible competitive antagonism of responses mediated by alpha adrenoceptors. The irreversible nature of this antagonism is responsible for the much longer duration of effect than with other alpha blocking drugs. Phenoxybenzamine has a greater affinity for the alpha$_1$ than the alpha$_2$ receptors. However, blockade of the alpha$_2$ receptors means that the release of noradrenaline from the adrenergic neurones is increased resulting in tachycardia and positive inotropic effects. In contrast to the haloalkylamines, imidazolines produce an equilibrium-competitive antagonism of the actions of noradrenaline at the alpha receptor and they do not show any selectivity for the alpha$_1$ or alpha$_2$ receptors. Tachycardia is therefore prominent after administration of phentolamine (see Figure 9.13).

The quinazoline derivatives, prazosin and doxazosin, have different haemodynamic effects to those of phenoxybenzamine and phentolamine. Postural hypotension is less common and the increases in heart rate, contractile force and plasma renin activity are less prominent. Some of these differences may be related to differences in the characteristics of pre-synaptic and post-synaptic receptors. Pre-synaptic alpha receptors limit the release of noradrenaline through a negative feedback loop (Figure 2.5). Phenoxybenzamine and phentolamine block the pre- and post-synaptic adrenoceptor antagonists and so enhance noradrenaline release. Increased heart rate, inotropic activity and renin release are related to stimulation of the beta receptors. Prazosin and doxazosin mainly block the post-synaptic alpha receptors and so lower blood pressure without causing beta adrenoceptor stimulation. Most post-synaptic receptors on smooth muscle are referred to as α_1 receptors and those which occur pre-synaptically are known as α_2 receptors. Prazosin and doxazosin are, therefore, referred to as alpha$_1$ receptor antagonists and phenoxybenzamine and phentolamine as non-selective alpha receptor antagonists.

Non-selective alpha adrenoceptor antagonists have a limited role in cardiovascular pharmacology. Phentolamine is now used only in hypertensive crises when there is excess alpha stimulation such as occurs in phaeochromocytoma, withdrawal of an alpha$_2$ agonist or hypertensive crises induced by monoamine oxidase inhibitors. Phenoxybenzamine is only used to treat phaeochromocytoma before and during surgery. Selective alpha antagonists, especially doxazosin, are used widely as a second- or third-line agent in the management of essential hypertension. They are effective in reducing blood pressure long term and do not induce sympathetic activation at normal doses.

Beta adrenoceptor antagonists

In general, beta adrenoceptor antagonists have greater structural similarity to their corresponding agonists than alpha adrenoceptor antagonists. This accounts for their increased specificity as blocking agents and the observation that some activate the beta receptors (partial agonist activity). The effect, however, is usually modest in comparison to the full agonist. Structural differences between agonists and antagonists can be identified.

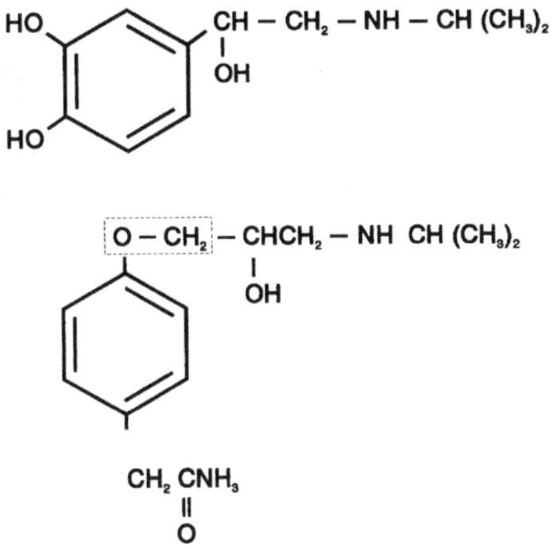

Figure 2.6. Comparison of the structures of isoprenaline, a beta agonist, and atenolol, a beta adrenoceptor antagonist, showing the oxymethylene bridge between the aromatic nucleus and the ethanolamine side chain on the antagonist.

An oxymethylene bridge between the aromatic nucleus and an ethanolamine side chain is a feature of almost all beta adrenoceptor antagonists (Figure 2.6). Those with membrane stabilising activity have some structural similarities to local anaesthetics. No clear structural differences, however, exist between beta$_1$ selective and non-selective agents.

The most important actions of the beta adrenoceptor antagonists are on the cardiovascular system. They decrease heart rate, myocardial contractility, cardiac output and conduction velocity within the heart. These effects are most pronounced when sympathetic activity is high or when the heart is stimulated by circulating agonists. The actions of beta adrenoceptor antagonists on blood pressure are complex. After acute administration there is little alteration in blood pressure as peripheral resistance increases to compensate for the reduction in cardiac output. Chronic administration results in a sustained reduction in blood pressure, probably due to alterations in baroreceptor activity and inhibition of renin release from the kidney.

Presynaptic beta adrenoceptors potentiate the release of noradrenaline from synaptic neurones, but the role of receptor antagonists in lowering blood pressure at this site is unknown. Some beta blockers produce additional vasodilatation which may contribute to their ability to lower blood pressure. Labetalol and carvedilol have additional alpha$_1$ adrenoceptor blocking effects while celiprolol has beta$_2$ receptor agonist activity and other vasodilating effects which are unrelated to activity at the adrenergic receptors.

Alpha adrenoceptor agonists

Alpha adrenoceptor agonists used in the treatment of cardiovascular disease are divided into two groups, alpha$_1$ and alpha$_2$ selective agonists. Alpha$_1$ agonists increase peripheral vascular resistance and blood pressure. The clinical utility of alpha$_1$ agonists such as methoxamine and phenylephrine is very limited, but they are occasionally used to treat severe hypotension. Alpha$_2$ agonists have greater clinical potential, but their use in treating hypertension has declined over the last 10 years due to the high incidence of adverse effects on the central nervous system and rebound hypertension on drug withdrawal. Clonidine and alpha methylnoradrenaline, the major active metabolite of methyldopa, appear to lower blood pressure by stimulating the alpha$_2$ adrenergic receptors in the cardiovascular control centres of the nervous system. This results in overall reduced sympathetic activity within the brain. Intravenous infusion of clonidine causes an acute increase in blood pressure apparently by activating the post-synaptic alpha$_2$ receptors in vascular smooth muscle. Clonidine also stimulates parasympathetic outflow which may account for some of the bradycardia observed with the drug.

Beta agonists

Beta adrenergic agonists are used in several clinical situations. Beta$_2$ agonists are widely employed in the treatment of bronchoconstriction in patients with obstructive airways disease and beta$_1$ agonists have a limited role as acute inotropic agents. Beta$_1$ agonists exert opposite effects to beta$_1$ adrenoceptor antagonists: direct myocardial stimulation which increases the strength of ventricular contraction, increased heart rate and a variable effect on the peripheral vasculature depending on whether the compound has alpha$_1$, beta$_2$ or other additional properties on vascular smooth muscle. Beta$_1$ agonists are occasionally used for the short-term treatment of cardiac decompensation occurring after cardiac surgery or following an acute myocardial infarction. Dobutamine is usually the preferred agent. It increases cardiac output, stroke volume and heart rate with minor effects on peripheral vascular resistance. All beta$_1$ agonists are arrhythmogenic and may increase the size of an acute myocardial infarction. Beta$_1$ agonists with additional alpha effects such as noradrenaline will increase peripheral resistance and afterload. Increased blood pressure is therefore at the expense of increased cardiac work so that cardiac output is likely to decline. Other drugs such as isoprenaline stimulate the beta$_2$ receptors and produce beneficial peripheral vasodilatation and reduction in afterload. However beta$_2$ stimulation also increases the risk of hypokalaemia with its arrhythmogenic potential. Another serious problem is that prolonged and vigorous beta stimulation leads to receptor down-regulation and diminished inotropic responses with time.

Other cardiovascular drugs which act at G-protein coupled receptors

One of the most promising areas of cardiovascular drug research is the development of agents which compete with endogenous peptides at the receptor. Although these substances are often peptides themselves, orally active non-peptide drugs are now available. The two best examples are the angiotensin receptor and endothelin antagonists.

Drugs acting at the angiotensin receptor

The effect of angiotensin II is exerted through specific cell surface receptors. Two subtypes AT_1 and AT_2 have been identified. The AT_1 receptor has a high affinity for losartan and related biphenyl tetrazole derivatives and a low affinity for PD 123177 and related 1-benzyl spinacine derivatives. In contrast the AT_2 receptor has a high affinity for PD123177 and a low affinity for losartan. To date, all the pharmacological effects of angiotensin II seem to be mediated by the AT_1 receptor and no clear functional role has been defined for the AT_2 receptor despite wide distribution in foetal tissues.

Attempts to develop angiotensin II receptor antagonists over 20 years ago resulted in a series of peptide analogues which were effective antagonists of the angiotensin II receptor. The best known of these was salarasin, 1-sarcosine, 8-isoleucine angiotensin II which was used extensively to investigate interactions with the renin angiotensin and related systems in experimental animals. Unfortunately, these agents were not orally active and they all had considerable partial agonist activity. Molecular modelling of these structures, however, gave rise to the hypothesis that a successful antagonist would have to closely mimic the pharmacophore of angiotensin II (Figure 2.7). Through a series of stepwise modifications a potent orally active and selective non-peptide angiotensin II receptor antagonist, losartan, was developed (Figure 2.7).

Losartan, by blocking the AT_1 receptor produces effects which are opposite to those of angiotensin II; peripheral vasodilatation, reduced blood pressure, decreased aldosterone and catecholamine release, and reduced growth-promoting effects in vascular smooth muscle and cardiac muscle. Unlike ACE inhibitors, angiotensin$_1$ receptor antagonists do not increase vasodilatory prostaglandins and kinins and are not associated

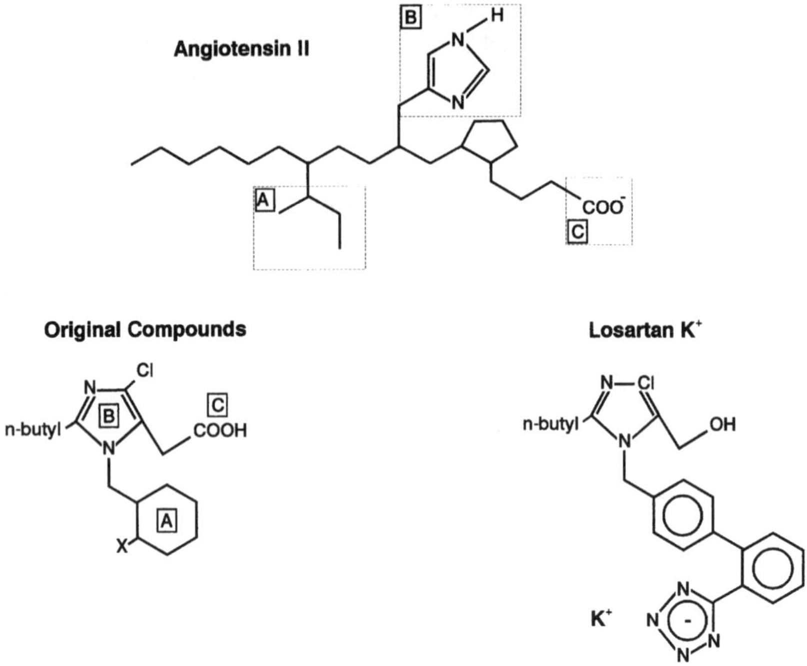

Figure 2.7. Structural relationships between sections of the angiotensin II molecule A, B, C and angiotensin II receptor prototypes. Modified from Timmermans *et al.* Angiotensin II receptors and angiotensin II receptor antagonists. *Pharmacological Reviews*, 1993, 45: 205–251.

with cough. Losartan and three other angiotensin II receptor antagonists, valsartan, candesartan and irbesartan, are now licensed for use in the treatment of hypertension, but their clinical role has still to be fully evaluated. They should prove to be as effective as ACE inhibitors in heart failure and hypertension, but with a lower incidence of cough and angioedema.

Drugs acting at the endothelin receptors

The vascular endothelium produces a number of vasoconstrictor substances known as the endothelins. Three peptides have been identified: endothelin 1, 2 and 3 each consisting of 21 amino acids. Endothelins 2 and 3 are produced in a variety of different tissues but endothelin 1 is only detected in vascular endothelial cells. Two receptors for endothelins ET_A and ET_B have been proposed according to their relative binding affinities of the agonists. Endothelin 1 has greater affinity for the ET_A receptor than endothelin 2 which in turn has greater affinity than endothelin 3. All three

Table 2.2. Binding characteristics of the endothelin receptor antagonists

	ET_A receptor	ET_B receptor
BQ123	+	−
FR139317	+	−
BMS182874	+	−
BQ788	−	+
Bosentan*	+	+
Ro462005	+	+
SB209670	+	+

*Orally active non-peptide.

have equal affinity for the ET_B receptor. It seems likely, however, that there is at least one other receptor and that multiple receptor subtypes will be identified in the near future.

Endothelins stimulate platelet aggregation and induce vasoconstriction. Like thromboxane A_2 they oppose the effects of nitric oxide and prostacyclin. They also function as mitogens and growth promoters for a variety of cells and induce bronchospasm when inhaled or injected intravenously. Several receptor antagonists have recently been developed (Table 2.2). BQ123, a derivative of a peptide isolated from *Streptomyces miskiensis* resembles the C terminal portion of endothelin and has been shown to be a selective antagonist of the ET_A receptor, while IRL 1038 has recently been shown to antagonise the ET_B receptor *in vivo*. PD142893, a linear hexapeptide analogue derived from the C terminal of endothelin 1 is a non-selective competitive receptor antagonist. The most exciting development, however, and one which could have major clinical implications, is the synthesis of an orally active non-peptide, non-selective endothelin 1 antagonist, Bosentan. This drug has a potential role in hypertension, heart failure, angina pectoris, acute myocardial infarction and peripheral vascular disease. Favourable haemodynamic effects have been described in patients with congestive cardiac failure at least in the short term.

Cardiovascular drugs acting as enzyme inhibitors

A variety of cardiovascular drugs produce their pharmacological effects by inhibiting enzymes involved in metabolic pathways or those controlling ion exchange on the cell surface. Examples of enzyme inhibitors acting on metabolic pathways include angiotensin converting enzyme inhibitors which prevent the conversion of angiotensin I to angiotensin II, phosphodiesterase inhibitors which prevent the breakdown of cyclic AMP, HMG Co enzyme A reductase inhibitors which inhibit cholesterol synthesis in the liver and cyclooxygenase inhibitors, notably aspirin, which reduce thromboxane synthesis in the platelet. Digoxin, on the other hand, inhibits the enzyme $Na^+/K^+ATPase$ on the cell surface increasing intracellular sodium and calcium and extracellular potassium concentration. Acetazolamide, a diuretic acting on the proximal convoluted tubule inhibits the enzyme carbonic anhydrase present in the brush border of the tubular cells. This results in a marked reduction in bicarbonate reabsorption with secondary loss of sodium and potassium ions due to increased delivery of non-reabsorbable sodium bicarbonate to the ascending loop of Henle, distal tubular cells and collecting ducts.

Site specificity and selectivity

Some drugs produce their pharmacological effect by inhibiting enzymes involved in very specific physiological processes. Inhibitors of HMG co-enzyme A reductase selectively inhibit the co-enzyme and effectively reduce LDL and VLDL cholesterol (see Figure 7.5). To date, these drugs appear to have a specific effect on cholesterol biosynthesis and there is no evidence that the adverse effects on the liver or skeletal muscle occur as a result of enzyme inhibition at these sites. Other drugs produce their pharmacological and toxicological effects by inhibiting more than one enzyme. The principal action of ACE inhibitors is to reduce the formation of angiotensin II, a powerful constrictor peptide by inhibiting its conversion from an inactive peptide, angiotensin I. However, another important action of the ACE inhibitors is to prevent the degradation of the potent vasodilator kinin peptide, bradykinin, to form inactive metabolites (see Figure 9.7). This results in secondary increases in vasodilator prostaglandins and nitric oxide production. This additional activity may contribute to the antihypertensive and vasodilator activity and may be responsible for the cough and angioedema which sometimes occur with these compounds.

Although agents such as theophylline and caffeine have been known for some time to have weak non-specific inhibitory effects on cyclic GMP and cyclic AMP phosphodiesterase, it was not until the 1980s that a number of isoenzyme sub-class specific inhibitors became available (Table 2.1). Cardiac muscle contains all known phosphodiesterase isoenzyme families. Of those listed in Table 2.1 the most commonly used inhibitors are those which are selective for the cyclic GMP inhibited, cyclic AMP phospho-diesterase (type III). These agents combine the potentially useful haemodynamic effects of inotropic activity and peripheral vasodilatation, while other selective phosphodiesterase inhibitors have inhibitory effects on platelet function or pure vasodilator activity.

Aspirin provides a good example of an enzyme inhibitor which although not specific for platelet cyclooxygenase, produces a selective platelet effect related to the relative abundance of the endoperoxides in the platelet and accessibility to the enzyme in different tissues. In platelets the major cyclooxygenase product is thromboxane A_2, a labile inducer of platelet aggregation and potent vasoconstrictor. Aspirin prevents the formation of thromboxane A_2 by covalently acetylating a serine residue near the active site for cyclooxygenase, the enzyme responsible for the production of the endoperoxide precursor of thromboxane A_2. Since platelets do not synthesise new proteins, the action of aspirin on cyclooxygenase is permanent and lasts for the life of the platelet. Useful antiplatelet effects can be achieved with doses as low as 30 mg and there is no evidence that higher doses are more effective. Higher doses are potentially less efficacious because there is a greater effect of prostacyclin formation. Inhibition of this endoperoxide has the opposite effect to thromboxane inhibition, but most prostacyclin is manufactured by the vascular endothelium which has the ability to regenerate cyclooxygenase. The site of action may also have an important impact on the action of angiotensin converting enzyme inhibitors. Local renin–angiotensin systems have been identified in blood vessels, adrenals, kidney, heart and brain. Reducing circulating angiotensin II accounts for most of the acute vasodilator and antihypertensive effects, but inhibition of ACE in vascular and cardiac tissues may contribute to the prevention of muscle hypertrophy and the long-term haemodynamic effects.

All cardiac glycosides are potent and highly selective inhibitors of the active transport of sodium and potassium across cell membranes by binding to the alpha sub-unit of the enzyme $Na^+/K^+ATPase$. This results in a reduction in the rate of active sodium extrusion and a rise in cytosolic sodium. This increased concentration reduces the transmembrane sodium gradient stimulating the extrusion of intracellular calcium during cardio-myocyte repolarisation (see Figure 6.2). As a result increased amounts of calcium are taken into the sarcoplasmic reticulum to be made available for the contractile proteins during the subsequent cell depolarisation cycle. Increased intracellular calcium accounts for the additional inotropic activity of digitalis and some of its antiarrhythmic activity: increased spontaneous (phase 4) rate of diastolic depolarisation and delayed after depolarisation. The inhibitory effect of the cardiac glycosides on $Na^+/K^+ATPase$ is not specific for cardiac muscle, but it is only at high dose that widespread enzyme inhibition produces important extra cardiac effects.

Cardiovascular drugs as ion channel antagonists on the cell membrane

A number of antiarrhythmic drugs produce their pharmacological effect by blocking ion channels on the cell membrane. Experimental evidence strongly supports the view that drugs which block the ion channels bind to specific receptor sites on the ion channel protein to modify its function and decrease the flux of that ion. The ions, sodium, potassium and calcium are principally affected.

When sodium channels are blocked in cardiac tissue the threshold for excitability and the conduction velocity in fast response tissues is generally decreased. Blockade of the sodium channels is a principal feature of class I antiarrhythmic drugs. Most available potassium channel antagonists interact with potassium channels involved with control of pacemaker activity, resting potential and the duration of the cardiac action potential. No drug, however, is available which specifically blocks only the potassium channels without interacting with beta adrenoceptors (sotalol) or other channels (amiodarone and quinidine). Amiodarone and sotalol appear to be at least as effective in blocking the sodium channels.

A large group of drugs referred to as the calcium channel antagonists produce their major electrophysiological effects by blocking the L-type (long lasting, high voltage activated) Ca^{2+} channels in slow response tissues of the sino-atrial and atrioventricular nodes, cardiac and vascular smooth muscle (Figure 2.8). Dihydropyridines such as nifedipine, widely used in the treatment of angina and hypertension, preferentially block calcium channels in vascular smooth muscle. Their cardiac effects, increased heart rate and inotropic effect, are mostly indirect and related to reflex sympathetic activity. Verapamil and diltiazem, on the other hand, selectively block calcium channels in cardiac smooth muscle cells at

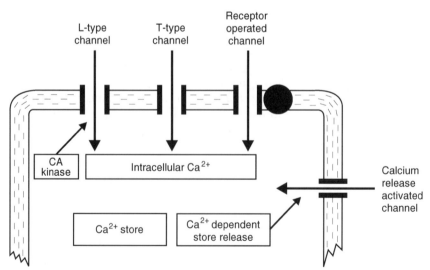

Figure 2.8. Types of calcium channels regulating cellular function. L-type: long lasting; T-type: transient, voltage operated.

standard therapeutic doses. Unlike the dihydropyridines the heart rate usually slows. Another important antiarrhythmic action is a reduction of the ventricular rate in atrial flutter and fibrillation.

Mibefradil is a member of a new class of calcium antagonists, the tetradol derivatives, which selectively blocks the T-type (transient, low voltage activated) calcium channels (Figure 2.8). This compound relaxes the coronary arteries without reducing myocardial contractility and blood pressure. Although an effective antihypertensive and antianginal agent in short-term studies, the drug is a potent inhibitor of oxidative metabolism and interacts with a variety of cardiovascular drugs, particularly the HMG co-enzyme A reductase inhibitors.

Actions of cardiovascular drugs not mediated by receptors

If a receptor is defined as a macromolecule which interacts with a drug, then several drugs appear to act by other mechanisms. Certain drugs interact specifically with small molecules which are commonly produced by the body. Vitamin C, vitamin E and probucol are free radical scavengers which bind to reactive metabolites which are thought to contribute to the process of atherogenesis. Recent evidence suggests a useful role for vitamin E in the prevention of myocardial infarction and cardiovascular events in patients with established coronary heart disease. Some clinically inert compounds such as mannitol can be given in amounts which are sufficient to increase the osmolarity of body fluids and alter the distribution of body water. Depending on the clinical situation, this property can be used to expand the circulating blood volume, promote diuresis or reduce cerebral oedema.

3 Cardiovascular Clinical Pharmacology: Rational Dose Selection and the Time Course of Drug Action

Introduction

The aim of rational drug prescribing is to achieve the maximum clinical effect with the minimum number of adverse effects. To attain this goal it is necessary to consider the principles of pharmacokinetics and pharmacodynamics. Pharmacodynamics are concerned with the concentration–effect relationships, while pharmacokinetics relate to the processes of absorption, distribution and elimination and how these factors alter the drug concentrations at the receptor (Figure 3.1).

Clinical pharmacology is based on the hypothesis that there is a relationship between the therapeutic and toxic effects of a drug and its concentration in a readily accessible site usually the plasma. For most cardiovascular drugs there is a relatively poor relationship between the plasma concentration and effect. This does not necessarily weaken the basic hypothesis but illustrates the need to consider the nature of the concentration–time relationship and the presence of other factors such as the formation of active metabolites. Knowing these relationships, allows the clinician to adjust therapy for a variety of pathological and physiological factors in the individual patient.

Pharmacokinetics

The two most important basic measurements in the discipline of pharmacokinetics are the clearance, a measure of the body's ability to eliminate a drug, and the apparent volume of distribution which is a measure of the apparent space in the body available to contain the drug.

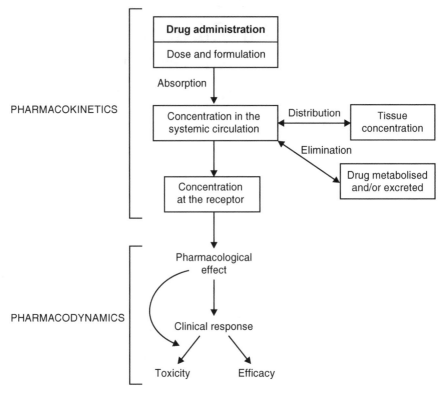

Figure 3.1.   Factors influencing the action of a drug.

Apparent volume of distribution

The apparent volume of distribution (V_d) relates the amount of drug in the body to the concentration (C_0) in the blood or plasma at time zero:

$$V_d = \frac{\text{Amount of drug in the body}}{C_0}$$

It is clear from the volumes listed in Table 3.1 that for several cardiovascular drugs the volume exceeds any physical volume within the body. Those drugs which have very large volumes of distribution will have much higher concentrations in the extracellular tissue than in the vascular compartment. Drugs which are confined to the vascular compartment have the smallest volumes of distribution, i.e. 0.04 l/kg. Of practical importance, drugs with large volumes of distribution such as amiodarone, digitoxin and digoxin have high tissue binding, distribute slowly and a loading dose may be required if a rapid effect is required.

Table 3.1. Pharmacokinetic values of some commonly used cardiovascular drugs

Drug	Oral bioavailability (%)	Urinary excretion (%)	Protein binding (%)	Clearance (l/hour per 70 kg)	Volume of distribution (l/70 kg)	Half-life (hours)	Effective concentrations
Atenolol	56	1	50	40	10	6	
Captopril	65	38	30	50	57	2	
Digitoxin	90	32	97	0.23	38	70	> 10 ng/ml
Digoxin	70	60	25	8	440	39	> 0.8 ng/ml
Diltiazem	44	4	80	50	220	4	—
Enalapril	95	90	55	9	40	3	> 0.5 ng/ml
Frusemide	60	66	100	8.5	8	1.5	—
Nifedipine	50	0	100	30	55	1.8	
Procainamide	83	67	16	36	130	3	3–14 mg/l
Propranolol	26	0	87	50	270	4	
Quinidine	80	18	90	20	190	6	2–6 mg/l
Verapamil	22	3	90	83	350	4	—

Clearance

The clearance of a drug (*Cl*) is the ratio of the rate of elimination by all routes to its concentration (C) in a biological fluid, usually the plasma.

$$Cl = \frac{\text{Rate of elimination}}{C}$$

Alternatively, it can be defined as the volume of fluid which is totally cleared of drug per unit time. One of the advantages of using clearance as a measure of drug elimination is that total body clearance can be calculated by adding the clearances of the individual eliminating organs.

$$Cl_{\text{total}} = Cl_{\text{renal}} + Cl_{\text{liver}} + Cl_{\text{other}}$$

Other tissues of elimination include the lungs, blood and muscle. Atenolol, digoxin, frusemide and most ACE inhibitors are almost entirely excreted in the urine, and renal clearance can be calculated by estimating the amount excreted in the urine and measuring the concentration in the plasma.

Within the liver, drug elimination occurs by a process of metabolism. The rate of metabolism is greatly influenced by genetic and environmental factors. Pharmacogenetic differences are seen in the acetylation of procainamide and hydralazine and the hydroxylation of metoprolol and several other beta adrenoceptor antagonists. Patients who are slow acetylators have higher concentrations for a given dose and are therefore at greater risk of toxicity. This defect seems to be related to reduced amounts of the enzyme and is inherited as an autosomal recessive trait (Figure 3.2). Genetically determined defects in oxidative metabolism are also transmitted as autosomal recessive traits and occur in about 3–10% of Caucasians. In affected individuals, the cytochrome P-450-dependent oxidation of metoprolol, bufuralol and other beta adrenoceptor antagonists is impaired.

A variety of environmental factors influence the metabolism of a number of cardiovascular drugs. Cigarette smoking increases the metabolism of theophylline and several beta blocking drugs. Enzyme-inducing drugs which include various hypnotics, tranquillisers, anticoagulants, insecticides and anticonvulsants accelerate the metabolism of various drugs. Patients who routinely take enzyme-inducing drugs require higher doses of drugs whose oxidative metabolites are less active than the parent compound. Cardiovascular drugs which have been reported to be affected include quinidine, digitoxin, felodipine, verapamil, propranolol and metoprolol. Stopping an enzyme-inducing drug can result in excessive pharmacological effect. An enzyme-inducer can often induce its own metabolism as well as

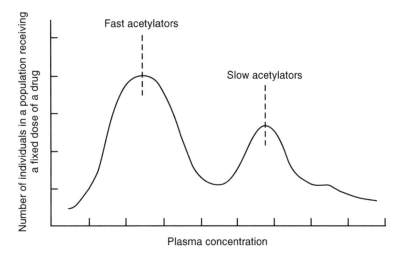

Figure 3.2. Distribution of plasma concentrations of drugs which are metabolised by acetylation, showing a clear bimodal distribution and the division into slow and fast acetylators. Reproduced from Evans, D. A. P., Manley, K. A., McKusick, V. A. Genetic control of isoniazid metabolism in man. *B. Med. J.* 1960; 2: 485 and is reproduced by permission of the BMJ.

the metabolism of other drugs. Thus, continued use of some drugs can result in progressive loss of effect.

Some drugs can inhibit oxidative enzyme activity and lead to toxic effects with drugs which have narrow therapeutic indices. Cimetidine, a potent enzyme inhibitor, has been shown to inhibit the metabolism of warfarin, amiodarone, metoprolol, propranolol, labetalol, diltiazem and nitrendipine, and so increase their pharmacological effect.

Various drugs require conjugation with endogenous substrates such as glutathione, glucuronic acid and sulphate for their inactivation. If two drugs are conjugated by the same system, then the faster reacting drug can deplete the endogenous conjugating agent and impair the metabolism of the slower reacting drug. If the slower reacting drug has a steep dose–response relationship (Figure 3.3) and a narrow therapeutic index, then increased pharmacological effect and increased toxicity can occur.

Acute and chronic liver diseases can alter the metabolism of several cardiovascular drugs. These conditions include cirrhosis, haemochromatosis, chronic active hepatitis, biliary cirrhosis and acute viral or drug-induced hepatitis. Liver cancer has also been reported to impair hepatic drug metabolism. Of particular interest is the effect of cardiac disease which, by reducing liver blood flow, can impair the metabolism of drugs such as lignocaine whose metabolism is flow-dependent. The hepatic clearance of this drug is almost equal to hepatic blood flow.

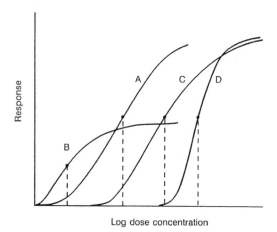

Log dose concentration

Figure 3.3. Dose–response relationships. Potency: A and B are more potent than C and D because smaller doses are required to produce 50% of maximum effect $(ED_{50})^*$. Efficacy: Drugs A, C and D have equal maximum efficacy which is greater than B. Curve D represents a steep dose–response relationship compared to A, B and C. The responses at the top of this curve may be excessive and cause clinical problems, e.g. coma caused by a sedative drug. *Alternatively the EC_{50} can be used i.e. the plasma concentration required to produce 50% of maximum effect. Reproduced from Kenakin, T. P., Bond, R. A. and Bonner, T. I. Definition of pharmacological receptors. *Pharmacological Reviews*, 1992; 44: 351–362. Reproduced with permission of The American Society for Pharmacology and Experimental Therapeutics.

Non-hepatic disease can also alter drug metabolism. Chronic chest disease is associated with impaired hydrolysis of procainamide, and hypothyroidism increases the half-life of digoxin and several beta adrenoceptor antagonists.

Elimination

For most drugs, clearance is constant over the therapeutic plasma concentration range, i.e. the rate of metabolism is directly proportional to the plasma concentration.

$$\text{Rate of elimination} = Cl \times C$$

This is commonly referred to as 'first-order' elimination kinetics.

Saturation kinetics

For certain drugs which demonstrate saturation or capacity-limited elimination – phenytoin, aspirin and ethanol, the clearance varies with the plasma concentration. At high dose the metabolic pathways are saturated. At these concentrations the rate of elimination is independent of the plasma concentration and if dosing exceeds the elimination capacity, steady-state plasma concentrations will not be achieved. Plasma levels will continue to rise as the dosing continues.

Elimination half-life

The elimination half-life is defined as the time taken to reduce the total amount of drug in the body by half during the period of elimination. This value is directly proportional to the apparent volume of distribution and inversely proportional to the clearance in a single compartmental model.

$$t_{1/2 \text{ (terminal)}} = \frac{0.7 \times V_D}{Cl}$$

where 0.7 is an approximation of the natural logarithm of 2.

The elimination half-life is a useful measurement since it indicates the time required to achieve 50% of steady-state or to decrease 50% from steady-state plasma concentrations after starting or stopping a particular drug (Figure 3.4). This provides information about the most appropriate frequency of drug administration. Cardiovascular drugs with long elimination half-lives include amiodarone ($\approx$ 30 days), digitoxin ($\approx$ 5 days) and digoxin ($\approx$ 2 days). Normally these drugs are given once daily but could be administered less frequently. Captopril, nifedipine and diltiazem have short half-lives and need to be given in divided doses. It is, however, important to be aware that elimination half-lives do not always reflect changes in drug clearance. For example, patients with chronic renal failure have reduced renal clearance of digoxin and smaller volumes of

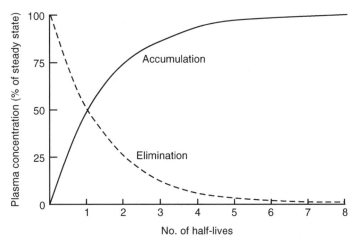

Figure 3.4. Plasma concentrations during drug accumulation and elimination.

distribution. The increase in digoxin half-life is therefore not as great as would be expected as a result of changes in renal function alone.

Drug accumulation

Accumulation occurs when drugs are given in repeated doses. In theory, it takes an infinite period to eliminate all of a drug. In other words, if the dosage interval is less than four half-lives, accumulation will occur. Accumulation is inversely proportional to the fraction of the dose removed during each dosage interval. A convenient index of drug accumulation is the accumulation factor:

$$\text{Accumulation factor} = \frac{1}{1 - \text{fraction remaining}}$$

For a drug given every half-life, the accumulation factor would be 2. Under these circumstances the maintenance dose could be defined as half the loading dose every half-life. The accumulation factor also predicts the ratio of the steady-state concentration to the value obtained after the first dose. Therefore, for a drug given every half-life, the value at steady state is twice the value after the first dose (Figure 3.4). Accumulation is clearly more likely to occur with drugs which have long elimination half-lives such as amiodarone and digitoxin, when the half-lives are prolonged due to impaired renal or hepatic function and when the drugs are given at intervals shorter than their half-lives.

Bioavailability

Bioavailability is defined as the percentage of unchanged drug which reaches the systemic circulation following drug administration. Although any route of administration can be considered, most information relates to oral administration. For intravenous administration bioavailability is 100%. Oral bioavailability depends on drug formulation, gastrointestinal absorption and first-pass metabolism in the liver or gut wall.

Absorption

The majority of drugs are incompletely absorbed from the gastrointestinal tract. For example, 70% of the dose of digoxin given orally reaches the systemic circulation mainly due to incomplete absorption. In part this is due to metabolism by bacteria within the intestine. Some drugs are too hydrophilic, e.g. atenolol, or too lipophilic to be absorbed easily from the gut and consequently have low oral bioavailability.

First-pass metabolism

Following absorption from the gut, the portal vein delivers the drug to the liver before entry into the systemic circulation. A drug can be metabolised in the gut wall or occasionally within the portal circulation, but most frequently this occurs within the liver. The effect of first-pass metabolism on bioavailability is usually expressed in terms of the extraction ratio (*ER*)

$$ER = \frac{Cl_{\text{liver}}}{\text{Blood flow liver}}$$

The systemic bioavailability of a drug (*F*) can be predicted from the fraction of drug absorbed and the extraction ratio

$$F = f(1 - ER)$$

It could be argued that therapeutic plasma levels could be achieved with high extraction drugs if a large enough dose were administered. However, following oral administration the levels of drug metabolites would be higher than after the intravenous route and, if active, could contribute to drug toxicity. For example, lignocaine and verapamil have similarly low oral bioavailability ($\approx 20\%$). Unlike verapamil, lignocaine is never given orally because the metabolites have significant central nervous system toxicity. Other cardiovascular drugs with high extraction ratios include glyceryl trinitrate, hydralazine, isosorbide dinitrate, morphine and prazosin. These drugs when administered orally show marked inter-subject variation in bioavailability, largely due to differences in hepatic function and liver blood flow. In patients with hepatic dysfunction shunting of blood past hepatic sites of elimination will result in substantial increases in drug bioavailability but reduced formation of active metabolites for pro drugs such as enalapril and most ACE inhibitors. By contrast, drugs such as digitoxin and theophylline with low extraction ratios will be largely unaffected. Hepatic first-pass metabolism can be avoided to a considerable degree by using the sublingual, transdermal and, to a lesser degree, the rectal route of administration. Using these routes, there is direct access to the systemic circulation.

The time course of drug effect

Immediate effects

For several drugs the effects of drug therapy can be directly related to plasma concentrations. However, because the relationship between drug concentration and effect is non-linear (Figure 3.3), the effect will not always be directly proportional to the drug concentration. For example, if the ACE

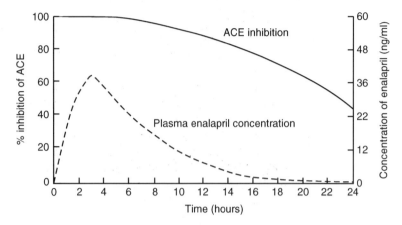

Figure 3.5. Relationship between percentage ACE inhibition and plasma concentration of enalapril.

inhibitor enalapril is administered once daily the degree of ACE inhibition remains high throughout most of the 24-hour period despite relatively low plasma concentrations of the drug (Figure 3.5). In other words, some drugs with relatively short half-lives such as enalapril and atenolol can be given once daily to maintain a 24-hour duration of effect provided trough concentrations exceed the EC_{50} (Figure 3.2).

Delayed effects

Changes in the magnitude of drug effect are frequently delayed in relation to changes in plasma concentrations. Short delays may be caused by the time required to distribute from the plasma to the site of action. This is well documented for digoxin, digitoxin and amiodarone. Longer delays may be due to the slow turnover of a physiological substance involved in the expression of a drug effect. A good example is provided by the anticoagulant warfarin which inhibits the enzyme vitamin K epoxidase. Although the inhibition of the enzyme is closely related to the plasma concentration of warfarin, it is the formation of the prothrombin complex of clotting factors which determines the anticoagulant effect. This complex has a half-life of about 14 hours and therefore the time to reach steady state and hence maximum anticoagulant effect is delayed.

Cumulative effects

Some drug effects are related to a cumulative rather than a rapidly reversible action. For example the pulmonary and hepatic adverse effects of amiodarone, the peritoneal, eye and skin manifestations of practolol and the cardiotoxicity of the antitumour antibiotics relate better to the cumulative dose than plasma concentrations.

Selection of appropriate dosage regimens

Rational therapeutics is based on the assumption that there is a dosage or plasma concentration range which will achieve the maximum or near maximum therapeutic effect with a low incidence of adverse effects. Commonly quoted therapeutic ranges are listed in Table 3.1 for a number of cardiovascular agents. The initial target concentration should be selected from the lower part of the range. In some cases the target concentration range will depend on the therapeutic objective. For example, the plasma concentrations of digoxin to control the ventricular rate in atrial fibrillation tend to be higher (1.5–2.5 ng/ml) while 1–2 ng/ml is usually adequate for patients with heart failure with sinus rhythm.

Maintenance dose

In clinical practice most drugs are administered to maintain relatively constant plasma concentrations. This is achieved by giving enough drug at each dose to replace the amount eliminated since the previous dose. If a drug is given as a continuous intravenous infusion (I) then the concentration at steady state (C_{SS}) is defined by the amount of drug infused per unit time and total plasma clearance (Cl).

$$C_{SS} = \frac{I}{Cl} \quad \text{or} \quad I = C_{SS}Cl$$

For oral therapy the dosage rate replaces the infusion rate and F represents the fraction absorbed.

$$\text{Dosing rate} = \frac{C_{SS} \times Cl}{F}$$

$$\text{Maintenance dose} = \text{dosing rate} \times \text{dosing interval}$$

When drugs are given by repeated oral therapy plasma concentrations oscillate around the steady-state value (Figure 3.6). The accumulation factor assumes that the drug follows a one-compartmental model and the absorption rate is much faster than the elimination rate. For calculation of peak and trough plasma concentrations these approximations are acceptable for most cardiovascular drugs.

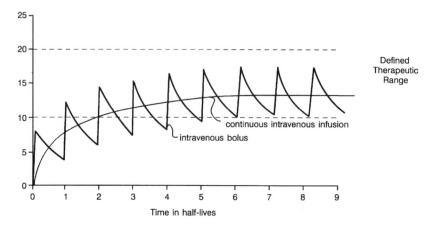

Figure 3.6. Relationship between maximum and minimum plasma concentrations (peak and trough) before and at steady-state following intravenous boluses given each half-life. The effect of giving a continuous infusion to achieve the same steady-state plasma concentration is illustrated.

Loading dose

When drugs have long elimination half-lives a loading dose may be required to achieve a more rapid pharmacological effect. If it is given as an intravenous bolus or is rapidly absorbed by another route, the initial concentration can be considerably higher than calculated. This is well illustrated with the drug lignocaine when used as an antiarrhythmic drug. Rapid intravenous bolus injection can result in toxicity soon after administration. Loading doses of this drug need to be given slowly or administered by repeated intramuscular injections.

The value of plasma concentration measurement in clinical practice

For a small number of cardiovascular drugs the relationship between steady-state plasma concentrations and clinical effects has been studied under relatively controlled conditions. Such drugs usually have narrow therapeutic indices—digoxin, digitoxin, quinidine and procainamide. The principal reason, however, for measuring plasma drug concentrations is because it is difficult to reach an optimum dosage schedule based purely on the clinical evaluation of drug response. It is therefore inappropriate to measure plasma concentrations when monitoring the effects of antihypertensive and anticoagulant drugs. It is debatable, however, how well the plasma concentrations of digoxin or digitoxin relate to clinical or toxic effect in patients with heart failure, and the antiarrhythmic drugs quinidine and procainamide are now rarely used in clinical practice. In general it is better to rely on clinical observation and judgement and use plasma concentration measurement sparingly especially since most of these so-called therapeutic ranges have been defined using clinical measures of effect and toxicity.

Poor drug compliance is a common cause of treatment failure. Those who measure plasma concentrations in an outpatient setting frequently find that concentrations remain low, despite adjustment of drug therapy. While other factors such as enzyme induction may be responsible, it is usually easy to identify the non-compliant patient, although taking medication on the day of the clinic visit can confuse the picture. For drugs with long elimination half-lives, measurement of steady-state plasma concentrations is a useful measure of drug compliance. Other indications for measuring plasma drug concentrations include the management of patients with poor or rapidly changing renal or hepatic function, those on complex combination therapies when drug interactions can cause problems, and in the management of drug overdose.

In conclusion, individual patients show a wide variation in response to the same dose of several cardiovascular drugs. Much of the variation in drug response is due to variations in pharmacokinetics which can be genetically determined or due to the effects of disease and other drugs. Drug dosage should be individualised to achieve the desired therapeutic response with a low incidence of adverse effects. For a small number of cardiovascular drugs, response and risk of toxicity relate better to steady-state plasma concentrations than dosage.

4 Drug Treatment of Angina Pectoris

Introduction

One of the best early descriptions of the syndrome of angina pectoris was given by William Heberden in 1772. "Those who are afflicted with it, are seized while they are walking, more especially if it be uphill, and soon after eating with a painful and most disagreeable sensation in the breast, which seems as if it would extinguish life, if it were to increase or to continue; but the moment they stand still, all this uneasiness vanishes."

It was over a century later that the important link between atherosclerosis and angina pectoris was established. This in turn led to the proposition that angina pectoris was related to reduced blood supply to the myocardium. Although myocardial ischaemia occurs when myocardial oxygen demand exceeds supply, the functional and electrocardiographic effects of ischaemia in the myocardium cannot be reproduced by hypoxia alone. The contractile activity of cardiac muscle depends on the availability of adenosine triphosphate produced by the myocardium. Although the production of adenosine triphosphate is critically dependent on the availability of oxygen, a more meaningful definition of myocardial ischaemia would be when the consumption of adenosine triphosphate exceeds its production. This results in anaerobic cellular metabolism and impaired myocardial contractility. The most common reason for this is the inability of blood flow in the coronary arteries to deliver oxygen and substrate for the given demand. When this imbalance is short-lived, ischaemia is transient and the condition of angina pectoris frequently results. If the process is sufficiently prolonged and myocardial necrosis occurs, then the clinical picture is that of a myocardial infarction.

The imbalance between blood supply and demand remains the basis for the events leading to the clinical syndrome of angina pectoris. The concept of fixed stenosis in diseased coronary arteries with reduced peripheral dilatory reserve has proved an inadequate explanation for several types of ischaemic conditions. Experimental and clinical data suggest that epicardial vessels, distal arterioles, collateral vessels and blood constituents all have important roles in the haemodynamic changes that occur following exertion. When sympathetic activity is increased, appropriate increases in blood flow occur in healthy regions of the heart. However, in potentially ischaemic areas blood flow is frequently reduced, not only because of fixed stenosis, but because of further narrowing in the epicardial arteries and distal arterioles. The reasons are unclear, but unopposed alpha$_2$ receptor activity and failure to produce an appropriate vasodilator response by the diseased endothelium appear to play a role.

Angina pectoris may also occur in the absence of increased sympathetic activity. In these situations pain is frequently triggered by disruption of a lipid-rich plaque and erosion of its fibrous cap. In its most extreme form this can result in extensive thrombosis, vessel occlusion and a myocardial infarction. A number of factors may act to limit the extent of the thrombosis, however, and result in unstable angina. These factors include the vessel diameter at the lesion site, the extent of coronary artery disease in other vessels, the geometry of the tear, the balance between dilator and constrictor effects, and between thrombotic and fibrinolytic activity. Occasionally angina at rest may occur in patients with normal coronary arteries due to coronary artery spasm. It may be related to local hypersensitivity to constrictor substances such as thromboxane A$_2$ or impairment of the normal vasodilator mechanisms.

Clinical presentation of myocardial ischaemia

Transient reversible myocardial ischaemia or angina pectoris can present in a number of different clinical settings (Table 4.1). In stable or classical angina, chest pain is precipitated by exertion, emotion or following meals, occurs in a reproducible manner and settles when the precipitating factors are no longer operating. These patients sometimes describe pain at rest, or in bed at night which wakens them from sleep, and occasionally a variable amount of exercise is required to induce the chest pain but these additional

Table 4.1. Syndromes associated with reversible myocardial ischaemia

With coronary artery disease	With normal coronary arteries
Stable angina on exertion	Variant angina
Stable angina on exertion and at rest	Syndrome X – reduced vascular reserve
Angina with varying threshold	Left ventricular hypertrophy
	–aortic stenosis
	–hypertension
Variant angina	–obstructive cardiomyopathy
Unstable angina	Coronary anomalies and arteritis (rare)
Silent myocardial ischaemia	

features are constant and reproducible. Much less frequently the typical chest pain of myocardial ischaemia occurs at rest in the absence of fixed coronary artery narrowing. This is often referred to as Prinzmetal's angina and appears to be related to coronary artery spasm.

Some patients with a history of stable angina pectoris can experience a sudden worsening of symptoms. Pain occurs more frequently, lasts longer and is often not relieved reliably by previously effective therapy. This syndrome is often referred to as unstable angina and may on occasions be so severe as to resemble a myocardial infarction sometimes referred to as the "intermediate" syndrome. Finally, there is growing evidence that a number of patients with obstructive coronary artery disease experience episodes of myocardial ischaemia in the absence of pain. These episodes probably have the same prognostic and haemodynamic significance as true angina pectoris.

Stable angina pectoris

The majority of patients with angina pectoris have this condition. Pathologically, almost all patients have atherosclerotic narrowing in one or more of their coronary arteries. Increases in heart rate, blood pressure, myocardial tension and contractility increase myocardial oxygen demand and increase the risk of developing chest pain (Figure 4.1). In patients with nocturnal pain and in those who have a variable threshold of exertion to

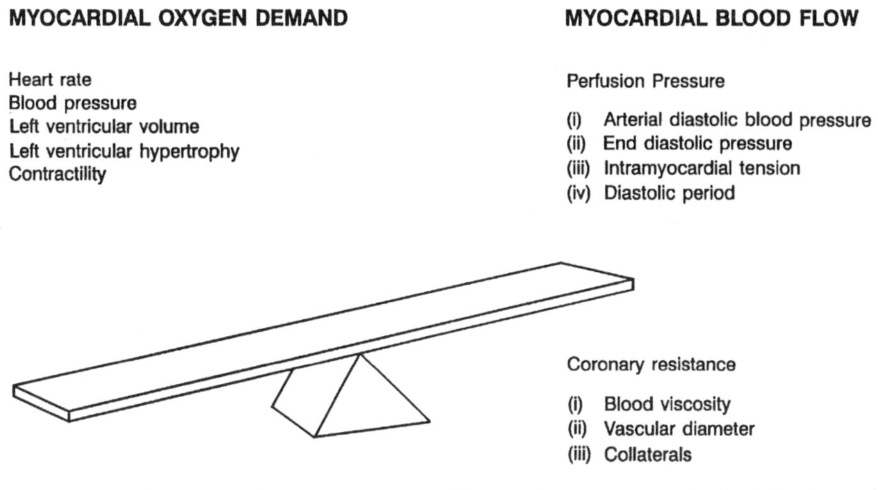

MYOCARDIAL OXYGEN DEMAND

Heart rate
Blood pressure
Left ventricular volume
Left ventricular hypertrophy
Contractility

MYOCARDIAL BLOOD FLOW

Perfusion Pressure

(i)   Arterial diastolic blood pressure
(ii) End diastolic pressure
(iii) Intramyocardial tension
(iv) Diastolic period

Coronary resistance

(i)   Blood viscosity
(ii) Vascular diameter
(iii) Collaterals

Figure 4.1.   Factors influencing myocardial supply and demand. Modification of Ross, R. S. Pathophysiology of coronary circulation. *British Heart Journal*, 1971; 33: 173–184. Reproduced with permission.

precipitate chest pain, coronary artery spasm, platelet aggregation at sites of vessel narrowing, and reduced vasodilator reserve in the distal coronary vasculature, play a role in addition to fixed stenosis.

Unstable angina pectoris

Patients with unstable angina tend to have severe atheromatous coronary artery disease and primary reduction in coronary blood flow is the principal underlying cause in the majority of patients with unstable angina pectoris. Ischaemic episodes, especially those occurring at rest may result from platelet plugging of already stenosed coronary arteries and local activation of vasoconstrictor substances, especially thromboxane A_2. Autopsy findings have revealed embolisation of thrombotic fragments to the distal segments of the coronary circulation. These probably contribute to the condition of severe unstable angina or intermediate syndrome and although small areas of infarction do occur, these are insufficient to cause increases in cardiac enzymes.

Variant angina pectoris

In addition to his description of classical stable angina pectoris, Heberden described an identical pain which occurred at rest rather than on exertion: "Some have been seized while they are standing still, or sitting, also upon first waking out of sleep". The episodes of chest pain tend to recur at approximately the same time of day and often in the early hours of the morning. During the episodes of pain, ST segment elevation is frequently seen on the electrocardiograph. A variety of arrhythmias accompany the chest pain – atrioventricular block, ventricular extrasystoles, tachycardia and fibrillation. In most situations, the pain responds readily to sublingual glyceryl trinitrate with resolution of the electrocardiographic findings. Although most of these patients have complete occlusion of one of the major coronary arteries, a small group of patients with normal coronary arteries also develop the condition.

Possible mechanism of coronary artery spasm

No clear trigger factors for the development of coronary artery spasm have as yet been identified. There is no evidence of increased sensitivity of vascular smooth muscle to noradrenaline, but there may be local hypersensitivity to and increased release of local constrictor substances such as thromboxane A_2 and endothelin I. Diseased vessels with impaired endothelial function produce less nitric oxide and the balance of vasoactive hormones tends to favour coronary vasoconstriction. Other proposed mechanisms include changes in pH, release of histamine, calcium activation, platelet aggregation and local production of endothelins and vasoconstrictor prostaglandins.

Thromboxane A_2 aggregates platelets and is a potent endogenous vasoconstrictor. It is rapidly degraded to a stable inert metabolic, thromboxane B_2. Prostacyclin on the other hand is an effective inhibitor of platelet aggregation and relaxes vascular smooth muscle. It is produced by the vascular endothelium and although it lasts somewhat longer than thromboxane A_2, it is degraded to its inactive form 6-keto $PGF_{1\alpha}$ within 2–3 minutes. Animal experiments have revealed that during periods of reduced coronary blood flow, clumps of platelets accumulate on the narrowed segment of the vessel. This results in cyclical reductions in coronary blood flow which can be prevented by antiplatelet drugs. There can be little doubt that a link does exist between vasospasm and platelet activation. Aggregating platelets release thromboxane A_2, a powerful vasoconstrictor. Also repeated vasoconstriction of the coronary arteries can lead to intimal damage. This in turn can result in platelet activation, thromboxane A_2 production and further vasospasm. Thus, it seems likely that thromboxane A_2 is involved in triggering vasospasm and/or perpetuating spasm once it has occurred.

Rare syndromes of myocardial ischaemia

1. Reduced vasodilator reserve.
2. Pathology in the smaller coronary arteries.

The coronary arteries dilate under normal circumstances as the work done by the myocardium increases to maintain adequate blood supply to the heart muscle. As in other regions of the circulation, the arterioles account for the main resistive component in the coronary circulation. Under ischaemic conditions, the distal coronary arterioles are normally maximally dilated. Under certain conditions, however, these smaller vessels fail to dilate appropriately and a condition of "reduced vasodilatory reserve" has been described. The significance of this abnormal response in angina pectoris has still to be fully assessed. A similar explanation has been proposed to explain the condition referred to as syndrome X. These patients have exertional angina, ST segment depression during stress testing but normal large coronary arteries. It is suggested that the abnormality in these patients is due to structural or functional disturbance of the small angiographically invisible coronary arteries. To date, the relative importance of this condition as a cause of ischaemic chest pain has still to be clarified since it relies on demonstrating that the large coronary arteries are entirely normal.

Rationale for the use of drugs in angina pectoris

Vast quantities of energy are required to maintain normal cardiac function. Mitochondria, the site of oxidative metabolism, and synthesis of adenosine triphosphate constitute 25–40% of the total volume of ventricular myocardial cells in the human heart. As a result, the heart requires a large and continuous supply of oxygen and cannot sustain an oxygen debt for more than a few seconds without resulting in significant myocardial dysfunction. To achieve this, the heart requires a very high blood supply which is out of all proportion to its mass. Since oxygen extraction from blood passing through the left ventricle is almost maximal, increased myocardial demand has to be met by increases in coronary blood flow. On the other hand, decreases in coronary blood flow or increased oxygen demand without increases in oxygen supply will result in myocardial ischaemia.

Control of coronary blood flow and the role of drug therapy

The two basic determinants of coronary blood flow are the perfusion pressure which is the inflow pressure for coronary flow and the coronary vascular resistance. Inflow pressure is defined as the difference between the pressure in the aorta and the intra-myocardial pressure. Not only does aortic pressure vary throughout the cardiac cycle but contraction and relaxation of the ventricular myocardium alters the phasic flow in the coronary arteries. Coronary blood flow is reduced during systole due to direct contraction of muscle fibres beside the inter-myocardial vessels and to indirect compression of the coronary vasculature produced by changes in the ventricular chamber pressures. Three principal factors influence coronary vascular resistance: blood viscosity, the length of the vessel and the diameter of the lumen. Since viscosity and vessel length are usually unaffected, the main determinant of vascular resistance is the cross-sectional area of the coronary vessels. Advanced atherosclerosis interferes with the regulation of coronary blood flow by adding fixed resistance in series with the resistance vessels. As already discussed, further narrowing can result from vasoconstriction beyond the region of fixed stenosis. As a result of compression during systole, the subendocardium is more sensitive to the effects of coronary artery narrowing and is the area most vulnerable to myocardial ischaemia.

In most clinical situations, drug therapy has little or no effect on coronary blood flow. In ischaemic syndromes, largely due to fixed stenosis, organic nitrates probably have little effect on total coronary flow although coronary artery dilatation may occur in some areas. Improved regional flow to ischaemic areas would clearly be beneficial although there is doubt about their effects on collateral coronary and subendocardial vessels where blood supply tends to be poorest. Coronary artery dilatation probably accounts for most of the beneficial effects in patients with chest pain due to coronary artery spasm. It has recently been suggested that glyceryl trinitrate like nitric oxide (endothelium-derived relaxing factor), inhibits platelet aggregation. There is some evidence that aggregation occurs in the presence of the sulphydryl donor N-acetylcysteine, but it is unclear whether this is due to the organic nitrate, the sulphydryl donor or the interaction between the two compounds acting from outside the cell.

The principal effect of the beta adrenoceptor antagonists is to reduce oxygen consumption although animal experiments suggest that propranolol improves coronary blood flow to ischaemic areas. There is no confirmation that this effect occurs in patients with angina pectoris.

The vasodilating properties of the calcium channel antagonists are not confined to the systemic arteries but also affect the coronary arteries so that under certain clinical conditions oxygen supply to the myocardium may increase. It is probably this property which makes the group particularly beneficial in the treatment of angina pectoris in which arterial spasm plays a major role although their effects in unstable angina have been disappointing. Occasionally the calcium channel antagonists precipitate the pain of angina by dilating coronary vessels supplying relatively normal myocardium and away from ischaemic areas.

Cyclical reductions in coronary blood flow are known to occur in vessels with fixed stenosis probably due to the accumulation of platelet aggregations in areas of severe stenosis and reduced blood flow. This cyclical flow can be attenuated by antiplatelet drugs such as aspirin, and is one of the principal reasons why these drugs are effective in unstable angina.

Factors influencing myocardial oxygen demand and the role of drug therapy

Myocardial oxygen requirements increase when there is an increase in heart rate, contractility, arterial blood pressure or ventricular volume (Figure 4.1). Other factors which play a part are the basal metabolic rate, activation of contraction and fibre-shortening and the thickness of the ventricular wall. In general, most antianginal treatment is directed at reducing myocardial oxygen demand.

Organic nitrates decrease venous pressure and reduce left ventricular volume with a small effect on systemic vascular resistance and hence blood pressure. These two effects combine to decrease ventricular wall tension, a major determinant of myocardial oxygen requirements. Although nitrates induce a reflex increase in heart rate and myocardial contractility which tends to increase myocardial oxygen demand, this is overshadowed by the reduction in ventricular wall tension. There is also some evidence that nitrates alter the haemodynamic responses to exercise. Peak systolic and end-diastolic pressures are reduced as is the response of the ischaemic myocardium to adrenergic stimulation.

Beta adrenoceptor antagonists reduce heart rate particularly after exercise, myocardial contractility and systemic blood pressure. The net effect is a reduction in myocardial oxygen demand although in some clinical situations, notably in patients with incipient heart failure, decreased myocardial contractility can lead to ventricular enlargement and increased oxygen consumption.

As a result of inhibiting calcium ion entry into cardiac and vascular smooth muscle cells, myocardial contractility and systemic blood pressure are reduced. The effect on heart rate is more variable. Nifedipine and other dihydropyridine calcium antagonists increase heart rate due principally to secondary beta adrenergic stimulation. Diltiazem tends to reduce heart rate while verapamil has the greatest depressant effect on the sino-atrial and atrioventricular nodes. In general, drugs which decrease resting heart rate tend to be more effective in angina pectoris than those which increase heart rate, but they are more likely to precipitate heart failure in "at risk" patients.

Silent myocardial ischaemia

Silent myocardial ischaemia has been defined as the presence of transient myocardial ischaemia without associated chest pain in patients with coronary artery disease. The frequency of silent ischaemia has been shown to be about three times that of symptomatic ischaemia and its presence has an adverse effect on survival. The pathophysiology of silent ischaemia is essentially the same as symptomatic myocardial ischaemia and results from an imbalance of myocardial oxygen supply and demand. The treatment of myocardial ischaemia is, therefore, directed at lowering myocardial oxygen demand and/or increasing oxygen supply. Several early studies suggested that antianginal therapy, used to treat painful myocardial ischaemia, was also useful for silent ischaemia, but the value of pharmacological treatment in this condition has recently been disputed.

Comparative studies and selection of the most appropriate therapy

Recent comparative studies suggest that beta adrenoceptor antagonists are more effective than nifedipine in the treatment of chronic stable angina (Figure 4.2). The combination, however, proved more effective than either agent given separately. Although calcium channel antagonists can prevent coronary artery spasm and may improve the ability of the myocardium to withstand ischaemia and reperfusion injury, they do not improve the

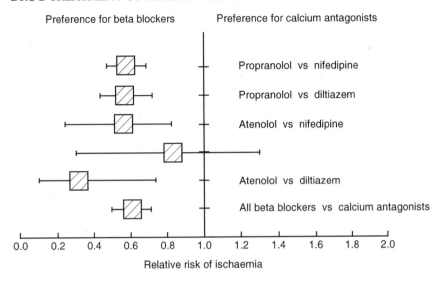

Figure 4.2. A comparison of beta blockers and calcium antagonists in angina pectoris. (Odds ratios ±95% Confidence Intervals)

prognosis in unstable angina and short acting nifedipine has recently been shown to have an adverse impact on the incidence of myocardial infarction. The beta adrenoceptor antagonist, metoprolol, had no effect on survival and improvement was only seen when metoprolol was combined with nifedipine. In contrast, aspirin has little effect on the incidence of recurrent ischaemia in patients with unstable angina but has a major impact on the risk of developing a myocardial infarction (see Figure 5.5).

Nitrates

In 1867, Thomas Brunton, a young house physician at the Edinburgh Royal Infirmary, was studying the effects of angina on blood pressure as measured by the newly introduced sphygmomanometer. Angina pectoris was associated with a rise in blood pressure and venesection resulted in a fall in blood pressure and relief of chest pain. He reasoned that amyl nitrite, a drug which was known to lower blood pressure, might be helpful in relieving the pain of angina pectoris. Brunton obtained a sample of amyl nitrite and poured it on a cloth for his patient to inhale. Within a minute the severe chest pain disappeared and the patient remained pain-free for several hours. Over the next few years Brunton satisfied himself that other nitrites had similar effects. He also examined the effects of nitroglycerine, a compound which had recently been synthetisised by Alfred Nobel for its explosive properties. However, it was 12 years later that William Murrel, a registrar at the Westminster Hospital, published his first report in the *Lancet* on the value of nitroglycerine (glyceryl trinitrate) in the treatment of angina. Much larger doses were required to produce a clinical effect when given orally compared to the buccal or sublingual route.

Mode of action

Nitrate-induced relaxation of vascular smooth muscle is mediated by the intracellular release of nitric oxide. Nitric oxide stimulates soluble guanylate cyclase, resulting in an increase in intracellular cyclic guanosine monophosphate which in turn causes smooth muscle relaxation. An intact endothelium is required for the activity of several vasodilator substances, notably acetylcholine and serotonin. Nitrates, on the other hand, produce vasodilatation whether or not endothelium is present. Nitrates, therefore, provide an exogenous source of nitric oxide which bypasses the endothelium and acts directly on vascular smooth muscle. Sulphydryl (SH) groups are required for the stimulation of guanylate cyclase and vascular tolerance to the action of organic nitrates occurs when the SH groups are oxidised by excess exposure to nitrate groups (Figure 4.3). Nitrates have greater venous than arterial effects, probably because the venous endothelium produces less nitric oxide and the nitrate receptors are up-regulated more than in arterial smooth muscle.

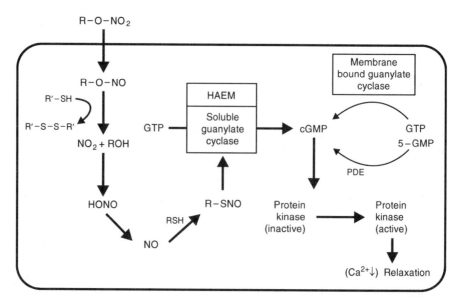

Figure 4.3. Proposed cellular actions of organic nitrates.

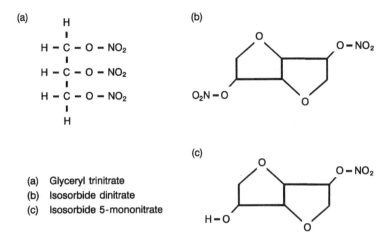

(a) Glyceryl trinitrate
(b) Isosorbide dinitrate
(c) Isosorbide 5-mononitrate

Figure 4.4. Clinical structures of organic nitrates.

Preparations and nitrate pharmacokinetics

Glyceryl trinitrate (Figure 4.4) and other short-acting nitrates have been the mainstay of the treatment of angina pectoris for over a century. The haemodynamic and therapeutic effects of glyceryl trinitrate last for about 30 minutes so various attempts have been made in recent years to prolong the duration of effect of this group of compounds. In addition to sublingual preparations, oral, chewable, transdermal, transmucosal and intravenous forms are now available.

Sublingual glyceryl trinitrate

Pharmacokinetics. Oral bioavailability is poor because of extensive hepatic first-pass metabolism. The clinical effects occur within 1–2 minutes and last 30 minutes to 1 hour. Peak plasma levels occur around 2 minutes and the elimination half-life is about 7 minutes (Table 4.2). Sublingual glyceryl trinitrate tablets should be administered initially at the smallest available dose (300 µg) and then increased until a maximum of 1200 µg if necessary. The drug should be taken as early as possible after the onset of angina or preferably used prophylactically before activities which are likely to cause the chest pain, such as walking uphill, emotional upset and sexual intercourse. If chest pain persists, doses of glyceryl trinitrate can be repeated at 5-minute intervals until pain relief is achieved. Clearly, if treatment is unsuccessful, medical advice should be sought. Patients frequently do not take their glyceryl trinitrate promptly because they

Table 4.2. Pharmacokinetic values of commonly used organic nitrates

	Glyceryl trinitrate	Isosorbide dinitrate	Isosorbide mononitrate
Duration of action	3 minutes–24 hours*	4–6 hours	1–10 hours
Time to onset of action	1–60 min*	20–30 minutes	<20 minutes
Time to peak	2 minutes (iv)	0.5–2 hours	0.5–3 hours
Plasma half-life	7.5 minutes (iv)	5 hours	4–5 hours
Metabolism	Very rapid and nearly complete hepatic metabolism	Very rapid and nearly complete hepatic metabolism	No significant metabolism
Oral bio-availability %	—	10–40%	Almost 100%
Excretion	Renal as metabolites	Renal as metabolite isosorbide mono nitrate	Renal unchanged

*Depends on the preparation.

believe it to be an addictive analgesic or develop severe headache and hypotension from taking too large an initial dose. At present buccal aerosol administration is preferred. Glyceryl trinitrate tablets have a limited life span of about 6 weeks and need to be kept in light-protected bottles. Metered dose aerosols allow very rapid buccal absorption and almost immediate effect. Each aerosol contains 200 doses of 400 μg per dose. Patients should be warned not to inhale the spray or use it near a naked flame.

Buccal glyceryl trinitrate

In this preparation, glyceryl trinitrate is impregnated into an inert polymer matrix which allows diffusion of the compound from the tablet and across the buccal mucosa. The tablet surface rapidly develops a gel-like coating which forms a surrounding seal and allows the tablets to adhere to the mucosal surface of the mouth. Absorption occurs provided the tablet remains intact. Chewing the tablet negates the pharmacological effect if rapidly swallowed, but can result in a large amount of the drug being absorbed if retained inside the mouth. Buccal nitrate formulation has an onset of action comparable to that of sublingual glyceryl trinitrate, but achieves its maximum effect about 30 minutes later. The preparation retains its pharmacological activity for up to 6 hours provided it remains inside the mouth. It is generally well tolerated and provides satisfactory pain relief. Tolerance has been reported less frequently than with transdermal formulations.

Transdermal nitrates

The use of transdermal glyceryl trinitrate was described as early as 1955, but this route of administration did not become popular until the mid-1970s when a sustained therapeutic effect could be demonstrated. Transdermal glyceryl trinitrate patches are available in different sizes and doses. Patches 5–30 cm^2 in area contain 2–5 mg/cm^2 in different vehicles to permit the timed release of the drug over 24 hours. Transdermal isosorbide dinitrate patches are also available.

Despite initial claims that effective 24-hour control could be achieved with transdermal nitrates, the majority of clinical studies have been unable to demonstrate prolonged improvement with chronic therapy. Apart from intravenous use, it is the route of administration most commonly associated with nitrate tolerance, and although transdermal preparations are now available with built in "nitrate-free interval", there is little to recommend this method of nitrate delivery.

Oral nitrates

Despite extensive first-pass hepatic metabolism, isosorbide dinitrate (Figure 4.4) improves exercise tolerance for up to 3 hours in patients with angina pectoris following a single dose and for up to 5 hours during chronic therapy (Table 4.2). The duration of effect in the prevention of chest pain is more variable and continuous administration throughout the 24-hour period tends to promote tolerance. To prevent this, a nitrate-free interval lasting at least 8 hours is now recommended during chronic therapy to reduce the risk of tolerance developing.

The active metabolite of isosorbide dinitrate, isosorbide 5′ mononitrate (Figure 4.4) is also available for oral prophylaxis. This preparation is not subject to significant first-pass metabolism in the liver and so its oral bioavailability is higher than that of the dinitrate. Plasma nitrate levels are also less variable with the mononitrate and the optimum dose range consequently is narrower. Tolerance can also occur with this preparation.

Sustained release preparations of isosorbide dinitrate and isosorbide mononitrate are also available. Matrix sustained-release formulations result in reduced peak plasma levels, prolonged absorption and longer duration of effect. Sustained release capsules contain micropellets with a rate-controlling membrane that allows two-stage delivery of the drug. Initially, 30% of the drug is released and the remainder as the maintenance dose. Chewable tablets can also be used to prevent or abort an acute attack of angina. Normally one or two tablets should be chewed until completely dissolved and then swallowed during an attack or before an expected attack.

Intravenous nitrates

Intravenous glyceryl trinitrate is very effective in the management of patients with severe unstable angina. The starting dose of 5–10 μg/minute can be increased to 200 μg/minute or higher depending on the clinical course. Intravenous therapy administered over a 5-day period, reduced the number of episodes of angina at rest and the need for pain relief in the form of sublingual nitrate or morphine. However, recent evidence has confirmed that this form of therapy has no impact on the long-term morbidity and mortality. Since glyceryl trinitrate has a short elimination half-life, intravenous therapy allows for rapid and effective dose adjustment. However, the doses required for pain relief vary widely and there appears to be little useful correlation between the infusion rate, plasma concentrations and haemodynamic effects. One reason for problems with dose adjustment is the administration of the drug through infusion sets made of polyvinyl chloride. In this situation the haemodynamic effects are reduced during the first few hours when the plastic is becoming saturated with the drug. Clearly this type of administration set should not be used in clinical practice.

Intravenous isosorbide dinitrate can be used as an alternative preparation which effectively relieves angina at rest at a dose of 1.25–5.0 ng/hour. It is unclear why intravenous therapy is more effective than full doses of oral therapy, although plasma concentrations are 10 times greater than the same dose given orally, reflecting the low oral bioavailability of this formulation of organic nitrate. Limited evidence suggests that provided large enough doses of isosorbide dinitrate are used to achieve the same plasma concentrations, equally effective results can be achieved with the oral route.

Nitrate tolerance

Despite considerable debate over the last 40 years, tolerance is now generally accepted as an important clinical phenomenon. Tolerance to the effects of organic nitrates has been demonstrated in the peripheral vasculature and attenuated clinical responses have been observed in patients with angina pectoris and congestive cardiac failure. In one early study, the hypotensive effect of oral isosorbide dinitrate was reduced within 48 hours of drug administration but was restored after a drug-free interval of 10 hours. These findings have been confirmed with intravenous and transdermal glyceryl trinitrate. Responses to a continuous infusion of glyceryl trinitrate in patients with congestive cardiac failure are markedly reduced within 48 hours. In contrast, tolerance was not observed when 12-hour infusions were followed by drug-free periods lasting 12 hours. Apart from the intravenous route, transdermal nitrates are the most likely preparations to be associated with tolerance. A substantial number of studies have reported partial or complete loss of effect within 24 hours following the use of transdermal nitrates.

Studies in patients with angina pectoris and congestive heart failure suggest that if plasma nitrate levels are subtherapeutic for a period of at least 8 hours, tolerance does not appear to develop. This knowledge has led to the introduction of nitrate dosage regimens which include a "nitrate-free interval" or "nitrate holiday". This treatment regimen is not without problems. At the end of this period without drug therapy, exercise time may be reduced and a group of patients experience increased angina episodes during this form of intermittent therapy. Since these problems are likely to occur, it is important to maximise other antianginal therapy to ensure good control during the nitrate-free interval.

Four principal explanations have been advanced to explain the phenomenon of nitrate tolerance: sulphydryl depletion, neurohormonal activation, plasma volume expansion and increased free radical activity. The most popular theory is depletion of the sulphydryl groups necessary for the conversion of organic nitrates to nitric oxide (Figure 4.3). Although there is some evidence that sulphydryl donors, such as N-acetylcysteine and large doses of captopril, may reverse nitrate tolerance, depletion of sulphydryl groups has not been demonstrated in vascular tissue showing nitrate tolerance and donors can improve nitrate responses in normal vascular smooth muscle. The experimental evidence for increased levels of vasoconstrictor hormones – noradrenaline, angiotensin II, endothelin I, etc., is also conflicting and like volume expansion is more likely to be a problem in congestive heart failure. Overall, ACE inhibitors, adrenoceptor antagonists and diuretics have little impact on nitrate tolerance. Finally, recent animal data suggest that tolerance to glyceryl trinitrate is associated with increased production of the superoxide anion and can be reversed by antioxidant administration – vitamin E, hydralazine and N-acetylcysteine.

Comparative pharmacokinetics

The pharmacokinetics of the three principal nitrate preparations are summarised in Table 4.2. The use of organic nitrates is strongly influenced by the presence of a high capacity, hepatic organic nitrate reductase which inactivates the drug. As a result, the bioavailability of most orally administered organic nitrates is very low. Because of very high systemic clearance, plasma concentrations of glyceryl trinitrate vary widely and can be altered by exercise, high ambient temperature and changes in cardiac output. If therapeutic effect is required rapidly then the sublingual or intravenous administration is required. Isosorbide dinitrate and mononitrate have lower systemic clearances and larger apparent volumes of distribution so that their half-lives and duration of effect are longer. Isosorbide dinitrate is partially metabolised while the 5′ mononitrate is unaffected. The principal metabolites have longer elimination half-lives but are less effective vasodilators. Excretion of the metabolites is mainly through the kidney.

Adverse effects

The major acute toxic effects of the organic nitrates are direct extensions of therapeutic vasodilatation – orthostatic hypotension, tachycardia and throbbing headache which tend to be more marked when combined with alcohol and other vasodilator drugs. Occasionally excessive tachycardia occurs in response to hypotension and the severity of the angina may be increased. Glaucoma, once thought to be a contraindication, is not aggravated by the use of these drugs, but nitrates continue to be avoided in patients with raised intracranial pressure. Nitrate groups react with haemoglobin to produce methaemoglobin but the amounts formed are very small and rarely of clinical significance.

Interactions and contraindications

Phenobarbitone increases the metabolism of glyceryl trinitrate but the effect is unlikely to be clinically important. In contrast, ethanol acts as an enzyme inhibitor and increases the drug's vasodilator activity. The hypotensive effects of tricyclic antidepressants are increased when they are used with organic nitrates and preliminary data suggest that indomethacin inhibits the peripheral vasodilator effects of the nitrates probably by reducing prostaglandin E_2 synthesis. Recent information suggests that the phosphodiesterase V inhibitor sildenafil is contraindicated in patients receiving organic nitrates. Sudden reductions in blood pressure have been reported with this combination.

A variety of cardiovascular diseases are contraindications or relative contraindications to the use of nitrate therapy. In angina pectoris related to hypertrophic obstructive cardiomyopathy, nitrates may aggravate outflow obstruction and could compromise diastolic filling in constrictive pericarditis and cardiac tamponade. For similar reasons, nitrates may cause deterioration in patients with tight mitral stenosis or in those following a major right ventricular infarction.

Nicorandil

Mode of action

Nicorandil (Figure 4.5) is a novel antianginal agent which combines two vasodilator mechanisms: potassium channel activation (Figure 4.6) and

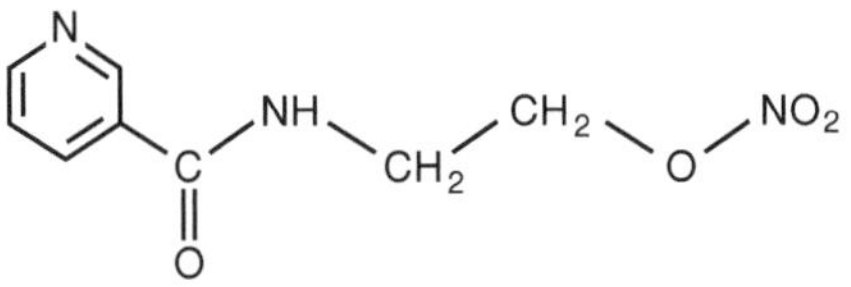

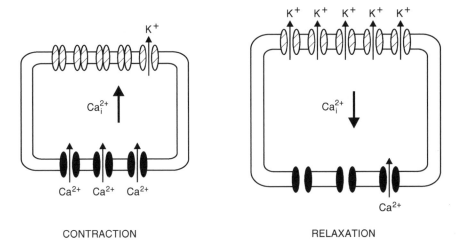

Nicorandil

Figure 4.5. Clinical structure of nicorandil.

CONTRACTION   RELAXATION

Figure 4.6. Schematic representation of the mechanism of action by which K^+ channel openers relax vascular smooth muscle cells. Increased potassium efflux results in reduced intracellular calcium and muscle relaxation.

increased cyclic guanosine monophosphate (cGMP) production in vascular smooth muscle. It dilates normal and stenotic segments of coronary arteries and systemic veins reducing preload and afterload. The effect on stenotic coronary arteries seems to be greater than that of organic nitrates. The net result is decreased oxygen consumption and increased coronary blood flow. These effects are not all due to the nitrate moiety, since the induction of nitrate tolerance by pretreatment with glyceryl trinitrate causes minimal effects on vascular haemodynamics, and to date tolerance to nicorandil has not been described. Although nicorandil has been shown to accelerate repolarisation and reduce action potential duration in animal models, electrophysiological studies have not demonstrated any detrimental nodal or ventricular activity in patients. Finally nicorandil has been reported to inhibit ADP induced platelet aggregation *in vitro*. The importance of this property is, however, unknown.

Pharmacokinetics

Nicorandil is well absorbed by the oral route with no significant first-pass metabolism resulting in an oral bioavailability of more than 75%. It undergoes hepatic metabolism and the parent compound and its metabolites are mostly excreted in the urine. No adjustments are required in liver or renal failure.

Clinical effects

Nicorandil has been shown to be effective in relieving the symptoms of angina pectoris, improving exercise duration and reducing the number and severity of chest pain in stable, unstable and variant angina. In addition there is some preliminary evidence that nicorandil can reduce post-ischaemic reperfusion injury in patients undergoing valve surgery and provide short-lived symptomatic improvement in patients with heart failure.

Adverse effects and interactions

Like the organic nitrates, headache is the most common adverse effect. The reported incidence varies from 20 to 50% and is most commonly seen when large doses are used as initial therapy. The drop-out rate at this stage may be as high as 10%. After 1 month, the incidence of headache is considerably less. Other infrequently reported adverse effects include dizziness, malaise, palpitations, nausea, vomiting, flushing and fatigue. At higher doses, hypotension and tachycardia may occur. There are no significant inter-actions reported so far with nicorandil with the exception of beta adrenoceptor antagonists which potentiate the drug's effect on lowering blood pressure.

Beta adrenoceptor antagonists

Mechanism of action in angina pectoris

Classically beta receptors are divided into the $beta_1$ receptors found largely in heart muscle and the $beta_2$ receptors found in bronchial and vascular smooth muscle. There are also significant populations of $beta_2$ receptors in the myocardium and other possible receptor subtypes, notably the $beta_3$ receptors. The exact roles for the cardiac $beta_2$ receptors and the $beta_3$ receptors have not been accurately defined. Beta adrenoceptor antagonists antagonise the effects of catecholamines at the beta receptors by occupying the receptors and competitively reducing catecholamine receptor

Table 4.3. Classification of beta adrenergic antagonists

Without partial agonist activity		With partial agonist activity			Dual action
					Alpha blocker or vasodilator activity
Non-selective	Beta$_1$ selective	Non-selective	Beta$_1$ selective	Beta$_2$ selective	
Propranolol	Atenolol	Pindolol	Acebutolol	Celiprolol (? beta$_1$ ISA)	Labetalol
Sotalol	Metoprolol	Oxprenolol	Prenalterol		Celiprolol
Timolol	Bisoprolol	Alprenolol	Xamoterol		Carvedilol
Nadolol	Betaxolol				

occupancy. Drugs which block the beta$_1$ receptor (Table 4.3) reduce oxygen demand by reducing heart rate, especially after exercise, myocardial contractility and systemic blood pressure.

Although beta adrenoceptor antagonists are now considered to be the first-line therapy for the long-term symptomatic management of angina pectoris, almost a fifth of patients fail to respond. This may be because coronary artery spasm has a major role, the underlying disease is so severe that pain occurs at low heart rates, or that because of excessive negative inotropic effects the left ventricular end-diastolic pressure increases and sub-endocardial flow is reduced.

Choice of beta blocker

All drugs which antagonise the beta$_1$ receptor appear to be equally effective in the treatment of angina pectoris provided equipotent doses are chosen. Two properties may influence the choice of drug therapy – beta$_1$ selectivity and partial agonist activity. It is doubtful whether partial agonist activity confers a major advantage in the management of angina pectoris, but agents with this property may be less likely to affect the peripheral circulation. This property may also protect against congestive cardiac failure, bradycardia and depression of atrioventricular conduction. These potentially useful properties are counterbalanced by the consideration that intrinsic sympathomimetic activity is probably undesirable in angina which occurs at rest or after minimal exercise. Although beta$_1$ selectivity offers some theoretical advantage by not blocking the cardiac β_2 receptors which oppose vasoconstriction due to alpha receptor stimulation, no clinical superiority has been demonstrated. The incidence of adverse effects due to beta$_2$ blockade: airways obstruction, reduced peripheral circulation and prolonged hypoglycaemia is, however, reduced.

Similarly, drugs with additional alpha blocking activity are no more efficacious than classic beta blockers in the treatment of angina pectoris.

Selection of patients

The nature of angina and the presence of other diseases may influence the choice of a beta adrenoceptor antagonist. Patients with bradycardia at rest may benefit from a drug with partial agonist activity while a beta blocker without this property would be preferable in a patient with angina at rest. Patients with asthma, insulin-dependent diabetes or peripheral vascular disease are less likely to develop problems with $beta_1$ selective agents, although other types of anti-anginal therapy would be preferable if problems arise. In general, there is little to choose between the different beta adrenoceptor antagonists in terms of efficacy, and the advantages of $beta_1$ selectivity and partial agonist activity have rarely been shown convincingly in clinical trials.

Pharmacokinetics and dose adjustment

One important aspect of the chemistry of beta adrenoceptor antagonists is lipid and water solubility. Water-soluble drugs such as atenolol, sotalol or nadolol tend to undergo less metabolism, demonstrate less plasma level variability, have longer elimination half-lives and fewer effects on the brain. The highly lipid soluble drugs such as propranolol, oxprenolol and penbutolol frequently demonstrate first-pass hepatic metabolism, greater plasma level variability, shorter half-lives and a higher incidence of disturbed sleep (Table 4.4).

Non-selective beta blockers without ISA

In this sub-group, propranolol and timolol are lipophilic and sotalol and nadolol are hydrophilic. Propranolol and timolol are hepatically metabolised, have short half-lives and are short-acting unless special formulations are used. Sotalol and nadolol are not metabolised to any degree and have long elimination half-lives making them suitable for once-daily administration. For most bioavailability tends to be low (Table 4.4) either because absorption with hydrophilic agents is low or because first-pass metabolism with lipophilic agents is high.

Beta_1 selective beta blockers with ISA

Atenolol is hydrophilic, incompletely absorbed, renally excreted unchanged with a relatively long half-life and suitable for once-daily

Table 4.4. Pharmacokinetic values of beta adrenoceptor antagonists

	Acebutolol	Atenolol	Bisoprolol	Celiprolol	Labetalol	Metoprolol	Oxprenolol	Pindolol	Propranolol	Sotalol
Duration of action (oral)	12–24 hours	24 hours	24 hours	24 hours	12 hours	8–12 hours (24 hour*)	6–12 hours	8–24 hours	6–24 hours*	24 hours
Time to onset of action	≈ 1 hour	≈ 1 hour	1–3 hours	0.5–1 hour	1 hour	1 hour	1 hour	1 hour	1–2 hours	1 hour
Time to peak effect	1–4 hours	2–4 hours	≈ 2 hours	2–3 hours	1–2 hours	1–2 hours	1 hour	1–3 hour	2–3 hours	2–3 hours
Plasma half-life	7–10 hours (Parent+ metabolites)	6–9 hours	10–12 hours	5–6 hours	3–6 hours	3–4 hours	2 hours	2–5 hours	3–6 hours	7–15 hours
Metabolism	Extensive to diacetolol	Less than 10%	Some hepatic metabolism	Almost none	Extensive to glucuronide	Extensive	Extensive to several metabolites	Extensive to hydroxy metabolites	Extensive to several metabolites	Not metabolised
Oral Bio-availability %	20–60	≈ 50	≈ 90	30–70	30–40	50	20–75	80	≈ 30	90
Excretion	Renal and biliary	Renal	Renal	Renal and biliary	Renal and biliary	Renal	Renal	Renal	Renal	Renal

*Sustained release.

administration. Metoprolol is extensively metabolised with a short half-life so that special formulations are required to produce suitable once-daily preparations.

Beta blockers with partial agonist activity

Most members of this subgroup are lipophilic and undergo extensive metabolism. Acebutolol and xamoterol are hydrophilic agents and although they are metabolised, they have relatively long elimination half-lives.

Dual-acting beta blockers

Drugs in this group, celiprolol and labetalol are lipophilic and have significant first-pass hepatic metabolism. Their half-lives are relatively short although celiprolol produces a sustained antihypertensive effect for up to a day.

Dose adjustment

Although a good relationship between plasma drug concentration and reduction of an exercise tachycardia does exist, for most beta adrenoceptor antagonists this does not always relate easily to the clinical situation. Plasma concentration measurement is rarely helpful in dose adjustment. It has been suggested that a resting heart rate of 50–60 beats/minute represents adequate beta blockade. This is often a poor guide since the rate varies widely between individuals and is largely determined by vagal rather than sympathetic activity. If the drug has partial agonist activity, then resting heart rate is clearly of no clinical value. Exercise heart rate is a better measure of drug effect, but does not lend itself to routine assessment of patients in the clinical setting. Dose adjustment must, therefore, depend on assessing the severity and duration of the chest pain and increasing the dose until the maximum benefit is obtained or until important adverse effects occur.

Adverse effects

A variety of minor adverse effects occur with propranolol due to high lipid solubility and central nervous system penetration—sedation, sleep disturbance and depression. Rash, fever and allergic manifestations are rare. The major adverse effects relate to predictable effects due to $beta_2$ adrenoceptor blockade. Non-selective agents tend to make obstructive airways disease worse and mild asthma can become severe after $beta_2$ blockade. While $beta_1$ selective drugs tend to have less effect on airways resistance than non-selective agents, they should be used cautiously, if at all, in patients with reversible airways obstruction.

Beta adrenoceptor antagonists depress myocardial contractility and excitability. In patients with marked impairment of myocardial function, cardiac output is largely dependent on increased sympathetic activity. Removal of this activity can result in cardiac decompensation even at low dosage. Severe congestive cardiac failure has occurred in some patients. Almost 5% of patients on propranolol develop symptoms closely resembling those of Raynaud's disease or complain that their claudication is worse. This is in part due to unopposed alpha stimulation resulting from beta$_2$ blockade, but reduced cardiac output can contribute in patients with ischaemic heart disease.

Catecholamines increase glycogenolysis and increase blood glucose levels. In addition, lipolysis is enhanced and free-fatty acids are released from adipose tissue. Beta blocking drugs (especially non-selective) antagonise these metabolic effects. Hypoglycaemic reactions have been reported during treatment with beta adrenoceptor antagonists in diabetics receiving insulin and in healthy volunteers receiving sulphonylureas. Of greater clinical importance is their effect in reducing the normal adrenergic responses to hypoglycaemia. This tends to prolong the duration of the hypoglycaemia and makes the diagnosis of drug-induced hypoglycaemia more difficult. The incidence of this condition is unknown and many patients on insulin and beta blockers do not develop the condition. In general, beta$_1$ adrenoceptor antagonists are preferred to non-selective drugs in insulin and non-insulin-dependent diabetes.

Other adverse effects of beta adrenoceptor antagonists include nausea, constipation, diarrhoea and skin rashes. These are usually mild and only rarely necessitate drug withdrawal. Renal function occasionally deteriorates during treatment probably due to reduced renal blood flow. Occasionally hypotension and/or marked bradycardia results in vertigo, syncope or orthostatic hypotension necessitating withdrawal or dose reduction.

Interactions

The combination of beta blockers and anaesthetic agents or class 1 antiarrhythmic drugs can cause severe cardiac depression. Non-steroidal anti-inflammatory drugs tend to reverse the antihypertensive effects of most antihypertensive drugs, including beta blockers. Verapamil and other drugs which depress atrioventricular conduction can cause hypotension, heart failure and bradycardia. Rebound hypertension seems to be more severe if clonidine and a beta blocker are stopped at the same time than if a beta blocker is suddenly discontinued on its own.

Rebound hypertension

Accumulated evidence suggests that patients with coronary heart disease are at increased risk of developing sudden deterioration in their clinical condition following withdrawal of beta adrenoceptor antagonists. Severe hypertension and prolonged chest pain can occur, especially in patients who have been on large doses. The mechanism of this effect is uncertain, but probably involves "up-regulation" of the beta receptors and increased sensitivity to circulating catecholamines. Patients should be warned of the dangers of stopping the drugs suddenly and in those in whom withdrawal is necessary, gradual tapering of the dose is recommended.

Calcium channel antagonists

Mode of action in angina pectoris

Verapamil, the first clinically useful member of the calcium channel antagonists was discovered as a result of attempts to synthesise more active analogues of papaverine, a vasodilator alkaloid from the opium poppy. This group of compounds acts by inhibiting post-excitation influx of calcium through the L-calcium channels in the cell membrane into myocardial cells and the cells of vascular smooth muscle. This interferes with the action of calcium-dependent ATPase which is required for the energy needs of cardiac and smooth muscle contraction (Figure 4.7). The overall effect is a reduction in myocardial contractility and dilatation of vascular smooth muscle. These agents selectively block the calcium channels and leave the sodium channels relatively unaffected. Therefore, myocardial contractility is reduced while myocardial depolarisation is largely unaltered. In patients with angina pectoris, the overall effect is to reduce myocardial oxygen demand and reflex tachycardia is rarely a problem. The vasodilating effects are not confined to the systemic arteries, and effects on the coronary arteries have also been described in certain conditions. Calcium channel antagonists tend to be useful in coronary artery spasm and overall oxygen supply to the myocardium can be increased. However, like other coronary vasodilators angina pectoris is occasionally aggravated as a result of redistributing blood away from ischaemic areas.

High affinity binding sites for calcium antagonists are present on the alpha$_1$ sub-unit. Since different groups of calcium channel blockers recognise different binding sites, these drugs are classified according to the chemical structures which facilitate their binding to the different sites (Table 4.5). The relative binding will determine whether these agents have greater effects on vascular smooth muscle, cardiac muscle or conducting tissue. Therefore, although these drugs have a common mode of action, they differ significantly with respect to myocardial contractility, systemic

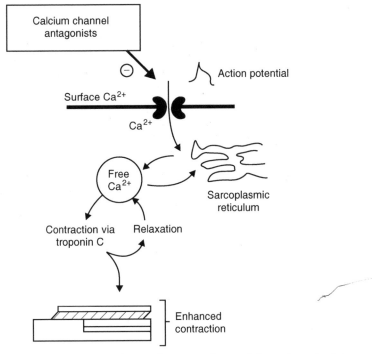

Figure 4.7. Role of calcium in smooth muscle contraction and the action of calcium channel antagonists.

vascular resistance, coronary vasodilatation, venomotor tone and anti-arrhythmic activity (Table 4.6).

Nifedipine produces a very rapid and marked decrease in blood pressure with an increase in heart rate due to secondary sympathetic stimulation. These effects occur within a few minutes of oral administration, peak at about half an hour and last for 3–4 hours. By contrast, the vasodilator effect of diltiazem occurs about 15 minutes after oral ingestion, reaches a maximum at 3 hours and lasts for 6–8 hours. Unlike nifedipine, diltiazem reduces heart rate and has little or no effect on myocardial contractility but can depress nodal activity. Verapamil has the greatest depressant effect on the sino-atrial and atrioventricular node and can exert a significant negative inotropic effect, especially in patients with poor cardiac reserve (Table 4.7).

Stable angina

Calcium channel antagonists as a group are effective in the long-term management of chronic stable angina. A number of studies have

Table 4.5. Properties of the three main groups of calcium channel antagonists

Type	Group	Examples	Principal action
I	Phenylalkylamines	Verapamil	*Cardiac:* Depressed AV conduction (***) Depressed myocardial contractility (***) *Vascular:* Vasodilatation (**)
II	Dihydropyridines	Nifedipine Amlodipine Nicardipine	*Cardiac:* Depressed myocardial contractility (*) *Vascular:* Vasodilatation (***)
III	Benzothiazepine	Diltiazem	*Cardiac:* Depressed AV conduction (***) Depressed myocardial contractility (*) Vasodilatation (**)

*Slight effect.
**Moderate effect.
***Marked effect.

Table 4.6. Comparative haemodynamics of the calcium channel antagonists used to treat angina pectoris

Property	Verapamil	Diltiazem	Nifedipine	Nicardipine	Amlodipine
Heart rate	↓	↓	↑	↑	—
Cardiac output	↓	↓	↑	↑	↑
Inotropic effect	↓↓	↓	↓	↓	—
Coronary artery tone	↓	↓	↓	↓	↓
Peripheral vascular resistance	↓	↓	↓↓	↓↓	↓↓
Reflex sympathetic activity	—	—	↑	↑	—
AV conduction	↓↓	↓	—	—	—
AV refractory period	↑↑	↑	—	—	—
Blood pressure	↓	↓	↓	↓	↓

↑= increase.
↑↑= greater increase.
↓= decrease.
↓↓= greater decrease.

Table 4.7. Effects of different calcium channel antagonists on electrocardiographic intervals

Electrocardiographic intervals	Bepridil	Verapamil	Nifedipine	Diltiazem
RR interval	↑	—	↓	↑
QRS interval	↑	—	—	—
QTc interval	↑	—	—	—
PR interval	↑	↑↑	—	↑

↑ = increase.
↑↑ = greater increase.
↓ = decrease.

demonstrated an increase in exercise duration and a significant delay in the onset of pain for all the commonly used agents. Verapamil's antianginal efficacy is similar to that of diltiazem and both are more efficacious than nifedipine and most other dihydropyridines as monotherapy. Aggravation of chest pain is also more likely to occur with nifedipine than the two other drugs, probably related to the greater increases in heart rate. Diltiazem and verapamil are as effective as beta adrenoceptor antagonists as mono-therapy, but the dihydropyridines appear to be less efficacious. On the other hand, a combination of a beta blocker with nifedipine is effective therapy for the treatment of stable angina pectoris. It is less likely to cause problems in patients following a myocardial infarction and those with conduction abnormalities than a combination of a beta adrenoceptor antagonist with verapamil or diltiazem.

Unstable angina

Although all three main groups of calcium antagonists have been shown to be effective in variant angina and early studies suggested a special role in patients with coronary artery spasm, their use in unstable angina has been disappointing. Recent evidence suggests that patients treated with the calcium channel antagonist, nifedipine, for unstable angina have an excess of cardiovascular events compared to a control population. Calcium channel antagonists can be used to treat angina pectoris, but beta adrenoceptor antagonists and nitrates are probably more effective despite the theoretical disadvantages.

Antiatherosclerotic effects of calcium channel antagonists

Animal studies have shown that calcium ions may mediate several of the metabolic processes involved in the progression of atherosclerosis. Calcium channel antagonists appear to prevent the entry of calcium into vascular tissue which precedes the development of necrosis. Eighty milligrams of nifedipine daily reduced the rate of new coronary lesions by 28% compared to placebo over a 3-year period, and 90 mg nicardipine produced a 40% reduction in minimal lesions over a 2-year period. In neither study, however, were there significant effects on the frequency of existing lesion progression or regression. At present calcium channel antagonists cannot be recommended in preference to other antianginal drugs because of possible antiatherosclerotic properties.

Pharmacokinetics and dosage adjustment

Verapamil

Verapamil undergoes extensive biotransformation with the N-demethylated form as the only active metabolite. Oral absorption is rapid and almost complete, but bioavailability is low due to extensive first-pass metabolism (Table 4.8). The oral doses required to produce a clinical effect in angina pectoris (up to 480 mg daily) are therefore much higher than the doses required intravenously. Plasma concentrations vary widely between patients and there is no simple relationship between plasma concentrations and effect.

Diltiazem

Following oral administration of diltiazem, over 90% of the drug is absorbed but bioavailability is about 40% due to high first-pass metabolism to desacetyldiltiazem which has about 40% of the activity of the parent compound. Reported half-lives of diltiazem in healthy volunteers range from 4 to 7 hours.

Nifedipine and other dihydropyridines

Nifedipine in capsular form is almost completely absorbed after oral administration although somewhere between 45 and 68% reaches the systemic circulation because of first-pass metabolism. Peak plasma levels are reached within 2 hours and the drug remains detectable for up to 6 hours after standard dosage. The hypotensive effect is apparent 30 minutes after an oral dose and within 5 minutes after a sublingual or 'bite and swallow' dose. The duration of effect following standard formulation is variably reported to be between 4 and 12 hours.

Nifedipine undergoes almost complete hepatic oxidation to three pharmacologically inactive metabolites which are excreted in the urine. Some studies have shown a relationship between plasma nifedipine concentrations and heart rate, but this is of little clinical relevance.

Table 4.8. Pharmacokinetic values of calcium channel antagonists

	Amlodipine*	Diltiazem*	Felodipine*	Isradipine*	Lacidipine	Nicardipine*	Nifedipine*	Nisoldipine*	Verapamil*
Duration of action (oral)	>24 hours	8–12 hours[†]	>24 hours	12 hours	8–12 hours	4 hours	4–12 hours[†]	8–12 hours	6 hours
Time to onset of action	1–2 hours	0.5–3 hours[†]	1–2 hours	20 minutes	30 minutes–1 hour	30 minutes	30 minutes–1 hour	30 minutes–1 hour	30 minutes–1 hour
Time to peak effect	6–12 hours	2–11 hours[†]	3–5 hours	2 hours	1–2 hours	1–2 hours	1–3 hours*	1–2 hours	1–5 hours[†]
Plasma half-life	30–50 hours	4–7 hours[†]	8 hours	2–6 hours	≈ 8 hours	8 hours	6–11 hours*	2–13 hours	3–12 hours
Metabolism	Extensive hepatic metabolism to inactive metabolites	Extensive hepatic metabolism	Extensive hepatic metabolism to inactive metabolites	Extensive liver first pass metabolism	Extensive first pass metabolism in the liver	Extensive first pass metabolism but no active metabolites	Extensive hepatic oxidation to three inactive metabolites	Extensive hepatic metabolism to inactive metabolites	Extensive metabolism to nor-verapamil which is pharmacologically active
Oral bio-availability %	60	40	15	20	—	35	40–70	<10	20–35
Excretion	Metabolites via bile and kidney	Metabolites via the kidney	Metabolites via the kidney	Metabolites via bile and kidney	Metabolites via the kidney	Metabolites via the kidney	Metabolites via the kidney	Metabolites via the kidney	Metabolites via the kidney

*Licensed for use in angina patients.
[†]Sustained release.

Nicardipine is also rapidly and completely absorbed after oral administration with peak concentrations occurring between 20 minutes and 2 hours. The vasodilatation lasts for 2–6 hours and as with other dihydropyridines the drug has a low systemic bioavailability of between 7 and 40%, depending on the dose. The plasma elimination half-life is relatively short. As a result the drug needs to be given three times daily.

Amlodipine has a much longer elimination half-life than other dihydropyridines and has a slower onset of action probably related to lower lipid solubility. Absorption is slow with peak plasma concentrations after 6–12 hours. The bioavailability is about 60% and the metabolites are inactive. Once-daily drug administration is therefore satisfactory.

Adverse effects and drug interactions

Verapamil is well tolerated during chronic therapy. Symptoms such as dizziness, headache, constipation and nausea can occur but usually disappear with continued therapy. Verapamil has been successfully combined with a variety of cardiovascular drugs, but caution should be exercised when co-administering verapamil with a beta blocker, particularly in patients with conduction abnormalities as heart block may result. Vasodilator effects do occur but are less common than with the dihydropyridines. Patients with atrial fibrillation or flutter and the Wolff–Parkinson–White syndrome may develop ventricular tachycardia because verapamil may enhance conduction across the anomalous pathway. In patients with poor ventricular function, verapamil should be avoided or used only if heart failure is well controlled. Allergic reactions, gingival hyperplasia and gynaecomastia are all unusual adverse reactions to verapamil.

Diltiazem is a very well tolerated calcium channel antagonist. Vasodilator effects (headache, flushing, hypotension and pedal oedema) do occur, but they are relatively uncommon and are less than with nifedipine. Constipation and bradycardia also rarely occur. Patients with slow heart rates or prolonged PR interval should be observed closely since there is a risk that they may develop second or third degree atrioventricular block (Table 4.7). Occasionally severe interactions with beta blockers have been reported, leading to bradycardia, hypotension and congestive cardiac failure. This is more likely to occur in patients with pre-existing conduction defects and left ventricular dysfunction.

Nifedipine is the prototype peripheral vasodilator and as such it has a high incidence of flushing, tachycardia, hypotension and peripheral oedema. Although a measure of tolerance does develop, a relatively high percentage of patients discontinue their therapy because of these adverse effects. The effects are dose-related and the lower doses now available have a substantially lower incidence. Worsening of angina and gingival hyperplasia have also been reported. Dihydropyridines may aggravate poor cardiac reserve but this is less than with verapamil.

The most common adverse effect of amlodipine is oedema. Dizziness, flushing, headache and sweating do occur but less than with nifedipine. It is probably safe in patients with poor left ventricular function and preliminary evidence suggests that it may be useful in the treatment of heart failure due to congestive cardiomyopathy. In patients with angina, ischaemic pain may be exacerbated. The adverse effects of nicardipine are similar to those of nifedipine.

Antiplatelet drugs

Aspirin

Platelet aggregation is now considered to play a major role in the pathophysiology of unstable angina pectoris. Aspirin inhibits adenosine diphosphate-induced platelet aggregation and collagen-induced release of adenosine triphosphate, serotonin and platelet antiheparin activity factor. Most importantly, however, aspirin rapidly and irreversibly acetylates the cyclooxygenase enzyme in platelets, preventing the formation of thromboxane A_2. As a result platelets are unable to synthesise new enzymes to replace those which are inactivated and platelet function is not restored until new platelets enter the circulation. The effect, therefore, lasts 4–7 days after a single oral dose. Aspirin also inactivates cyclooxygenase in the vascular endothelium which could reduce the anti-aggregatory effect of prostacyclin. However, vascular cyclooxygenase can be resynthesised within hours especially if low doses of aspirin are used. The platelet effects therefore predominate, and the net result is a prolonged inhibitory effect on platelet aggregation.

Clinical indications for aspirin

Aspirin has been shown to provide acute and long-term protection of major cardiac events during and after an episode of unstable angina pectoris. Aspirin has not been shown to reduce the number of ischaemic episodes or relieve pain during an episode of unstable angina. The optimal dose has not been agreed. Doses ranging from 325 to 1300 mg daily have been shown to be effective in patients with unstable angina casting some doubt on the "prostacyclin-thromboxane balance" theory. A dose of 40 mg is required for maximum suppression of platelet aggregation and beneficial effects have now been reported with doses as low as 75 mg. Given the presently available evidence the choice would seem to be between doses of 300 and 75 mg daily.

Adverse effects

In patients with unstable angina who receive standard doses of aspirin (325–1300 mg daily) up to 50% of patients complain of gastrointestinal symptoms – dyspepsia, nausea and vomiting. Gastrointestinal bleeding occurs in about 7% with frank melaena in about 1% and haematemesis in about 0.1% over a 1-year period of treatment. Reduced dosage and intermittent therapy reduces the incidence of adverse effects.

Drug interactions and contraindications

Although most non-steroidal anti-inflammatory drugs attenuate the antihypertensive effects of diuretics and most antihypertensive drugs, aspirin does not appear to share this property. The risk of aspirin-induced gastrointestinal bleeding is increased by alcohol, corticosteroids, non-steroidal anti-inflammatory drugs and warfarin. Aspirin decreases the urinary excretion of uric acid and urate levels should be monitored if the patient is receiving thiazide diuretics or has a previous history of gout. Aspirin is best avoided in patients who have haemophilia, a history of gastrointestinal bleeding, peptic ulcer or evidence of bleeding from other sites. Allergy to aspirin is usually an absolute contra-indication.

Abciximab

Abciximab is a monoclonal antibody which inhibits platelet aggregation and thrombus formation. It acts by antagonising the IIb/IIIa receptor on the platelet membrane. This receptor, when activated, undergoes a conformational change and binds fibrinogen which then cross-links platelets and causes aggregation. It is the final common pathway in platelet aggregation irrespective of the pathway of activation and, therefore, represents a logical therapeutic target. Abciximab is not specific for the IIb/IIIa receptor and may block platelet mediated thrombin generation and inhibit ATP release. Although the plasma half-life is short, receptor binding is not reversible and this produces a longer duration of effect.

Abciximab is indicated for use by invasive cardiologists as an adjunct to heparin and aspirin in preventing ischaemic complications in their risk patients undergoing percutaneous transluminal coronary angioplasty. There is also preliminary evidence that abciximab and other drugs which antagonise the IIb/IIIa receptor eptifibatide and tirofiban, may be of value in reducing the number of ischaemic events in severe unstable angina. Bleeding with or without thrombocytopaenia is the principal adverse effect.

Anticoagulants

Heparin

Since thrombin activation is an important mechanism in the pathogenesis of unstable angina, heparin has been widely employed during an acute severe episode of unstable angina. Heparin produces its anticoagulant effect by binding to and activating antithrombin III which reduces thrombin generation and fibrin formation. Three major trials have confirmed the value of continuous intravenous heparin in patients with severe unstable angina. The number of ischaemic episodes and major cardiovascular events – acute myocardial infarction and sudden death were reduced. During the period of treatment the incidence of recurrent angina was reduced, but to date no long-term efficacy data are available.

Low molecular weight heparins

Unfractionated heparin has a number of disadvantages. It binds to plasma proteins which compete with its binding to antithrombin. This produces variability in the dose–response relationship and contributes to the syndrome of heparin resistance. Heparin also binds to endothelial cells and macrophages and is responsible for the dose-dependent elimination of the drug. Heparin also binds to platelets and this contributes to the bleeding complications during long-term therapy. To overcome these problems standard heparin, which is composed of molecular masses of 2000–30 000 Da, has been fractionated to form molecular masses of 2000–6000 Da. These low molecular weight heparins bind less to plasma proteins and endothelial cells and therefore do not share the pharmacokinetic limitations of unfractionated heparin. In contrast to heparin, they have more predictable clinical responses, longer durations of effect and a lower incidence of microvascular bleeding. Alteparin reduces the risk of death or myocardial infarction in patients with unstable angina and is at least as effective as unfractionated heparin. Enoxaparin is also more effective than aspirin in reducing the incidence of death, acute myocardial infarction and severe unstable angina.

Low molecular weight heparins seem to represent a significant improvement over unfractionated heparin. Overall they appear equivalent to or better than standard therapy, can be administered without monitoring and have a lower incidence of bleeding complications.

Other vasodilator drugs

Drugs with alpha blocking activity

Coronary artery vasospasm is mediated via the alpha adrenoceptors, so selective and non-selective alpha adrenoceptor antagonists have been used to treat angina pectoris. To date, however, alpha blockers have not been shown to be useful in the management of stable or unstable angina and drugs such as labetalol which have alpha and beta blocking activity, are no more effective than drugs which are pure beta adrenoceptor antagonists.

Angiotensin converting enzyme inhibitors

There are several theoretical reasons why ACE inhibitors might be of value in the treatment of angina pectoris. There is experimental evidence that they improve endothelial function, attenuate sympathetic vasoconstriction in patients with coronary artery disease, reduce the risk of nitrate tolerance and prevent vascular hypertrophy. In addition, they delay the development of symptomatic heart failure in patients with impaired left ventricular function. To date the studies using ACE inhibitors in patients with angina pectoris have been inconclusive and larger controlled trials are needed to define their role in this condition.

Bepridil

Bepridil is a calcium channel antagonist with direct negative chronotropic and inotropic actions. In contrast to other calcium channel antagonists the drug displays modest peripheral vasodilatation and antihypertensive activity. Its plasma elimination half-life is between 1 and 2 days and the drug is effective when given once daily. Results from short-term clinical trials have shown that bepridil is as effective as other calcium channel antagonists and propranolol in reducing the frequency of anginal attacks and the consumption of glyceryl trinitrate in patients with stable angina. Bepridil is also more effective than nifedipine in improving exercise performance in patients with stable angina. The adverse effects profile is similar to established calcium antagonists, but the drug causes a rate-dependent prolongation of the QTc interval (Table 4.7) which predisposes to the development of *torsade de pointes*. The drug should, therefore, be avoided in patients with hypokalaemia, those receiving other drugs which prolong the QT interval or with congenital prolongation of the QT interval. The results of further studies are required before this drug can be recommended for general clinical use.

Mibefradil

Mibefradil is a calcium channel antagonist which selectively blocks the T channels in nodal tissue and vascular smooth muscle. T-type channel blockade with mibefradil results in reduced blood pressure and heart rate with a low incidence of the adverse effects commonly associated with calcium channel antagonists. Leg oedema, and depressed myocardial contractility are rarely observed.

In hypertensive patients, mibefradil has similar or superior efficacy to other calcium antagonists and improves exercise tolerance, frequency of chest pain and consumption of glyceryl trinitrate in those with angina pectoris. The drug is well tolerated but in June 1998 mibefradil was withdrawn because of a high incidence of interactions with commonly used cardiovascular drugs which are metabolised through the cytochrome P450 pathway.

5 Drug Treatment of Acute Myocardial Infarction

Introduction

Acute myocardial infarction is the single leading cause of death in Europe and the United States. However, mortality has been declining in most Western societies over the past two decades by about 2% per year. Primary prevention and advances in the management of acute myocardial infarction have probably contributed substantially to this decline in mortality.

Since coronary thrombosis occurs in almost all cases of myocardial infarction, therapies to lyse the clot and to prevent further clot formation have proved to be the most effective interventions in this condition. Thrombolytic therapy reduces cardiovascular mortality by about 25% and low dose aspirin confers a similar reduction in mortality of 23%. Other important aspects of management include pain relief, management of arrhythmias and the treatment of hypovolaemia, heart failure and acute hypotension.

Pain relief

Morphine given by slow intravenous injection at a dose of 5–10 mg combines a potent analgesic effect with beneficial haemodynamic properties. A vasodilator effect on the arteries and veins reduces afterload and preload and so decreases myocardial oxygen demand. In patients with hypovolaemia and reduced filling pressure, marked decreases in blood pressure can occur. The peripheral vasodilator effects have been attributed to a number of mechanisms including the release of histamine and central depression of vasomotor-stabilising mechanisms. No consistent effects on cardiac output are observed and the electrocardiograph is unaffected. Other important acute adverse effects include respiratory depression, which is due to central nervous system depression, and vomiting which is more likely to occur if the patient is moved soon after drug administration.

Management of arrhythmias

Atropine given as bolus injections of 0.3 mg up to a maximum of 2.0 mg is useful in the management of bradyarrhythmias with atrioventricular block which are particularly common after an inferior myocardial infarction. Atropine may also be helpful in sinus or nodal bradycardia with hypotension or when there are multiple ventricular ectopic beats related to severe bradycardia. Small doses and careful monitoring are important since reduced parasympathetic activity can unmask latent sympathetic overactivity and predispose to tachyar-rhythmias including ventricular tachycardia and fibrillation. Prophylactic atropine for uncomplicated bradycardia has therefore been largely abandoned.

Sinus tachycardia frequently occurs in the early stages after an acute myocardial infarction due to increased sympathetic activity. This can increase myocardial oxygen demand and predispose to more serious tachyarrhythmias. Pain and anxiety relief, correction of hypovolaemia and treatment of underlying heart failure are frequently successful, but beta adrenoceptor antagonists are safe and effective provided the patients are carefully observed. Trials using beta adrenoceptor antagonists have confirmed a 15% reduction in acute phase mortality and a 25–30% reduction in late phase mortality. These small but real benefits suggest that intravenous beta blockade should be used even in the absence of factors such as sinus tachycardia and hypertension. Reduced heart rate is associated with a limitation of infarct size. Early beta adrenoceptor antagonist administration can be usefully combined with thrombolytic therapy. The combination reduces recurrent infarction and ischaemia and the presence of the beta blocker reduces the risk of cerebral haemorrhage following tissue plasminogen activators.

Type I antiarrhythmic drugs have largely been abandoned for the prophylaxis and therapy of early post-infarction ventricular arrhythmias. Beta adrenoceptor antagonists seem to be more effective in this situation. Treatment of left ventricular failure and electrolyte disturbances will also reduce the risk of serious dysrhythmias. Atrial fibrillation, flutter and paroxysmal supraventricular tachycardia are usually transient but can be recurrent and cause haemodynamic problems. Precipitating factors such as hypoxia, heart failure, pericarditis and acidosis require treatment. If the patient has heart failure, intravenous adenosine can be highly effective while verapamil or a short-acting beta adrenoceptor antagonists can be used in those who have no clinical evidence of heart failure. Increasing vagal tone may sometimes be useful in paroxysmal atrial tachycardia while cardioversion and atrial overdrive pacing may be required in resistant cases.

Management of heart failure

There are special problems caused by the development of heart failure in the context of an acute myocardial infarction. Loop diuretics, in particular frusemide, when given intravenously can induce peripheral vasoconstriction resulting in an acute deterioration in cardiac output. In addition, when pulmonary oedema is present excessive diuresis can result in marked reductions in the left ventricular filling pressures and it is advisable in these situations to carefully monitor the preload using a Swan–Ganz catheter or bedside echocardiographic recordings. Similarly, potent vasodilator drugs such as sodium nitroprusside are best avoided unless there is frequent monitoring in an intensive care unit. Short-acting glyceryl trinitrate or angiotensin converting enzyme inhibitor would seem to be preferable.

In patients with low cardiac output and without signs of pulmonary or peripheral congestion it is essential to exclude hypovolaemia which is frequently diuretic induced or due to the presence of a right ventricular infarction.

The most effective treatment in this situation is an inodilator or the combination of dobutamine with an ACE inhibitor. Careful haemodynamic monitoring is again required in an intensive care facility. Nitrates are usually best avoided since their main action is to reduce preload. Inotropic support by digoxin remains controversial. The benefits are small even in patients with overt heart failure and should only be used in those not responding adequately to diuretics and ACE inhibitors except when fast atrial fibrillation is present.

Acute reperfusion therapy

An increase in the blood supply to the myocardial is the most effective method of reducing infarct size and preventing myocardial ischaemia. Intravenous thrombolytic therapy is now regarded as the most effective intervention for patients with evolving myocardial infarction especially when ST segment elevation denotes ischaemia. Numerous trials have demonstrated reduced mortality compared to placebo and the benefits appear greatest when the treatment is initiated within 6 hours of the onset of symptoms (Figure 5.1).

Thrombolytic therapy

Four thrombolytic agents are currently available for the management of acute myocardial infarction: streptokinase, alteplase, anistreplase and

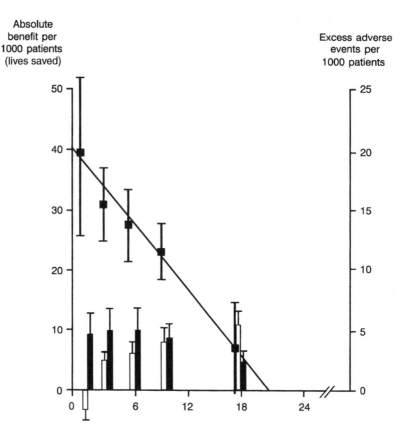

Figure 5.1. The relationship between the effectiveness and adverse effects of thrombolytic therapy and the time from the onset of suspected myocardial infarction. Reproduced from *The Lancet*, 1994; 343: 311–322. Fibrinolytic Therapy Trialists: ■ haemorrhagic complications; □ non-haemorrhagic complications. © by The Lancet Ltd. reproduced with permission.

reteplase. These agents differ in their clearance, fibrin selectivity, plasminogen binding and potential to cause allergic reactions (Table 5.1). In the United Kingdom streptokinase is usually the drug of first choice because of its low cost but this practice has been changed somewhat since the results of the GUSTO-1 trial (Table 5.2). In the United States alteplase is more frequently used as first line. There is a general consensus, however, that alteplase and related compounds are preferred in patients who have previously received streptokinase because the presence of antibodies

Table 5.1.   Characteristics of the different thrombolytic agents

Drug	Streptokinase	Alteplase	Anistreplase	Reteplase
Fibrin selective	–	+	–	+
Plasminogen binding	Indirect	Direct	Indirect	Direct
Fibrinogen breakdown	++++	++	+++	++
Hypotension	+	–	+	–
Allergic reactions	+	–	–	–

Table 5.2.   Comparison of mortality rates expressed as percentages in the major trials comparing streptokinase and alteplase

Trial	No. of patients	Mortality (%)	
		Streptokinase	Alteplase
GISI-2	12 490	8.6	9.0
ISIS-3	41 299	10.6	10.3
GUSTO-I	41 021	7.3	6.3*
INJECT	6 000	9.4	8.9[†]

GISI—Gruppo Italiano per lo studio della supravenza n'ell' infarcto miocardico.
ISIS—International study of infarct survival.
GUSTO—Global utilisation of streptokinase and tPA for occluded arteries.
INJECT—International joint efficacy comparison of thrombolytics.
*Accelerated tissue plasminogen activator.
[†]Reteplase.

reduces the effectiveness of thrombolysis and increases the risk of allergic reactions. Other advantages over streptokinase include earlier onset of action and better long-term results in non-anterior infarction. On the other hand streptokinase is preferred in hypertensive patients because of the lower risk of cerebral haemorrhage.

Mode of action

Despite earlier views to the contrary, it is now well established that a myocardial infarction is most frequently due to a thrombosis in the coronary artery supplying that region of cardiac muscle. The localised vascular occlusion occurs initially as a result of endothelial damage, platelet aggregation and subsequently by the activation of the coagulation proteins involved in the clotting cascade (Figure 5.2). This eventually results in the development of sufficient thrombin to convert fibrinogen into fibrin. After

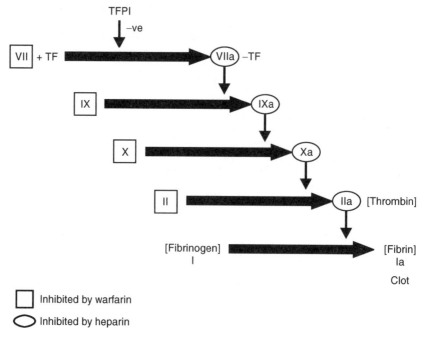

Figure 5.2.   Final stages of the clotting cascade.

cross-linkage, fibrin forms a thrombus at or near the original site of endothelial damage. Soon after formation, the thrombus constitutes an active environment in which fibrin continues to form and the fibrinolytic mechanisms are activated (Figure 5.3). At this point the patient may exhibit the signs of unstable angina or those of a myocardial infarction. The rationale for using thrombolytic therapy is to increase the amount of plasmin locally available to dissolve the clot to inactive fragments while at the same time minimising the increased risk of bleeding due to high levels of circulating plasmin.

Plasmin which is responsible for the degradation of fibrin and fibrinogen is formed from its inactive precursor, plasminogen. Under appropriate conditions this is achieved by an enzyme tissue type plasminogen activator which circulates in a pre-enzymatic form. Fibrinolytic therapy produces its effect by inducing additional plasminogen activation which is usually short acting and rapidly returns to normal levels when the treatment is withdrawn (Figure 5.3). The thrombin time usually returns to less than twice the normal value within a few hours, but the prothrombin time can be prolonged for periods up to 24 hours as a result of reduced fibrinogen and other clotting factors.

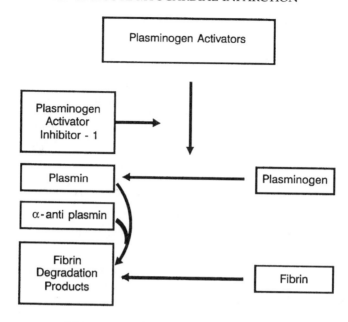

Figure 5.3. Plasma fibrinolytic system.

Streptokinase

Streptokinase, which is extracted from beta-haemolytic streptococci, activates plasminogen indirectly by forming a complex with it. The plasmin which is formed as a result of the interaction acts on fibrinogen and fibrin to form degradation products and is inhibited by $alpha_2$ antiplasmin. High doses produce more complete plasminogen binding and reduced release of plasmin. Antistreptococcal antibodies are commonly present and the dose must be sufficient to overcome their effects. In the majority of patients 250 000 units is enough to overcome their activity while doses between 0.75 and 1.5×10^6 units are usually effective in the treatment of an evolving acute myocardial infarction. At these doses fewer life-threatening bleeding events occur than with alteplase or anistreplase. Small reductions in blood pressure and reduced blood viscosity seen with this compound can reduce myocardial work and have an oxygen-sparing effect.

Pharmacokinetics

Streptokinase is administered by the intravenous and intracoronary route. It has a short half-life of 10–15 minutes and is extensively metabolised. Other pharmacokinetic values are listed in Table 5.3.

Table 5.3. Pharmacokinetic values of the three commonly used thrombolytic agents

Drug	Streptokinase	Anistreplase	Alteplase
Duration of action	Unknown	Unknown	Unknown
Time to peak action	≈60 minutes	90–120 minutes	90–120 minutes
Plasma half-life	10–15 minutes	90 minutes	5–8 minutes
Metabolism	Hydrolysis (almost complete)	Hydrolysis (almost complete)	Hydrolysis (almost complete)
Route of excretion	Unknown	Unknown	Unknown

Table 5.4. Advantages and disadvantages of the three commonly available thrombolytic agents

Drug	Advantages	Disadvantages
Streptokinase	Clinically proven value Relatively inexpensive	Antigenic Occasional allergic reaction Hypotension
Anistreplase	Clinically proven value Rapid effect with prolonged action	Antigenic Occasional allergic reaction Moderately expensive
Alteplase	Clinically proven value Non-antigenic Highly clot selective	Simultaneous heparin therapy required Short half-life Very expensive

Adverse effects and contraindications

Bleeding, symptomatic hypotension and allergic reactions represent the most common and serious reactions associated with streptokinase therapy. Bleeding can occur from any site but most major morbidity has been due to intracerebral haemorrhage. Post-streptokinase bleeding diathesis is particularly common in those patients who also receive heparin therapy, although the ISIS-3 trial indicated that severe bleeding was less common with streptokinase than the other two agents. Transient hypotension is a frequent finding during drug administration. Hypotension also occurs with streptokinase and other thrombolytic agents at the time of reperfusion associated with successful thrombolysis and recanalisation. Arrhythmias, including ventricular fibrillation, can occur at this time and contribute to the decrease in blood pressure. Allergic reactions (Table 5.4) including fever, rashes, serum sickness, polyneuropathy and rarely acute anaphylaxis occur in about 12% of patients treated. These are rarely seen with other thrombolytic agents and severe reactions are most likely to occur in patients who are re-exposed to the drug within a period of 6 months.

Patients treated with streptokinase also appear to be at increased risk of cardiac rupture. This occurs with all thrombolytic agents and the incidence can be reduced by the co-administration of a beta adrenoceptor antagonist. Patients with atrial fibrillation or left atrial enlargement due to mitral valve disease are at increased risk of cerebral embolisation. Other adverse effects include back pain, chills and headache.

Contraindications

Any condition which increases the risk of bleeding represents a relative or absolute contraindication to the use of streptokinase and other thrombolytic agents. Of particular interest is a history of previous cerebrovascular disease, a bleeding diathesis, haemorrhagic ophthalmic conditions, peptic ulcer and poorly controlled hypertension. Coexisting conditions for which streptokinase is contraindicated include acute pancreatitis, pericarditis, menorrhagia, bacterial endocarditis, pregnancy or recent delivery. A previous history of an allergic reaction to streptokinase, especially within the previous 3–6 months, is an absolute contraindication. Great care is also required when giving this drug to patients already receiving anticoagulants and antiplatelet drugs.

Interactions

The principal interactions are with anticoagulant and antiplatelet drugs. These increase the risk of unwanted bleeding and should be discontinued when thrombolytic therapy is initiated and reintroduced when treatment is finished.

Alteplase

Alteplase (tPA) is extracted from a human melanoma cell line or using recombinant DNA techniques. Although there is evidence for a higher immediate patency rate, there is little evidence that it is more effective than streptokinase in preventing deaths in the later post-infarction period. It is, however, associated with a lower incidence of allergic reactions, symptomatic hypotension and possibly a lower incidence of reinfarction. The elimination half-life of alteplase is shorter than streptokinase (Table 5.3) and stopping an infusion results in a return of plasma levels and major antithrombotic effect within 30–40 minutes.

Clinical use

A commonly used regimen in patients with an acute myocardial infarction is a 10 mg intravenous bolus followed by 50 mg in the first hour and 40 mg over the next 2 hours given as a continuous intravenous infusion. This can be given to all age groups, but more careful monitoring is required in the elderly because of the increased risk of bleeding.

Anistreplase

Anistreplase (anisolylated plasminogen streptokinase activator complex, APSAC) is a complex of streptokinase with human plasminogen. *In vitro* studies have demonstrated a thrombolytic potency 10 times greater than streptokinase and indicate that its thrombolytic action depends in large part on fibrin binding. Because of the slow dissociation of the streptokinase–plasminogen complex, the fibrinolytic activity lasts much longer than with streptokinase and alteplase. The clinical importance of this is unclear, although because it is effective as a single bolus it may be the agent of first choice for use outside hospital.

Current information suggests that the patency rate is less than alteplase but the risk of re-occlusion may be less. Effects on mortality are the same as with the other two thrombolytic agents but bleeding is more common than with streptokinase.

Clinical use

This is the simplest antithrombotic drug to administer. Normally 30 units are given intravenously over 4–5 minutes within 6 hours of a suspected acute myocardial infarction. This dose is also suitable for elderly patients, but again more careful monitoring for bleeding complications is required than for the younger age group.

Reteplase

Reteplase (r-PA, recombinant plasminogen activator) is a non-glycosylated deletion mutant of wild type tissue plasminogen activator. Overall, although easier to administer it does not provide any survival benefit in the treatment of acute myocardial infarction. Adverse effects, particularly the incidence of stroke, were identical to those observed with alteplase.

Combinations of thrombolytic therapy

Since 15% or more of patients treated with a single thrombolytic agent do not achieve successful coronary perfusion, various combinations have been used in an attempt to improve the response rate, the incidence of bleeding complications and to reduce cost. Small pilot clinical studies have suggested a synergism between thrombolytic drugs and this has resulted in a reduction in the total doses used. The combination of alteplase with streptokinase has been shown to be associated with greater early potency rates, lower occlusion rates and fewer total complications than standard doses of the individual drugs. Mortality rates, however, were largely unchanged and the risk of haemorrhagic stroke and other bleeding complications was increased with the combination. At present there is insufficient information to recommend combinations of thrombolytic agents.

Timing of thrombolytic therapy

An inverse relationship between survival and the time taken to initiate thrombolytic therapy after an acute myocardial infarction is well documented (see Figure 5.1). In addition the risk of cardiac rupture is greater the later thrombolytic therapy is started. After 6 hours, beneficial effects are hard to demonstrate and the risk of cardiac rupture is substantial. However, most of this information was derived from retrospective subgroup analysis of the large thrombolysis intervention studies and therefore lacked statistical power and was open to bias in interpretation. In two recent prospective studies, alteplase but not streptokinase was associated with a significant 27% reduction in 35-day mortality which was maintained for up to 1 year when treatment was initiated 6–12 hours after the onset of symptoms of a myocardial infarction. The overall conclusion seems to be that treatment should be initiated as soon as possible, preferably within the first hour after the onset of symptoms but that small benefits may occur with alteplase and possibly other thrombo-lytic agents between 6 and 12 hours.

These observations prompted the initiation of a series of small trials looking at the impact of pre-hospital administration of a variety of thrombolytic agents. Overall they demonstrated a small reduction in all cause mortality, but larger outcome studies are required before this practice can be widely recommended in the management of acute myocardial infarction.

Adjunctive therapy after thrombolysis

Given the previous success of isolated thrombolytic therapy the role of adjunctive strategies following thrombolysis is assuming increasing importance in the short- and long-term management of an acute myocardial infarction. The principal aims of such therapy are to help maintain coronary artery patency, prevent late reocclusion and ventricular dilatation and reduce myocardial ischaemic and infarct size.

Aspirin

Experimental and clinical studies have consistently implicated platelet thrombus formation as a major factor in preventing rethrombosis after successful thrombolysis. Clinical benefit is well documented in patients with suspected myocardial infarction whether or not thrombolytic drugs are used. However, the combination of aspirin and streptokinase reduced 5-week mortality by almost 20% more than streptokinase alone, probably by preventing reocclusion. Aspirin therapy should therefore be used in all patients who tolerate the drug after a myocardial infarction whether or not thrombolytic agents are used.

Heparin

Reocclusion after thrombolysis is related to increased thrombogenicity which is in part due to persistent vessel stenosis and partly to the presence of residual thrombus. Since the coagulation cascade and platelet activation is intimately involved in this process, heparin therapy should prevent thrombin production, platelet activation aggregation and deposition and so reduce the rate of reocclusion with its short- and long-term sequelae. Unfortunately a recent overview of randomised clinical trials concluded that the current evidence does not justify the routine addition of heparin in the treatment of an acute myocardial infarction and increases the risk of haemorrhagic stroke.

Warfarin

In the absence of clinical information comparing the long-term benefits of warfarin and aspirin and the clear benefits of aspirin, warfarin at present has no clear role in the routine long-term management of an acute myocardial infarction. In patients with established thromboembolic disease or those at higher risk of systemic embolisation, e.g. a large anterior infarction or atrial fibrillation, warfarin would be preferred to aspirin. At present there would seem to be no justification for combining warfarin with thrombolytic agents in any clinical situation.

New antithrombotic and antiplatelet agents

Several attempts have been made to increase the efficacy of plasminogen activators and/or prolong their duration of effect. Various deletion mutants of alteplase (tPA) have been produced but most have no greater thrombolytic activity than the parent compound; tPA from the saliva of the vampire bat is similar to human tPA but is more fibrin selective. Tests in man have not been performed. Several plasminogen activators consisting of various portions of tPA and urokinase type PA have been synthesised in an attempt to combine the fibrin selectivity of the two molecules. Again these have been shown to have no clear advantages over existing therapy. Staphylokinase, a 136 amino acid protein produced by certain strains of staphylococci has been shown to be more effective than streptokinase for dissolving platelet rich arterial graft thrombi and is less immunogenic. Early clinical studies appear promising.

Aspirin and heparin do not consistently prevent reocclusion. This could in part be due to the non-selective inhibition of anti-aggregatory as well as pro-aggregatory prostaglandins and the ineffectiveness of heparin as an inhibitor of clot associated thrombin. Several more specific approaches to platelet aggregation are currently being explored. These include specific thromboxane synthase inhibitors, serotonin antagonists, monoclonal platelet antibodies and antithrombin snake venoms. Another approach is to use selective thrombin inhibitors particularly hirudin and its derivatives or synthetically produced compounds. Some of these agents are more effective than aspirin or heparin in preventing arterial thrombosis, reocclusion and accelerating recanalisation. Unfortunately the risk of bleeding is very high. Improved thrombolytic therapy will therefore probably consist of more potent and specific plasminogen activators in combination with targeted anticoagulants and antiplatelet agents in the future.

Intravenous beta adrenoceptor antagonists

Although intravenous beta blockade as monotherapy reduces infarct size and decreases hospital mortality when used within 4–6 hours of an acute myocardial infarction it is only since the publication of the TIMI (thrombosis in acute myocardial infarction) trial that its value when combined with a thrombolytic drug (tPA) has been confirmed. Non-fatal reinfarction and recurrent ischaemic events occurred less frequently in patients who received 15 mg metoprolol immediately after an acute myocardial infarction as compared to those who received oral metoprolol 6 days after the infarction. The general recommendation therefore is that in patients receiving thrombolytic therapy, 15 mg metoprolol or 10–20 mg atenolol should be given intravenously in the first 4 hours after the onset of symptoms of an acute myocardial infarction.

Prevention of reperfusion injury

There is a wealth of experimental evidence detailing the changes and potential injury which occur as a result of coronary reperfusion. Well-documented events include mechanical "stunning", ventricular dysrhythmias, microvascular injury, free radical formation and possible myocardial cell necrosis. Although free radicals are formed following successful thrombolysis, clinical studies have been unable to show beneficial effects with free radical scavengers such as superoxide dismutase. At present the most effective way of reducing reperfusion injury is to limit the severity of ischaemic injury using beta receptor antagonists or non-dihydropyridine calcium channel antagonists if beta blockers are contraindicated.

Limitation of infarct size

Like angina pectoris, a myocardial infarction occurs as a result of an imbalance between myocardial oxygen supply and demand. It therefore appears logical to employ drug therapy which has proved beneficial in the management of angina pectoris. Other measures include the treatment of arrhythmias, hypoxia, heart failure, hypertension and tachycardia. Hypokalaemia is common after an acute myocardial infarction due in large part to catecholamine-induced movement of potassium into the myocardial cells and previous diuretic therapy. Timely correction of hypokalaemia should help prevent arrhythmias and myocardial dysfunction. Despite considerable experimental evidence for a variety of pharmacological interventions in reducing infarct size, definite clinical evidence is largely elusive.

Nitrates

Until two decades ago glyceryl trinitrate was contraindicated in patients with an acute myocardial infarction. Subsequent canine and later patient studies confirmed that glyceryl trinitrate or sodium nitroprusside given intravenously at low dose in the 48-hour period following an acute myocardial infarction not only improved performance in left ventricular failure but also limited ischaemic injury, infarct size and infarct related complications. Recent studies with more prolonged nitrate therapy spanning the healing phase of an acute anterior Q wave infarction produced further limitation of left ventricular remodelling and helped preserve myocardial function. Disappointingly, however, the recently completed ISIS-4 mega trial failed to demonstrate any beneficial effect on survival with long-term nitrate therapy.

Beta adrenoceptor antagonists

Some of the beneficial effects of early beta adrenoceptor blockade seen with metoprolol and atenolol are probably due to limitation of infarct size and there is some evidence that a small beneficial effect occurs.

Calcium channel antagonists

Calcium channel antagonists have a very limited role in limiting infarct size. Nifedipine (and probably all other dihydropyridine calcium antagonists) are contraindicated. Nifedipine when administered in the very early stages of an acute myocardial infarction is associated with increased mortality. On the other hand, diltiazem and verapamil may help prevent early reinfarction.

Magnesium

Based on the assumption that magnesium deficiency is a common manifestation of an acute myocardial infarction and that high levels of magnesium alter platelet function, reduce catecholamine production and inhibit calcium entry into cells, intravenous magnesium has been used in patients with acute myocardial infarction to limit infarct size and to improve long-term prognosis. Reduced mortality was suggested in earlier studies, but long term survival was not altered in the ISIS-4 trial. Routine magnesium administration in patients following an acute myocardial infarction cannot be recommended.

Glucose–insulin–potassium therapy

Metabolic support using glucose insulin and potassium was shown to reduce in-hospital mortality following an acute myocardial infarction with and without thrombolytic therapy in two small studies. Its value in larger populations has not been studied, probably because of its low commercial potential.

Long-term therapy after an acute myocardial infarction

Treatment of associated risk factors

Stopping smoking, rehabilitation, exercise and rigorous management of hyperlipidaemia have all been shown to improve prognosis after a myocardial infarction. Until recently there was little information on the value of post-infarction blood pressure control. Diltiazem has now been shown to improve survival over a 4-year period, but because of its negative inotropic activity is contraindicated in patients with poor left ventricular function. It seems likely that it is the lowering of blood pressure which is important rather than the type of antihypertensive agent used. In view of the other beneficial effects of beta blockers and ACE inhibitors these agents would seem ideal in controlling blood pressure in this situation.

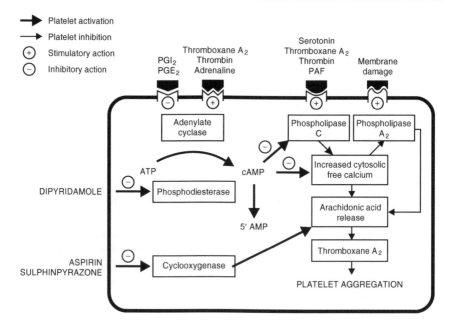

Figure 5.4. Proposed modes of action of aspirin, sulphinpyrazone and dipyridamole on platelet function.

Antiplatelet drugs

Aspirin

Mode of action. The principal effect of aspirin is inhibition of the enzyme cyclooxygenase in the platelet and vascular endothelium. Aspirin irreversibly acetylates cyclooxygenase for the lifetime of the platelet and activity is therefore not restored until new platelets are formed (Figure 5.4). Aspirin also inhibits cyclooxygenase in the vascular endothelium and theoretically could have a detrimental effect by reducing the anti-aggregatory effects of prostacyclin. The important factor, however, is that vascular cyclooxygenease can be resynthesised within a few hours. The observation that high dose aspirin appears to be as effective as low dose aspirin in inhibiting platelet function provides substantial weight to the argument that inhibition of endothelial prostacyclin is relatively unimportant. Aspirin has no effect on lipooxygenase or the synthesis of leukotrienes.

Chemistry and pharmacokinetics. Salicyclic acid is a simple organic acid with a pK_a of 3.0. Aspirin (acetylsalicylic acid) has a pK of 3.5. These values are important in aspirin overdosage since alkalinisation of the urine has a marked effect on drug elimination.

The salicylates are rapidly absorbed from the stomach and upper jejunum, yielding peak salicylate levels within 1–2 hours. High concentrations have a direct damaging effect on the gastric mucosa, which can be reduced by maintaining gastric pH above the pK_a value. After absorption aspirin is hydrolysed to salicylate and acetic acid by esterases in tissue and blood and largely excreted by the kidney as water-soluble conjugates (Table 5.5). At higher doses the metabolising enzyme systems are saturated and the drug displays "zero order" elimination kinetics. Aspirin also displays dose-dependent albumen binding.

Selection of preparation and dose. Aspirin is available in many different forms designed to reduce gastrointestinal adverse effects. Most buffered preparations do not contain sufficient alkali to prevent damage to the gastric mucosa and they have no advantages over conventional aspirin in terms of efficacy or adverse effects. Enteric coated preparations, which are mostly absorbed in the upper small bowel, have some advantages in reducing gastrointestinal effects but are more expensive, while the addition of drugs which reduce gastric acid secretion or act as prostaglandin analogues are of value in selected patients.

Despite numerous studies, the optimum maintenance dose of aspirin when used as an antiplatelet has not been clearly defined. Doses used in secondary prevention studies have ranged from 75 mg to 1000 mg daily, despite the fact that 20–40 mg provides effective inhibition of platelet

Table 5.5. Pharmacokinetic values of aspirin, dipyridamole and sulphinpyrazone

Drug	Aspirin	Dipyridamole	Sulphinpyrazone
Duration of action	Life of platelet	Unknown	≈10 hours
Time to peak action	Unknown	Unknown	1–2 hours
Plasma half-life	15–20 minutes	1–12 hours	3 hours
Metabolism	Hydrolysis in gut liver and blood to salicylic acid	Liver metabolism 20% entero-hepatic recirculation	Mostly to parahydroxy metabolite in liver
Oral bio-availability %	50–100 (depends on formulation)	25–70	Unknown
Excretion	Renal as salicylic acid and conjugates	Mostly biliary as glucuronide	Renal 40% unchanged 60% conjugates
Protein binding	> 90%	> 90%	> 90%

aggregation with minimal inhibition of prostacyclin biosynthesis. Until clearer clinical evidence on outcome is forthcoming, aspirin 75 mg or 300 mg daily should remain the preparations of first choice in the United Kingdom (81 mg and 325 mg in the United States).

The role of aspirin in secondary prevention.   A single daily dose as outlined above is recommended for all survivors of an acute myocardial infarction unless there are serious contraindications. A meta analysis of six aspirin post-myocardial infarction studies demonstrated beneficial effects on total mortality, cardiovascular mortality and recurrent infarction. There is no evidence that the combination with dipyridamole confers any additional benefit and the role of sulphinpyrazone remains undefined. Aspirin is of clear benefit in patients with good left ventricular function, in the elderly and those with coexisting cerebrovascular and peripheral vascular disease. Warfarin may be the preferred drug in high risk patients with anterior or apical myocardial infarction, left ventricular dysfunction and those with atrial fibrillation.

Adverse effects and contraindications.   At the low doses given for its antiplatelet activity the only major adverse effect of aspirin is gastrointestinal bleeding. Minor gastrointestinal symptoms are common and can be reduced by using an enteric-coated preparation or taking the drug with meals and/or antacids. Upper gastrointestinal bleeding is more commonly due to erosive gastritis than peptic ulcer and occurs in about 5% of patients treated. Other adverse effects at these doses include small increases in uric acid, hypersensitivity reactions including rashes, bronchoconstriction and anaphylaxis.

Aspirin intolerance, haemophilia, a previous history of a peptic ulcer and evidence of previous severe bleeding from any site are strong contra-indications. Relative contraindications include iron deficiency anaemia, gout, retinal haemorrhages and administration to patients who are receiving drugs likely to exhibit major interactions.

Interactions.   Although most non-steroidal anti-inflammatory drugs increase blood pressure and attenuate the effects of antihypertensive drugs and diuretics, there is no evidence that aspirin at low dose has these effects. In the recent HOT (Hypertension Optimal Treatment) study (see hypertension chapter, p. 231), no reduction in the antihypertensive effect was seen in the aspirin treated group of calcium antagonists and ACE inhibitors. Aspirin can interact with uricosuric agents and thiazide diuretics to precipitate an acute attack of gout. The risk of gastrointestinal bleeding is increased by alcohol, corticosteroid drugs, warfarin and other non-steroidal anti-inflammatory agents.

Dipyridamole

Mode of action. Dipyridamole has a number of pharmacological actions. It is a vasodilator due to its inhibitory effects on adenosine deaminase, it inhibits platelet adhesion to damaged blood vessels and reduces platelet aggregation by potentiating prostacyclin. It also inhibits phosphodiesterase (Figure 5.4) and the breakdown of adenosine in the platelet. It is more effective than aspirin in preventing platelet adhesion and less effective in reducing platelet aggregation.

Pharmacokinetics. The pharmacokinetics of dipyridamole is poorly defined and the bioavailability and elimination half-lives are very variable. No adjustment is necessary in patients with renal impairment, but because of the high biliary excretion reduced doses are advisable in patients with biliary obstruction (Table 5.5).

Clinical use and dosage. Dipyridamole has not been shown to improve survival in patients following an acute myocardial infarction. In combination with aspirin there is also no evidence of additional benefit. When used with anticoagulant drugs the combination appears useful in patients undergoing vascular grafts, in secondary stroke prevention and in patients with mitral valve disease. It is also more effective than placebo in reducing the risk of thromboembolism from prosthetic values.

Adverse effects and contraindications. Most of the adverse effects of dipyridamole are due to vasodilatation. These include flushing, headache, dizziness, hypotension and occasional increases in chest pain in patients with angina pectoris. Minor gastrointestinal symptoms may occur and rashes are relatively uncommon.

Interactions. Apart from increasing the risk of bleeding when combined with anticoagulants, thrombolytic and other antiplatelet drugs there are fewer major interactions with dipyridamole. There is some evidence that antacids can reduce its antiplatelet activity.

Sulphinpyrazone

Mode of action. Sulphinpyrazone is an anti-inflammatory drug related to phenylbutazone which has antiplatelet and uricosuric activity. Unlike aspirin its antiplatelet effect is reversible and its activity therefore is only present while it remains in the circulation.

Pharmacokinetics. The principal pharmacokinetic values are listed in Table 5.5. Despite a short elimination half-life of about 3 hours, the antiplatelet effect lasts for at least 10 hours. Patients with renal impairment are at increased risk of urate stone formation and worsening renal function.

Clinical use and dosage. The anturane reinfarction trial demonstrated a 32% reduction in cardiac mortality and a 43% reduction in sudden death compared with placebo over a 24-month treatment period following an acute myocardial infarction. The benefit was mainly due to reduced sudden death during the first 2–7 months, treatment having been started at about 1 month after infarction. Despite this, three factors have mitigated against the use of sulphinpyrazone after an acute myocardial infarction. First it is less effective and more toxic than aspirin, second it is more expensive and third there has been major doubt about the conduct, design and conclusions of the trial.

Adverse effects and contraindications. Major adverse effects of sulphinpyrazone include the development of acute gout, gastrointestinal bleeding and acute renal failure in patients with existing renal impairment. The formation of urate stones may also contribute to renal impairment. Hypersensitivity reactions including rashes, bone marrow depression, asthma and fever have also been described. The most commonly used dose is 800 mg/day given in four divided doses which is gradually titrated from a dose of 100 mg/day. Sulphinpyrazone is contraindicated in patients with active peptic ulceration, in severe renal or hepatic disease and in those with haemophilia or bone marrow depression. Patients with a known hypersensitivity to the drug oxyphenbutazone or phenylbutazone should not receive sulphinpyrazone.

Interactions. Sulphinpyrazone is very highly protein bound to plasma proteins and can displace other highly protein bound drugs from their binding sites. The clinical relevance of this type of interaction has probably been exaggerated in the past since higher free concentrations of a drug result in increased metabolism and renal elimination. However, it can be important for drugs such as warfarin, oral diabetic agents and phenytoin. As with other antiplatelet agents the risk of bleeding with anticoagulants and thrombolytic agents is increased. Other uricosuric agents can reduce the renal clearance of sulphinpyrazone and the action of insulin may be enhanced.

Clopidogrel

Clopidogrel is a selective, non-competitive, ADP platelet receptor antagonist that irreversibly inhibits ADP binding to platelet membrane receptors and the subsequent expression of GP11b/IIIa receptors. It has no inhibitory effect on cyclo-oxygenase and thromboxane A_2. A recent clinical trial suggested benefit in terms of preventing myocardial infarction, stroke and vascular death in patients with a recent myocardial infarction if administered between 2 and 35 days after the event. Preliminary studies have shown greater efficacy than aspirin in high risk populations with a lower incidence of gastrointestinal bleeding. At present it should be considered for post-myocardial prophylaxis in patients who are intolerant of aspirin.

Beta adrenoceptor antagonists

When administered during the period following an acute myocardial infarction beta adrenoceptor antagonists reduce the risk of sudden death and reinfarction. Timolol, metoprolol and atenolol are effective, while those drugs, which have partial agonist activity, are relatively ineffective, although in the high risk patients acebutolol reduced total and vascular mortality. Although these agents are widely used in patients following an acute myocardial infarction several questions about their use remain unresolved. It is not known whether low risk patients benefit from routine beta blocker administration as their prognosis is already excellent. The timing and selection has not been fully resolved, but early intravenous administration of a drug used in the successful post-infarction studies followed by oral therapy with the same drug would seem to be appropriate. Most clinicians would continue these drugs indefinitely especially in patients with angina pectoris and given the poor record of calcium channel antagonists following acute myocardial infarctions, beta blockers would be preferred to these agents except in those with severe obstructive airways or peripheral vascular disease. It is important to remember that those patients who appear to benefit most have the greatest number of contraindications, and approximately 50% of patients entering the various outcome studies were excluded.

Angiotensin converting enzyme inhibitors

New data suggests that angiotensin converting enzyme inhibitors may be of value in patients following an acute myocardial infarction. The SAVE (survival and ventricular enlargement) trial has demonstrated that captopril attenuated left ventricular enlargement, reduced the severity of congestive cardiac failure and improved survival in patients with asymptomatic left ventricular function following an acute myocardial infarction. Reinfarctions and the need for revascularisation procedures were also reduced by captopril therapy. Similar findings were evident in the AIRE (acute infarction ramipril efficacy) study in which there was a reduction in mortality and cardiovascular events in patients with clinically evident heart failure treated with ramipril following an acute myocardial infarction.

In contrast CONSENSUS II (Co-operative New Scandinavian Enalapril Survival Study) which evaluated enalaprilat/enalapril maleate in unselected patients with acute myocardial infarction was essentially negative for the beneficial effects of ACE inhibition. However, in this study the approach was different. Enalaprilat intravenously was given for a suspected myocardial infarction within 24 hours of the onset of chest pain and no assessment was made of left ventricular function. In two very large studies GISS-3 and ISIS-4, which involved unselected patients apart from those with hypotension, lisinopril revealed a small benefit which may have been due to inclusion of patients with left ventricular dysfunction.

Based on the current evidence, ACE inhibitor therapy cannot be recommended for all patients following an acute myocardial infarction. Only 20% of patients have prognostically important left ventricular dysfunction and it is these patients who should receive an ACE inhibitor, probably captopril or ramipril. Alternatively, all patients could receive an ACE inhibitor which could be discontinued later in those with good left ventricular function.

Calcium channel antagonists

Nifedipine is contraindicated in patients following an acute myocardial infarction mainly due to increased mortality in those with poor left

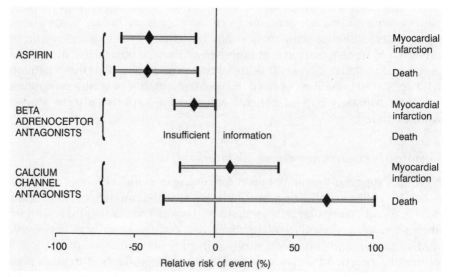

Figure 5.5.   Effect of aspirin, beta adrenoceptors and rapid-acting dihydropyridine calcium channel antagonists on the risk of death and myocardial infarction following a myocardial infarction. Adapted from Yusuf *et al.*, 1988.

Table 5.6. Effects of type I antiarrhythmic drugs on mortality after an acute myocardial infarction

| Class | No. of patients | % Deaths | |
		Active	Control
Quinidine 1a Procainamide Disopyramide	5 229	9.7	8.2
Lignocaine 1b Mexiletine Tocainide	14 013	4.3	4.0
Encainide 1c Flecainide Propafenone	2 538	7.4	6.0

ventricular function (Figure 5.5). Longer acting and more cardioselective dihydropyridines may be less likely to cause problems and have been used to improve myocardial blood flow after "stunning". Verapamil and diltiazem may help prevent early reinfarction especially in patients who have sustained a subendocardial or non-Q wave myocardial infarction and have good left ventricular function. Their main role would be in patients who are intolerant of beta adrenoceptor antagonists.

Antiarrhythmic drugs

Ventricular tachycardia and complex ventricular ectopic activity in the late hospital phase of an acute myocardial infarction are predictors of subsequent sudden death independent of left ventricular function. Unfortunately, the value of antiarrhythmic therapy in preventing sudden cardiac death is extremely doubtful. In the CAST (cardiac arrhythmias suppression trial) the type Ic antiarrhythmic agents, flecainide and encainide, given after an acute myocardial infarction, were associated with a threefold increase in mortality. A similar effect has been described with quinidine and in a follow-up study to CAST moracizine was stopped prematurely because of increased mortality in the treated group. An overview of the effects of type 1 agents showing increased mortality is illustrated in Table 5.6.

To date beta adrenoceptor antagonists without partial agonist activity and non-dihydropyridine calcium channel antagonists are the only antiarrhythmic agents which have beneficial effects on survival after a myocardial infarction, although preliminary data suggests that amiodarone may be useful. The value of digoxin remains controversial, but the drug should not be withheld at present from patients with atrial fibrillation and severe heart failure.

HMG Co enzyme A reductase inhibitors

Two recent large clinical trials have confirmed beneficial effects from lowering cholesterol with simvastatin and pravastatin after an acute myocardial infarction. In the 4S there was a 37% reduction in fatal and non-fatal reinfarction. This equates to 12 fewer reinfarctions per 1000 patient years of treatment, a somewhat greater benefit than that obtained with aspirin or beta adrenoceptor antagonists. In CARE[†] (cholesterol and recurrent events) the risk of reinfarction was reduced by 25%.

[†](CARE) Sacks, F. M., Pfeffer, M. A., Moye, L. A. *et al.* The effect of pravastatin on coronary events after myocardial infarction in patients with average cholesterol levels. *N. Eng. J. Med.*, 1996; 335: 1001–9.

6 Drug Treatment of Heart Failure

Definition

There is at present no satisfactory definition of the syndrome of congestive cardiac failure. It covers a spectrum of conditions ranging from asymptomatic left ventricular dysfunction to symptomatic ventricular failure. In pathophysiological terms it can be defined as the inability of the heart to deliver blood and hence oxygen at a rate necessary for adequate tissue metabolism despite normal or increased ventricular filling pressures. This standard definition implies a defect in systolic function, whereas abnormalities of diastolic function can and frequently do play an important part in the development of the syndrome. In addition, changes of arteriolar constriction and salt and water retention occur secondary to neurohormonal activation which in turn can contribute to the failure to deliver oxygen to the metabolising tissues. In clinical terms heart failure is defined as a syndrome characterised by dyspnoea, fatigue and oedema occurring as a consequence of inadequate delivery of oxygen and increased ventricular filling pressure. However, in some patients with left ventricular function these features may be absent.

Prevalence and incidence

The Framingham study estimated an annual incidence for congestive heart failure of 3.7 new cases per 1000 men and 2.5 per 1000 women. For both sexes aged 35–64 years, the incidence was 3 per 1000, but for those aged 65–94 years a much higher incidence of 10 per 1000 was recorded. In a recent survey of three general practices in the London area, 0.4% were considered to have heart failure in a population of over 30 000. In the London District Hospital study, congestive heart failure accounted for almost 5% of all admissions over a 6-month period, the vast majority being over the age of 65 years. Mortality associated with heart failure is high. In the Framingham study the probability of dying within 5 years of the onset of congestive heart failure was 62% for men and 48% for women, and several similar studies have confirmed this very poor prognosis. The mortality risk increases with the severity of the condition. In patients with left ventricular dysfunction without clinical evidence of heart failure the annual mortality rate is 5%, but

12.5% in patients with overt congestive heart failure. In patients with New York Heart Association, classes II and III, 1-year mortality rates have been quoted as 19.5%, while in patients with grade IV the rate may be as high as 60%.

Pathophysiology

Haemodynamic derangement occurring in heart failure can be considered in terms of three major determinants – contractility, preload and afterload.

Contractility

Myocardial contractility is defined as the force with which the ventricle can contract independent of heart rate, preload and afterload. It is a difficult value to consider or measure since in reality it is never independent of these factors. Until recently loss of contractility was equated with loss of functioning muscle due to infarction or cardiomyopathy. There is growing evidence, however, that the surviving muscle may show abnormal contractile responses. Inotropic responses of the remaining healthy muscle can be reduced due to down-regulation of the beta receptors resulting from exposure to high levels of circulating catecholamines, and high levels of hormones, neurotransmitters and other toxins may injure or even destroy remaining cardiac muscle. Alteration in calcium homeostasis, reduced sarcoplasmic reticulum function, impaired myocardial metabolism and mitochondrial function and abnormalities of the collagen interstitium have all been described in myocardial cells in the syndrome of congestive cardiac failure. These changes give rise to the concept of a self-perpetuating vicious cycle in which the compensatory mechanisms that are designed to restore cardiac function may result in further deterioration.

Preload

Preload describes the relationship between end-diastolic fibre stretch and muscle function in which an increase in stretch is associated with an increase in muscle function. It is determined by ventricular compliance and the end-diastolic pressure and the relationship with stroke volume is commonly known as the Frank–Starling curve illustrated in Figure 6.1. Preload is usually increased in congestive cardiac failure due to extra-cellular fluid volume expansion, venoconstriction and, in several cases, a decrease in ventricular compliance. Since the left ventricular function curve is depressed in congestive heart failure (Figure 6.1), an increase in preload does not result in significant increases in cardiac output and as the end-diastolic pressure rises, pulmonary oedema results. The coronary perfusion

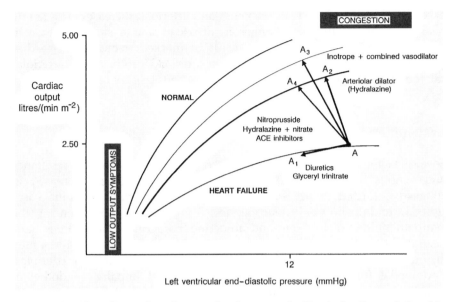

Figure 6.1. The effects of cardiovascular drugs on the Frank–Starling relationship in heart failure.

pressure (aortic diastolic pressure − left ventricular end-diastolic pressure) is also reduced in the presence of increased preload so that myocardial ischaemia, especially in the sub-endocardial regions, can increase.

Afterload

Afterload refers to the tension or force per cross-sectional area in the wall of the ventricle during ejection of blood from the ventricle or the wall tension that must be generated to maintain stroke volume. According to the Laplace's law, wall tension is proportional to the pressure during systole multiplied by the diameter of the chamber and divided by the thickness of the wall. If cardiac output is to be maintained in the presence of an increased systemic vascular resistance, then blood pressure must rise. The rise in pressure must be offset by a rise in wall tension during ejection, and afterload therefore rises.

Left ventricular systolic pressure is dependent largely on aortic impedance. This is mostly determined by systemic vascular resistance, although large artery compliance, blood viscosity, and intra-arterial blood volume contribute.

Hypertrophy of cardiac myocytes reduces the load per fibre and is initially successful in normalising wall stress, but may lead to impaired sub-endocardial blood flow. Eventually the increase in the ventricular diameter exceeds the increases in wall thickness and afterload increases. The failing heart is very sensitive to changes in afterload and a small increase in systemic vascular resistance can result in marked decreases in cardiac output. Conversely, a small decrease in afterload produced by arteriolar dilators can substantially increase cardiac output (Figure 6.1).

Systemic vascular resistance and vasoconstriction

Several factors combine together to increase systemic vascular resistance and venous tone. A variety of constrictor hormones are increased in congestive cardiac failure – noradrenaline, angiotensin II, arginine vaso-pressin, endothelin and neuropeptide Y. Increased activation of the sympathetic nervous system and autocrine/paracrine abnormalities have been described in vascular smooth muscle. Some of these substances may also act as growth factors leading to structural remodelling of arterioles. Endothelial function may also be abnormal and impaired endothelial-mediated vasorelaxation has been described in this syndrome.

Peripheral haemodynamics and regional blood flow

When cardiac output is reduced, blood is shunted away from non-critical tissues such as the skin to important organ beds such as the brain. Two important systems do not receive adequate blood supply – the kidney and skeletal muscle. This is an important factor in producing the cardinal manifestations of heart failure – fluid retention, dyspnoea, muscle fatigue and poor exercise tolerance.

Renal changes

Despite the decreases in renal blood flow, glomerular filtration rate is preserved at least until the syndrome is well advanced. This is thought to be achieved by the preferential vasoconstrictor effect of angiotensin II on glomerular efferent arteriolar tone. Removal of this effect can cause a fall in glomerular filtration rate so that ACE inhibitors and angiotensin II receptor antagonists can produce similar problems to those observed in renal artery stenosis. The significantly higher risk of renal artery stenosis due to atherosclerosis in this group of patients also increases the problem. Tubular reabsorption of sodium is increased as a result of the increased filtration fraction, and the effects of angiotensin II, aldosterone and increased sympathetic activity.

Muscle abnormalities

In addition to reduced muscle blood flow and electrolyte depletion, a variety of other abnormalities have been described in the muscles of patients with congestive heart failure. Alterations in fibre type, muscle enzyme activity, metabolism and muscle strength have been reported. Skeletal muscle fatigue is an important symptom of heart failure and reduced muscle protein synthesis occurs early in the syndrome. In advanced heart failure, muscle wasting associated with protein breakdown (cardiac cachexia) is well described.

Neuroendocrine abnormalities

As already discussed, the sympathetic nervous system, the renin–angiotensin–aldosterone system, arginine vasopressin and endothelin have potent renal effects leading to sodium and water retention and renal vasoconstriction. Aldosterone causes potassium and magnesium wasting. Some of these hormones such as angiotenin II and vasopressin may contribute to the intense thirst found in several patients with heart failure. In high concentrations there is growing evidence that angiotensin II and catecholamines may be directly cardiotoxic. Many other hormonal abnormalities have been described in congestive heart failure (Table 6.1). Drugs to reverse the vasoconstrictor and anti-natriuretic influences are likely to represent important therapeutic areas in the future.

Although most of the hormonal abnormalities occurring in heart failure can be detected early in the condition or even in asymptomatic left ventricular dysfunction, the great majority increase with the severity of the disease. There is good reason to suggest that neurohormonal derangements, once initiated in heart failure, then contribute to its pathophysiology and progression and are not just markers of disease. The long-term benefits of ACE inhibitors would lend weight to this conclusion.

Electrolyte abnormalities

Heart failure is characterised by a variety of plasma and cellular electrolyte abnormalities occurring partly as a result of neurohormonal stimulation and partly as a consequence of diuretic therapy. Cellular depletion of potassium and magnesium is common and relates to prognosis and risk of serious dysrhythmias. The increased intracellular sodium may contribute to wall "stiffness" and is probably a factor in the impaired vasodilatation seen in congestive cardiac failure.

Table 6.1.   Hormonal and other factors involved in congestive heart failure

---

Increased vasoconstrictor hormones
  Noradrenaline
  Angiotensin II
  Arginine vasopressin
  Neuropeptide Y
  Endothelin I
Increased vasodilator hormones
  Atrial natriuretic peptides
  Vasodilatory prostaglandins
  Dopamine
  Calcitonin gene-related peptide
  Substance P
Reduced vasodilator hormones
  Endothelium-derived relaxing factor (nitric oxide)
Other increased circulatory factors
  Opioid peptides
  Erythropoietin
  Natriuretic hormone (digitalis-like)

Impaired baroreceptor function

Many of the neurohormonal abnormalities seen in congestive cardiac failure occur secondary to abnormal baroreceptor function. Sympathetic nervous system activity is increased because of the inability of cardiopulmonary and mechanoreceptors to inhibit the vasomotor centres in this condition. Parasympathetic autonomic function is also abnormal in heart failure and decreased vagal tone is thought to contribute to the loss of heart rate variability and increased risk of ventricular arrhythmias.

Pulmonary and ventilatory abnormalities

Several pulmonary abnormalities, in addition to respiratory muscle weakness, have been reported in congestive cardiac failure. Patients with congestive heart failure ventilate more for a given workload than healthy controls, and demonstrate airways obstruction and abnormal patterns of breathing during sleep with arterial desaturation. Finally, cough, a metabolically demanding form of exercise is more common in patients with heart failure.

Rationale for the use of drugs in congestive cardiac failure

There are three main areas of therapeutic intervention in the treatment of heart failure: diuretics to reduce plasma volume and venous pressure, vasodilators to increase venous capacitance and reduce afterload and inotropic agents to enhance myocardial contractility. Recent evidence suggests that a significant percentage of patients with idiopathic, ischaemic and other forms of cardiomyopathy improve during therapy with beta adrenoceptor antagonists.

Diuretics, by reducing plasma volume and hence preload, help to relieve breathlessness caused by pulmonary congestion. They do not necessarily improve myocardial performance and reductions in filling pressure may on occasions result in reduced cardiac output. They can, however, improve myocardial performance indirectly by relieving pulmonary vascular congestion and increasing blood oxygenation. The loop diuretics, frusemide and bumetanide, are particularly valuable in acute pulmonary oedema since they increase venous capacitance and renal blood flow acutely. These effects occur independent of their diuretic activity and are usually shortlived. Transient haemodynamic deterioration has been reported following intravenous administration of frusemide in patients with chronic heart failure. An increase in mean arterial pressure, systemic vascular resistance and left ventricular filling pressure and a decrease in cardiac output have been described. These effects are not seen with equal diuretic doses of bumetanide and seem to be related to acute activation of the renin–angiotensin–aldosterone system and increases in circulating noradrenaline and vasopressin concentrations. Loop diuretics are also preferred to thiazide diuretics in the long-term management of heart failure because of a steep dose–response relationship and a lower incidence of adverse metabolic effects at high dose.

Organic nitrates act as potent venodilators and are beneficial in heart failure. Pulmonary capillary wedge and pulmonary artery pressure are reduced at rest and during exercise and stroke volume may increase or remain unchanged. Systemic and pulmonary vascular resistance tend to decrease. Nitrates are, therefore, most beneficial in patients with symptoms associated with pulmonary venous congestion such as orthopnoea, paroxysmal nocturnal dyspnoea and dyspnoea on exertion. Two large studies have also described beneficial effects on mortality when combined with the arteriolar dilator, hydralazine.

The ACE inhibitors produce a substantial fall in systemic vascular resistance and systemic blood pressure. Despite the fall in arterial blood pressure, heart rate remains unchanged or may even decrease. In patients with heart failure there is an increase in cardiac output. These drugs also produce considerable venodilatation with a reduction in pulmonary wedge and right atrial pressure. A number of other drugs – hydralazine, minoxidil and calcium channel antagonists reduce afterload, and prazosin, trimazosin and sodium nitroprusside alter preload and afterload. With the possible exception of hydralazine, none of these drugs has been shown to have any long-term clinical benefit in the management of heart failure, although preliminary data suggest that amlodipine may be effective in congestive cardiomyopathy.

In patients with chronic heart failure and depressed left ventricular systolic function, cardiac output generally increases following digitalis therapy. Although an increase in peripheral vessel tone occurs in healthy subjects, a reduction in arteriolar and venous tone has been observed in patients with heart failure. Increases in cardiac function can result in improvements in renal haemodynamics and increased diuresis.

Most other drugs which increase the force of cardiac contraction act directly or indirectly on the beta $_1$ adrenoceptors. All have been shown to have short-term increases in stroke volume and decreases in pulmonary and systemic vascular resistance. Filling pressure and myocardial oxygen consumption also tend to decline. Although clinical improvements have been described in short-term studies, long-term benefits are hard to demonstrate and increases in mortality have been described with milrinone, enoximone and xamoterol.

The use of diuretics in heart failure

The cardiovascular system in heart failure has a higher than normal left ventricular end-diastolic volume for a given ventricular performance. The inability of cardiac output to increase with effort results in underperfusion of the tissues, leading to increased fatigue and exertional dyspnoea. As cardiac performance declines the kidney responds by increasing sodium and water uptake within the tubule. As a result venous return to the heart is increased and the myocardial cells are exposed to increased stretch in order to increase stroke volume (Figure 6.1). Ultimately plasma volume expansion results in pulmonary vascular congestion and movement of fluid from the pulmonary capillaries into the alveoli causing pulmonary oedema.

Diuretics produce their beneficial effects by reducing plasma volume and venous return to the heart. As a result, the severity of breathlessness is reduced. Loop diuretics are particularly useful in acute pulmonary oedema. Intravenous frusemide, bumetanide and ethacrynic acid produce rapid reductions in plasma volume, and acute venodilatation may account for some of the beneficial effects on breathing before diuresis occurs. Diuretics also lower arterial blood pressure and can improve cardiac haemodynamics by decreasing afterload.

Mode of action of loop diuretics

Loop diuretics inhibit sodium and chloride in the thick ascending loop of Henle (see Figure 9.5). All are actively secreted by the proximal tubule and achieve high concentrations at the luminal membrane of the loop of Henle. Since these drugs are effective at doses well below the top of the dose–response relationship they are frequently referred to as "high ceiling" diuretics. The acute vascular effects are associated with acute activation of the renin angiotensin and prostaglandin systems.

Pharmacokinetics

The pharmacokinetic values of loop diuretics are summarised in Table 6.2. Frusemide has an elimination half-life ranging from 19 to 100 minutes. It is metabolised to the glucuronic acid conjugate in the liver and eliminated by the kidneys. The metabolism of ethacrynic acid also involves the formation of a glutathione conjugate which is further degraded to cysteine and mercaptopurine derivatives in the liver and nephron. Bumetanide is rapidly and completely absorbed from the gastrointestinal tract. Oral bioavailability is high in renal and hepatic disease, but in both conditions the elimination half-life is prolonged. Piretanide has a relatively short half-life of 30–50 minutes. In all respects, the pharmacokinetics are similar to frusemide.

Diuretic resistance in heart failure

Some patients with congestive heart failure become refractory to the effects of loop diuretics. This may occasionally be due to reduced intestinal

Table 6.2. Pharmacokinetic values of the loop diuretics

Drug	Bumetanide	Ethacrynic acid	Frusemide	Piretanide
Duration of action	4–6 hours (oral) 2–3 hours (iv)	6–8 hours (oral) 2–3 hours (iv)	5–7 hours (oral) 2–3 hours (iv)	4–6 hours (oral)
Time to peak action	1.25–1.5 hours (oral) <5 minutes (iv)	30 minutes (oral) <5 minutes (iv)	1–2 hours (oral) <5 minutes (iv)	<30 minutes
Plasma half-life	1.2–1.5 hours	0.5–1 hour	$\approx$19–100 minutes	30–50 minutes
Oral bioavailability (%)	85–95	72–96	50–60	50–60
Metabolism	Hepatic to at least five metabolites	Gluthathione conjugate degraded to cysteine and mercaptopurine in the liver	In part to glucuronide in the liver	Partial to five metabolites
Excretion	Renal–parent compound and metabolites	Renal	Renal	Renal

absorption but has also been observed when the drugs are given intravenously. In most cases this is due to increased absorption of tubular fluid at sites within the nephron not blocked by the loop diuretics. This type of diuretic resistance can often be reversed by using another diuretic which acts at a different site within the tubule, such as a thiazide diuretic or a related compound, metolazone. An alternative approach is to introduce an ACE inhibitor to increase cardiac output and renal blood flow.

Another group of patients are resistant to loop diuretics because of decreased delivery of sodium chloride to the diuretic sensitive sites related to increased reabsorption in the proximal tubule and reduced glomerular filtration. Water restriction and continuous infusions of the drugs may help overcome this type of resistance.

Special problems caused by loop diuretics in heart failure

Reduction of extracellular fluid volume is a common complication of loop diuretics in heart failure. These patients frequently experience gastrointestinal adverse effects such as nausea, vomiting and diarrhoea and may be unable to take enough salt and water to compensate for daily urinary losses. Volume depletion can lead to impaired renal function and contribute to the metabolic alkalosis which can accompany over-vigorous use of diuretics in heart failure. Both usually respond to dose reduction and/or administration of intravenous saline. The importance of hypokalaemia in hypertensive patients receiving thiazide diuretics will be discussed later.

In general, the risk of developing hypokalaemia and the need for potassium supplements or potassium-sparing diuretics is greater in patients with heart failure receiving loop diuretics than those receiving lower dose thiazide therapy for hypertension. This is particularly true in patients receiving digitalis therapy since hypokalaemia significantly increases the risk of toxicity. In general, exaggerated potassium loss is less likely if appropriate decreases in the extracellular fluid volume are achieved and hypokalaemia tends to be most pronounced in patients who take diuretics with a high fluid intake. In these patients restriction of salt and water intake helps to prevent excessive potassium loss. Spironolactone, triamterene and amiloride prevent potassium secretion in the distal and collecting tubules. These agents are effective when used in combination with loop and thiazide diuretics to reduce the loss of urinary potassium. Potassium-sparing diuretics are problematical in patients with renal impairment since severe hyperkalaemia can result.

Hyponatraemia is relatively common in patients receiving diuretics for heart failure especially if hypokalaemia is also present. This most commonly occurs in patients who drink water at a rate faster than the ascending limb can generate dilute urine. Potent loop diuretics also cause contraction of the extracellular fluid compartment and facilitate release of antidiuretic hormone to further enhance the development of hyponatraemia. Unlike thiazide diuretics which increase calcium reabsorption in the distal tubule, loop diuretics acutely increase calcium excretion. However, with chronic administration the calciuria returns to baseline values.

Loop and thiazide diuretics decrease the renal clearance of uric acid and elevate serum uric acid levels. In general chronic hyperuricaemia is less of a problem in cardiac failure treated with loop diuretics than with long-term use of thiazide diuretics in hypertension. Acute gout can, however, occur and it is important to remember that non-steroidal anti-inflammatory drugs can antagonise the effects of diuretics. The importance of carbohydrate intolerance and increased lipids is unknown in patients with heart failure. These effects appear less common with loop diuretics than thiazide diuretics.

The loop diuretics can cause dose-related hearing loss which is usually reversible. It most commonly occurs when large doses are used in the presence of impaired renal function or when combined with other nephrotoxic drugs such as the aminoglycoside antibiotics. Hypersensitivity reactions such as skin rashes, eosinophilia and interstitial nephritis are occasionally caused by frusemide therapy. These are probably related to the sulphonamide component and are much less common with ethacrynic acid. Acute pancreatitis, encephalopathy, gastrointestinal bleeding and liver function abnormalities have also been described with loop diuretics.

Contraindications to the use of loop diuretics in heart failure

Loop diuretics will clearly be problematical in patients with hypotension, hypovolaemia and severe renal impairment. Those with hepatic failure can develop encephalopathy if large doses are used to treat ascites. Acute urinary retention in men with prostatic hypertrophy is relatively common, particularly after intravenous administration in patients with acute pulmonary oedema. Clinically important interactions are listed in Table 6.3.

The use of vasodilator drugs in the treatment of congestive heart failure

The concept that drugs which relax vascular smooth muscle might have favourable effects on the clinical syndrome of heart failure arose from haemodynamic observations made in acute studies. During infusions of nitroprusside the elevated left ventricular filling pressure was reduced, the low cardiac output was markedly increased with little change in blood pressure or heart rate. A similar response was seen with other vasodilator

Table 6.3.   Interactions with loop diuretics

Lithium	Reduced renal clearance of lithium and increased risk of lithium toxicity
Non-steroidal anti-inflammatory drugs	Reduced diuretic and antihypertensive effects
ACE inhibitors	Prior use of diuretics predisposes to first-dose hypotension
Digoxin	Diuretic induced hypokalaemia increases the risk of digoxin toxicity
Warfarin	Risk of gastrointestinal bleeding is increased
Uricosuric agents and xanthine oxidase inhibitors	Reduce the effectiveness of anti-gout medication
Aminoglycosides	Increase the risk of nephrotoxicity when administered together

drugs such as alpha adrenoceptor antagonists or direct-acting vasodilators, hydralazine and minoxidil, but some differences appeared to be related to relative actions on the venous and arterial vasculature. Drugs which altered venous capacitance such as organic nitrates had more effect on cardiac filling pressure, while those which reduced arterial tone and thus impedance to left ventricular ejection had a more profound effect on cardiac output and stroke volume.

Preliminary studies using orally active vasodilator drugs confirmed favourable effects on left ventricular performance at least in the short term. However, the variability in response stimulated exploration of neuro-hormonal reflex control mechanisms as well as direct vascular effects. For example, ACE inhibitors produced greater reductions in blood pressure and less effects on cardiac output than nitroprusside and flosequinan, but produced smaller increases in heart rate than most other vasodilator drugs tested.

Clinical efficacy of vasodilators

Using exercise tolerance and assessment of symptoms as major endpoints, a variety of vasodilator drugs have been shown to exert beneficial effects in patients with heart failure in studies lasting up to 6 months. Angiotensin converting enzyme inhibitors, hydralazine and isosorbide dinitrate, flosequinan and some vasoselective calcium channel antagonists, have demonstrated favourable clinical effects and sustained reductions in vascular tone. For most vasodilator drugs the improvements in exercise time and oxygen consumption are maximal after 3–6 months and are usually quite modest. Quality of life as assessed by detailed questionnaires has also been shown to improve with vasodilator therapy, and provides a useful and less expensive method of assessing therapy in heart failure.

The effects of vasodilator drugs on mortality

Most deaths in heart failure occur suddenly in the absence of new symptoms or from progressive pump failure when symptoms are unresponsive to drug treatment. It is assumed that sudden death is due to the development of a terminal arrhythmia while the progressive syndrome is thought to be related to a gradual decline in left ventricular systolic function. To be effective in reducing mortality in heart failure, drugs would therefore have to prevent life-threatening dysrhythmias or have long-term beneficial effects on ventricular function. In the first long-term trial to assess mortality (vasodilator heart failure trial), patients with left ventricular dysfunction and reduced exercise tolerance receiving digoxin and a diuretic were randomly assigned to placebo, prazosin or a combination of hydralazine and isosorbide mononitrate. The combination produced a significantly lower cumulative mortality rate than placebo. In contrast, prazosin therapy had no clinical benefit or favourable effects on mortality. This occurred despite persistent vasodilator effects suggesting that reductions in preload and afterload were not sufficient to account for the long-term favourable effects of therapy. In keeping with this, a meta analysis performed in 1987 was unable to show any improvements in survival with direct-acting vasodilators. In addition, nifedipine has been shown to be less effective than placebo and there is no evidence for a beneficial effect on mortality with nifedipine and other calcium channel antagonists, with the possible exception of amlodipine.

The second important study relating mainly to mortality was the Co-operative North Scandinavian Enalapril Survival Study (CONSENSUS) published in 1987 in which enalapril, an ACE inhibitor, improved survival. In this study 253 patients were randomised to placebo or enalapril. The population was elderly with a mean age of 70 years and were receiving a variety of cardiovascular drugs including antiarrhythmic drugs, and warfarin. A 40% reduction in mortality involving grades 3 and 4 heart failure was observed after 6 months. Two other recently published studies have had a major impact on the management of heart failure. In the second veterans heart failure trial, isosorbide dinitrate/hydralazine was compared with enalapril in a controlled trial of men with an ejection fraction less than 45%. After 2 years there was a 25% mortality in the isosorbide/hydralazine group and an 18% mortality in the enalapril-treated group. The enalapril was more effective in reducing mortality than the vasodilator combination.

In the SOLVD (studies of left ventricular dysfunction) trial, 2569 patients in NYHA classes II and III and with ejection fractions <35% were randomised to placebo or enalapril. There was an overall reduction in mortality and a delay in the development of progressive heart failure. Enalapril also reduced the development of symptomatic heart failure in a second group of asymptomatic patients with ejection fractions less than 35%. A series of studies recently performed in patients with poor left ventricular function following an acute myocardial infarction, have demonstrated a reduction in mortality and a delay in the development of symptomatic heart failure with a variety of ACE inhibitors.

Possible mechanisms for the beneficial effects of ACE inhibitors in heart failure

Recent trials have clearly demonstrated that ACE inhibitors reduce morbidity and mortality in heart failure and delay the onset of symptomatic heart failure in patients with left ventricular systolic dysfunction and minimal symptoms. This beneficial effect is seen whether the treatment is started soon after a myocardial infarction or in patients with progressive heart failure. Most of the large heart failure studies with the exception of the CONSENSUS and SOLVD treatment trials, have recorded sudden death as the most common cause of death. This has generally been regarded as indicating the presence of a fatal dysrhythmia, but sudden death can be due to a variety of other factors including myocardial ischaemia and cardiac rupture.

Drug therapy with ACE inhibitors could alter the progression of heart failure in several ways. Therapy could reduce the rate of deterioration or "reset" the system so that the patient starts from an improved baseline without altering the rate of decline. Alternatively, ACE inhibitors could reverse to detrimental effects caused by diuretics resulting from neuro-endocrine activation. These possible mechanisms are not mutually exclusive and various combinations may be responsible.

ACE inhibitors are known to have beneficial haemodynamic effects in patients with heart failure. They reduce preload and afterload, decreasing systolic and diastolic wall stress and cardiac volumes. However, the combination of hydralazine and isosorbide dinitrate had superior haemo-dynamic effects to enalapril but was less favourable in reducing morbidity and mortality. It seems likely that the beneficial effects of ACE inhibitors relate to their neuroendocrine activity. ACE inhibitors reduce angiotensin II formation, aldosterone production and sympathetic outflow, and increase cardiac parasympathetic drive. In keeping with this hypothesis is the observation that those patients with the greatest activation of their renin angiotensin system are most likely to benefit from ACE inhibition. Recent evidence from the SOLVD sub-study suggests that ACE inhibitors might also reduce ventricular dilatation in heart failure patients and prevent or reduce ventricular enlargement after a myocardial infarction.

Pressure and volume overload are major risk factors in the development of cardiac arrhythmias. The numerous actions of ACE inhibitors, particularly their effects on cardiac volume, structure, pressures, electrolyte balance and autonomic function, are likely to have an important impact on the development of arrhythmias.

Clinical indications for ACE inhibition in heart failure

Patients with left ventricular systolic dysfunction represent a continuous spectrum ranging from asymptomatic patients to those with severe symptoms and signs of heart failure. In asymptomatic patients the primary goals are to prevent the development of symptomatic heart failure and delay the onset of death. In mild to moderate symptomatic heart failure, improving symptoms, reducing mortality and preventing the deterioration in ventricular function are all important. In severe heart failure the prognosis is very poor and improving the symptoms and quality of life are the primary aims.

It is now clear that ACE inhibitors should be given to all patients with reduced left ventricular systolic function unless there are clear contra-indications. It is no longer appropriate to wait until the appearance of the symptoms and signs of heart failure. The optimum dose has yet to be determined although beneficial results have been obtained with 20 mg enalapril, 150 mg captopril, 20 mg lisinopril and 10 mg ramipril. A recent study with lisinopril demonstrated a therapeutic advantage with high dose (32.5–35 mg) when compared to low dose lisinopril (2.5–5 mg) in terms of hospitalisations and all-cause mortality with no increase in adverse effects.

Special problems caused by ACE inhibitors in heart failure

There is little doubt that first-dose hypotension is more common in congestive cardiac failure than in patients with hypertension. In the CONSENSUS I study, 12% of the first 34 patients had to be withdrawn because of hypotension, so amendments were made to the protocol to reduce the risk. These included reduction of the dose, more careful selection of patients and avoiding patients with poor renal function. In the V-HeFT II study, symptomatic hypotension was seen in 28% of patients receiving enalapril and 5% had to be withdrawn from the study. This may well have been an underestimate since one in three patients were excluded from entry after the initial screen. In the SOLVD and SAVE studies, less than one-third of patients who were screened entered the trials, some being excluded because the initial blood pressure was too low. About 10% were sympto-matic from hypotension, but the overall incidence is unclear. The risk and duration of hypotension varies according to the drug selected. Captopril at the lowest available dose is preferred for first-dose therapy because of a short duration of effect and there is increasing evidence that perindopril has a lower incidence of first-dose hypotension than most other ACE inhibitors. Acute deterioration in renal function also occurs more commonly in patients with congestive cardiac failure than in those with essential hypertension. Decreases in blood pressure and blood volume related to diuretic therapy; atherosclerosis of the renal vessels with reduced renal perfusion and pre-existing renal disease, probably all contribute to the condition.

Use of organic nitrates in the treatment of heart failure

Haemodynamic effects

As already discussed, the principal effect of organic nitrates is to dilate the venous capacitance vessels and reduce right atrial pressure (Figure 6.1). This combined with a direct effect on the pulmonary arterial circulation results in a reduction in pulmonary artery pressures. The left ventricular filling pressure is also reduced and a direct effect on the resistance arterioles produces a modest but clinically important reduction in systemic vascular resistance. A small increase in cardiac output usually results. Of greater importance is the observation that oral isosorbide dinitrate improves maximum exercise time and oxygen consumption in patients with chronic heart failure. As already discussed, the combination of hydralazine and isosorbide dinitrate proved more beneficial than placebo or prazosin.

Effects on survival

The effect of nitrate therapy alone on survival in patients with chronic heart failure has never been studied and, therefore, the beneficial effects are unknown. When combined with hydralazine, the cumulative mortality at 1 year was reduced compared with placebo and prazosin, and the difference in mortality between the two groups persisted for 3 years. The annual mortality rate was slightly higher in patients with coronary artery disease. The hydralazine/isosorbide dinitrate combination was less effective than enalapril in reducing sudden death, but there was no difference between the two treatments in reducing mortality due to worsening heart failure. The combination of isosorbide dinitrate with hydralazine is not as effective as enalapril in reducing mortality, but this combination is a useful alternative in patients with chronic congestive cardiac failure who do not tolerate ACE inhibitors.

Special problems caused by organic nitrates in heart failure

Adverse effects

Although there is no information on the adverse effects of nitrate therapy when used alone in large groups of patients with heart failure, the results of the V-HeFT studies are helpful in understanding the limitations of directly acting vasodilator therapy: 17% of patients discontinued both study drugs, 5% discontinued hydralazine only and 10% stopped isosorbide dinitrate only. The combination was associated with a significantly higher incidence of headache than enalapril, while the enalapril caused more symptomatic hypotension and cough. At the final study visit 29% of patients had discontinued hydralazine and 10% had reduced the dose, while 31% had stopped their isosorbide dinitrate and 10% had reduced the dose. In comparison, 22% of patients receiving enalapril had discontinued their treatment and an additional 8% had reduced the dose.

Nitrate resistance

In a recent haemodynamic evaluation of 40 mg isosorbide dinitrate in a large group of patients with moderate to severe congestive cardiac failure, no haemodynamic effect was found in almost half the patients. The non-responders tended to have higher atrial pressures than responders and almost half the patients responded to an increase in dose. However, this left about one-quarter of the patients who failed to respond to doses as high as 120 mg, a value found in several other studies. Possible explanations include maximal dilatation of the capacitance vessels at the time of drug administration, impaired responsiveness of vascular smooth muscle due to sodium and water retention within the vascular wall, excessive vasoconstrictor activity and deficiency of sulphydryl groups within the vascular smooth muscle.

Nitrate tolerance

As in the treatment of angina pectoris, tolerance to the action of organic nitrates has been described in patients with congestive cardiac failure and is more likely to occur with transdermal and intravenous preparations and when the drug is given orally 4–6 hourly throughout the day. The development seems to be multifactorial. The most popular theory is that it is related to depletion of sulphydryl groups and can be reversed in most *in vitro* and some *in vivo* studies by the administration of sulphydryl donors. Activation of reflex vasoconstriction to offset the initial vasodilatory effects has also been suggested as a mechanism for early attenuation of the nitrate effect.

This mechanism is supported by animal studies which show that acute tolerance can be prevented by abolishing the compensatory reflexes and the increases in heart rate and plasma renin activity which accompany the development of tolerance. Finally, some investigators have described increases in intravascular blood volume following nitrate therapy in patients with congestive heart failure. Increases in blood volume may offset the vasodilatation and increased venous capacitance following nitrate therapy.

The clinical implications of nitrate tolerance and resistance in patients with heart failure are not entirely clear and the impact on exercise tolerance, symptoms and survival is unknown. Until such data are available, clear recommendations cannot at present be made. However, a reduction in left ventricular filling pressure is likely to have a favourable effect on symptoms and possibly survival since exercise tolerance and mortality have been shown to relate to this measurement. For these reasons, it seems justified to consider isosorbide dinitrate in patients with severe congestive heart failure and to increase the dose in those patients who show a poor response. As in the treatment of angina pectoris, the use of intermittent nitrate therapy allowing daily "nitrate-free" intervals of 8–12 hours seems prudent to prevent attenuation of the haemodynamic effects.

Use of hydralazine in the treatment of heart failure

Hydralazine is a potent, direct-acting vasodilator which causes smooth muscle relaxation of the arterial resistance vessels. It produces effective dilatation of the renal and peripheral vasculature, but has no major direct effect on the coronary arteries. Although hydralazine is alleged to have direct positive inotropic effects, this is mostly mediated by a reflex increase in sympathetic tone. In patients with chronic heart failure, hydralazine produces a decrease in systemic vascular resistance with a marked increase in cardiac output. Pulmonary vascular resistance also decreases but usually less than with the organic nitrates. Despite these acute beneficial haemodynamic effects, there is usually no improvement in exercise tolerance in the long term. Hydralazine when combined with isosorbide dinitrate improves the symptoms and signs of heart failure and improves survival. The contribution of hydralazine to this combination is unknown.

Role of sodium nitroprusside in the treatment of congestive heart failure

Sodium nitroprusside is a potent vasodilator which affects the arterioles and veins and is used intravenously to treat acute severe heart failure.

Nitroprusside reduces systemic vascular resistance and increases cardiac output. Potent venodilatation leads to reductions in atrial and pulmonary artery pressures. This drug is most valuable in patients with high left ventricular filling pressure and systolic pressures $\geqslant 100$ mmHg. In these patients there is a striking increase in cardiac output and a reduction in pulmonary capillary wedge and right atrial pressures. Nitroprusside is best administered with careful haemodynamic monitoring to avoid excessive reductions in arterial pressure and to record the reductions in right atrial pressure. The most common adverse effect in heart failure is symptomatic hypotension.

Use of inotropic agents in the treatment of heart failure

Introduction

Drugs with inotropic activity produce their effect by increasing the availability of intracellular free calcium to the contractile proteins within the myocardium. Increased sensitivity to calcium may also play a role. A variety of mechanisms can increase intracellular concentration. A transient increase in intracellular sodium is associated with increased calcium entry or calcium retention through the sodium–calcium exchange mechanism (Figure 6.2). Increased intracellular sodium concentrations may result from

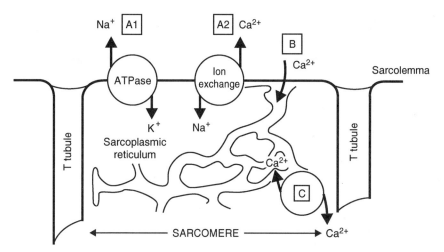

Figure 6.2. Possible sites of action of the cardiac glycosides: (A1) inhibition of the sodium/potassium pump; (A2) activation of the sodium/calcium exchanger; (B) increased permeability of the ion channel to calcium entry; (C) reduced uptake of calcium by the endoplasmic reticulum.

inhibition of sodium efflux or enhanced sodium influx through the fast sodium channel. Higher extracellular concentrations will then promote calcium influx across the sarcolemmal membrane and increase contractility. Increased calcium influx can occur by activation of the slow calcium channels or by increasing membrane permeability to calcium. This results in increased calcium concentrations within the cell. Alternatively, the calcium content may increase as a result of augmented release or reduced uptake of the substance from the sarcoplasmic reticulum.

Myocardial cyclic AMP (adenosine 3'-5' cyclic monophosphate) exerts an important regulatory influence on the level of intracellular calcium and hence the contractile state. Cyclic AMP production is mediated by the membrane-bound enzyme adenylyl cyclase which is regulated by stimulatory and inhibitory protein sub-units. Increased intracellular cyclic AMP activates a protein kinase which controls calcium fluxes across the sarcolemma. Increased release of calcium from the sarcoplasma reticulum and augmented reuptake and storage of calcium in the sarcoplasmic reticulum occurs when intracellular concentrations of cyclic AMP are elevated.

Increased cyclic AMP levels can also occur as a result of decreased degradation which is principally mediated by the enzyme phosphodiesterase. By inhibiting the activity of this enzyme, cyclic AMP concentrations increase, intracellular calcium rises and increased myocardial contractility results. The classification proposed by Katz for inotropic drugs is based on these cellular modes of action and is outlined in Table 6.4.

Rationale for the use of inotropic agents

The main aim of inotropic therapy is to provide support for the heart to maintain adequate organ perfusion. This can be achieved in low output or

Table 6.4.   Principal cellular modes of action of inotropic drugs

---

Drugs which increase cytosolic calcium
1.   Those that inhibit sodium efflux–cardiac glycosides
2.   Those that increase extracellular calcium–parathormone
3.   Those that promote calcium influx via the slow calcium channel–Bay-K-8644

Drugs which increase cyclic AMP levels
1.   Those that increase cyclic AMP production
     –Beta$_1$ adrenergic agonists, glucagon
2.   Those that decrease cyclic AMP breakdown
     –bipyridines, methylxanthines

Drugs which modify myofibrillary proteins
1.   Those that increase sensitivity to calcium–AR-L115 BS
2.   Those that modify myosin isoenzyme composition–thyroxine

---

congestive cardiac failure for short periods, but long-term beneficial effects are more difficult to demonstrate and mortality tends to increase.

At first glance the rationale for using inotropic agents in heart failure appears quite logical. If the failing heart cannot maintain the demands of the peripheral circulation because of impaired contractile function and depletion of cyclic AMP, a drug which increases cyclic AMP and enhances contractility by increasing intracellular concentration would seem to be an ideal choice. Two important strategies are used to increase cyclic AMP. A variety of drugs which stimulate the $beta_1$ receptor have been used to increase cyclic AMP production. Unfortunately the majority of these drugs, although producing short-term benefit, are associated with tolerance to their effects and increased incidence of arrhythmias.

The second group of agents has been equally unsuccessful. These are the phosphodiesterase inhibitors which increase cyclic AMP within the cell by inhibiting a group of enzymes which are responsible for its breakdown. Almost all these agents are associated with increased mortality during chronic treatment, probably due to the development of arrhythmias.

When one considers that advanced heart failure is a state of energy starvation in which catecholamine activity is already high and the beta receptors are down-regulated, it is perhaps not surprising that further stimulation is often unsuccessful or even harmful. Digitalis remains the only inotropic drug which is recommended for general clinical use. This agent acts as an inhibitor of $Na^+K^+ATPase$ and results in an improvement in myocardial contractility by increasing intracellular calcium concentrations. Digitalis has no beneficial or detrimental effect on overall mortality.

The digitalis glycosides

In 1785, William Withering reported the beneficial effects of digitalis in dropsy, although at the time he believed that it relieved the symptoms and signs of heart failure by acting on the kidney. In 1911, McKenzie observed that digitalis slowed the ventricular rate in atrial fibrillation and this remains the main indication for this group of drugs when there is associated heart failure. Although these properties have been described for some time the physiological and pharmacolgical effects have only recently been elucidated and the value of cardiac glycosides in patients with heart failure and sinus rhythm has only been confirmed within the last few years.

Preparations

A number of cardiac glycosides are presently in clinical use although in the United Kingdom and in the United States of America; almost all the prescriptions are for digoxin. Digitoxin, digitalin and digitalis are derived from the leaves of the purple foxglove (*Digitalis purpura*), lantoside C and deslanoside from *Digitalis lanata*, and ouabain from the seeds of *Strophanthus gratus*. Since digoxin is the most commonly used glycoside the majority of the information presented will refer to this preparation.

Digoxin

Pharmacokinetics

Digoxin (12-hydroxydigitoxin) is relatively well absorbed from the gastrointestinal tract although its absorption is influenced by a variety of factors. Decreased motility of the gastrointestinal tract is associated with enhanced absorption and increased motility with reduced absorption. Co-administration of cholestyramine, colestipol, kaolin, pectin and some antacids retard absorption, and neomycin and sulphasalazine interfere with absorption across the small intestine. Although plasma digoxin levels following oral administration have sometimes been reported to be reduced in patients with congestive cardiac failure, studies using tritiated digoxin have failed to demonstrate a decrease in bioavailability even in patients with severe right heart failure. Problems were reported over 20 years ago with preparations of variable oral bioavailability but these are now standardised and absolute bioavailability is maintained between 60% and 80%. Malabsorption syndromes and the presence of food appear to have little effect on overall oral absorption.

Digoxin is not extensively metabolised in humans. After absorption approximately 25% is protein bound. The drug, however, is avidly tissue bound resulting in a large apparent volume of distribution. The concentration of the glycoside in human cardiac tissue may be as high as 30 times of that in the plasma and bears a relatively constant relationship. Digoxin is also readily bound to skeletal muscle but adipose tissue contains little digoxin. Thus lean body mass rather than total body mass has been used to calculate the loading dose. Myocardial uptake of digoxin is influenced by the plasma concentrations of sodium and potassium. Hyponatraemia and hyperkalaemia reduce the concentrations of digoxin within the myocardial cells by altering the binding to the enzyme $Na^+K^+ATPase$.

Digoxin is principally eliminated from the body through the kidney. 60–90% being excreted unchanged in the urine and only a small fraction (15–20%) appearing in the faeces. Renal elimination occurs primarily by glomerular filtration although a saturable tubular secretory process also contributes. This can be demonstrated clinically by spironolactone which increases the concentrations of digoxin in plasma by inhibiting the secretory mechanism. The elimination half-life in healthy subjects with normal renal function is approximately 36 hours. In patients with congestive cardiac failure and reduced renal perfusion the elimination half-life is usually 2–4 days. Intestinal reabsorption of digoxin by the enterohepatic circulation is limited and represents approximately 6.5% of the administered dose. The principal pharmacokinetic properties of digoxin and digitoxin values are listed in Table 6.5.

Pharmacodynamics

Proposed cellular mode of action. It is generally agreed that the digitalis glycosides interact with $Na^+K^+ATPase$ in cardiac cells although other mechanisms may contribute to the increases in intracellular calcium (Figure 6.2). Inhibition of $Na^+K^+ATPase$ results in an increase in intracellular sodium. This increase in sodium reduces the release of calcium from the cell by the Na^{2+}/Ca^{2+} exchange mechanism and intracellular concentrations of calcium rise. Increased entry of calcium into the cell could also occur through the voltage-dependent calcium channels during the plateau phase of the action potential (Figure 6.2). A third possible mechanism is enhanced release of stored calcium from the sarcoplasmic reticulum (Figure 6.2). Finally, increased release or decreased uptake of endogenous noradrenaline could also be contributory.

Electrophysiological effects

Digitalis exerts a number of important electrophysiological effects directly on the heart and indirectly by interacting with the autonomic nervous system. Direct actions result in a prolongation of the cellular action potential and an increase in membrane resistance. This is followed by a period of shortening of the action potential and a decrease in membrane resistance, probably related to increased membrane potassium conductance due to increased intracellular calcium. Reduction in the length of the action potential probably contributes to the reduced refractoriness of the atrial and ventricular conducting tissue.

Table 6.5. Pharmacokinetic values and dosages of digoxin and digitoxin

	Digoxin	Digitoxin
Gastrointestinal absorption	60–85%	90–100%
Onset of action	15–30 minutes	30–120 minutes
Time to peak effect	1–5 hours	4–12 hours
Plasma elimination half-life	1–4 days	5–10 days
Therapeutic range	0.8–2.0 ng/ml	14–26 ng/ml
Principal route of elimination	Renal	Hepatic–renal
Recommended loading dose	1.0–1.5 mg	1.0–1.5 mg
Recommended maintenance dose	0.125–0.5 mg	0.05–0.2 mg

Indirect actions of the cardiac glycosides on the cardiac conducting system are largely mediated through the autonomic nervous system. In patients with heart failure, the heart rate tends to fall due to improvements in cardiac function and reductions in sympathetic tone. In the absence of heart failure, digitalis does not usually produce any reduction in heart rate and a small increase may be observed.

Reductions in atrioventricular nodal conduction is one of the major therapeutic effects of this group of compounds. Atrioventricular nodal conduction is reduced and the nodal effective refractory period is prolonged. These nodal effects result from a combination of increased cholinergic and reduced adrenergic effects, although a slight direct effect has been demonstrated in the denervated heart. On the other hand, the electrophysiological effects of digitalis on the Purkinje fibres and ventricular myocardium result in slight prolongation of the action potential and do not involve alteration in autonomic nervous system activity.

Interaction with the autonomic nervous system

At therapeutic concentrations the main effect of digitalis is to stimulate the parasympathetic nervous system and reduce sympathetic activity. At toxic concentrations, stimulation of the sympathetic nervous system can occur. The effect on vagal activity occurs by a variety of mechanisms. Alteration of the activity of the arterial baroreceptor, the cardiopulmonary receptors, the efferent vagal nerve pathways and the end-organ responses to vagal stimulation have all been described. These interactions with the autonomic nervous system have important clinical consequences. Excessive para-sympathetic activity can, under certain circumstances, reduce the direct inotropic effects and slow the heart excessively so that cardiac output decreases. Reduction in the ventricular response in atrial flutter and fibrillation results mainly from vagal effects on the atrioventricular node. In atrial fibrillation the effect of digitalis on the ventricular rate is greater at rest when the vagal tone is high, compared with exercise when sympathetic activity predominates. Large concentrations of digitalis increase sympa-thetic tone by increasing efferent nerve activity from the central nervous system and by altering peripheral catecholamine release and reuptake by the nerve endings. This contributes to the pro-arrhythmic effect of digitalis at high dose although adrenoceptor antagonists are ineffective in control-ling the arrhythmias due to digitalis overdose.

The clinical use of the cardiac glycosides in congestive cardiac failure

The role of the cardiac glycosides in the management of congestive cardiac failure has been plagued by controversy since William Withering's treatise on the foxglove in 1785. The nature of the controversy is well illustrated in a recent published survey of more than 2700 physicians who were involved in the treatment of heart failure. In this analysis about 60% considered digitalis to be effective in improving exercise tolerance, but only 30% thought it would prolong life. About one-third considered it to be a useful first-line agent in patients with congestive cardiac failure and sinus rhythm, and the remainder did not. Differences in opinion about the efficacy of digitalis are reflected by different prescribing patterns throughout the world. As documented in the SOLVD (studies of left ventricular function) register, 25% of patients in Belgium were receiving digitalis as compared with 41% in Canada and 49% in the United States of America. The clinical profile in the three groups was similar.

Recent questions have also been raised regarding the effect of digitalis on mortality, especially in patients with coronary artery disease who have had a recent myocardial infarction. To date these studies have been inconclusive.

Evidence for clinical efficacy in patients with heart failure and who are in sinus rhythm

Two principal methods have been used to determine the long-term efficacy of the digitalis glycosides (almost exclusively as digoxin) in patients with heart failure and sinus rhythm. The first technique was to withdraw the drug in a group of patients who have been receiving it for some time. In this type of study few patients deteriorate after the drug is discontinued provided patients show no clinical evidence of heart failure at the time of withdrawal. There are several reasons for this. In some patients digoxin was inappropriately prescribed, for example, to treat angina pectoris, peripheral oedema without other signs of heart failure and sinus tachycardia following an acute myocardial infarction. Many patients were receiving insufficient digoxin because the dose was inadequate or because of poor compliance. In patients with steady-state plasma concentrations below the therapeutic range, successful withdrawal was achieved in almost 100% of cases. Another possible explanation was that the reasons for the initial prescribing no longer applied; for example, digitalis prescribed for a supraventricular arrhythmia after an acute myocardial infarction or thyrotoxicosis is usually not required long term.

In order to assess accurately the value of chronic digoxin therapy various criteria need to be satisfied. All patients in whom assessment of withdrawal is to be made must have clearly documented congestive cardiac failure and evidence of poor left ventricular function. Patients should remain in sinus rhythm and there should be no previous history of atrial tachyarrhythmias. The studies should be randomised, have a placebo control and in the digoxin-treated group plasma concentration should be maintained within the defined therapeutic range. When these criteria are met, it appears that digoxin does exert a chronic beneficial effect in patients with heart failure and sinus rhythm, especially in those with poor left ventricular function as defined by an ejection fraction less than 0.35 and/or the presence of a third heart sound (Table 6.6).

Although withdrawal studies have provided us with useful information about the value of digoxin therapy in clinical practice, for accurate evaluation it is essential to assess the drug in randomised placebo-controlled studies preferably using a parallel group design. The major studies performed over the last 15 years are listed in Table 6.6. Overall, patients with congestive heart failure who are in sinus rhythm benefit from chronic digoxin therapy. The drug appears to be particularly useful in patients with marked left ventricular systolic dysfunction, cardiomegaly and congestive heart failure. These patients clearly demonstrate improvements in exercise capacity, improved measures of left ventricular function and beneficial effects on the clinical features of heart failure.

Table 6.6. Clinical trials of digoxin in heart failure with sinus rhythm

Study	No. of patients	Design features	Endpoints (digoxin vs placebo)
Fleg et al. (1982)	30	PDRFT	Decreased LVEDD. Decreased STI
Lee et al. (1982)	25	PDRFC	Improved heart failure score. Decreased LVEDD. Decreased CT ratio
Taggart et al. (1983)	22	PDRCL	Decreased STIs
Guyatt et al. (1988)	20	PDRFTC	Improved 6-minute walk. Reduced dyspnoea. Decreased CHF score. Decreased CT ratio. Increased echo FS.
Xamoterol Study (1988)	433	PDRFTC	Improved exercise tolerance. Reduced symptoms
Captopril–digoxin (1988)	300	PDRTC	Decreased diuretics in digoxin group. Increased EF. Fewer hospital admissions
Milrinone–digoxin (1989)	230	PDRTC	Increased exercise. Decreased diuretic use. Increased EF
Pugh et al. (1989)	44	PDRLTC	Decreased treatment failure. Decreased STIs

R – randomised. D – double-blind. P – placebo control. C – clinical endpoints. L – plasma levels. T – exercise testing. F – ejection fraction.

Table 6.7.   Digoxin and survival (retrospective database studies)

Study	No. of patients	Effect on mortality (digoxin vs control)
Moss et al. (1981)	812 (189)	NS
Ryan et al. (1983)	14 547 (2600)	NS
Madsen et al. (1984)	1599 (585)	NS
Bigger et al. (1985)	504 (229)	Higher mortality with increased digoxin levels NS after adjustment for AF and CHF
Byington et al. (1985)	1921 (250)	NS
Muller et al. (1986)	903 (281)	NS

NS – non significant. Figures in brackets refer to number of patients taking digoxin.

Effect of digoxin on survival

Although several inotropic agents have been shown to have a detrimental effect on mortality, a recent large placebo controlled study revealed no negative impact. Several studies have retrospectively evaluated the relationship between digoxin therapy and mortality, however (Table 6.7). Overall the data suggest that digoxin administration is not likely to be associated with an independent mortality risk, at least in patients with coronary heart disease. It seems much more likely that the patients on the drug had more severe heart failure, greater left ventricular dysfunction and a higher incidence of serious dysrhythmias. The Digitalis Investigation Group has recently published the results of their study on the effects of digoxin in patients with heart failure and left ejection fractions $\leqslant 45\%$. Deaths due to worsening heart failure and hospitalisations due to heart failure were reduced, but overall mortality was unaffected.

Dose–response characteristics of digoxin in heart failure

Although elevated steady-state plasma digoxin levels are more common in patients with drug toxicity, few data are available on the relationship between plasma concentrations and the therapeutic effect in patients with heart failure. Preliminary data from the PROVED (prospective randomised study of ventricular failure and efficacy of digoxin) and RADIANCE (randomized assessment of digoxin on inhibitors of the angiotensin converting enzyme) trials, have shed some light on this subject. Patients were divided into three groups: 0.5–0.9 ng/ml; <0.9–1.2 ng/ml; >1.2 ng/ml. All three groups were better than placebo in terms of exercise tolerance, but no dose–response relationship was determined and low plasma concentrations of digoxin appeared as effective as higher concentrations.

Concomitant digoxin and vasodilator therapy appears to be more effective than either therapy alone. This has been shown with a combination of isosorbide dinitrate and hydralazine, and with enalapril and captopril.

Atrial dysrhythmias

Digitalis remains the treatment of choice when heart failure is associated with fast atrial fibrillation. It decreases the ventricular response and helps to decompress the atrium in mitral stenosis. Increased ventricular filling associated with a slower ventricular rate improves haemodynamics. Conversion of atrial fibrillation to sinus rhythm with digoxin rarely occurs.

In atrial flutter, decreased atrioventricular conduction is associated with increased atrioventricular block and decreased ventricular response. Larger doses tend to be required to achieve the effect in atrial flutter compared to atrial fibrillation because of the decreased refractoriness of the AV node in atrial flutter. On occasions atrial flutter may be converted to atrial fibrillation with a further decrease in the ventricular rate. As in atrial fibrillation, combinations with beta adrenoceptor antagonists and calcium channel antagonists can achieve further decreases in the ventricular rate.

Digoxin can also be used to control paroxysmal atrial or atrioventricular tachycardia. The oral and intravenous administration of digoxin may abruptly terminate these attacks, but a variety of other drugs, notably verapamil, diltiazem and adenosine are more effective. Similarly, digoxin is occasionally effective in controlling supraventricular tachycardia associated with the Wolff–Parkinson–White syndrome, but other antiarrhythmic agents, notably types IA, IC and II drugs are usually preferred.

Acute myocardial infarction

Although there remain major doubts concerning the therapeutic efficacy and toxicity of the digitalis glycosides, these compounds continue to be widely used following acute myocardial infarction and the following tentative recommendations can be made. Digoxin should be used to control the rapid ventricular response in patients with atrial fibrillation after an acute myocardial infarction, especially if it is accompanied by evidence of heart failure. In patients with sinus rhythm and heart failure, digoxin should be reserved for those patients who do not respond adequately to a combination of diuretics and ACE inhibitors, or those with low ejection fractions and/or left ventricular chamber enlargement as indicated by a third heart sound or a large internal diastolic diameter. The inotropic effect of digoxin is small in comparison to most other inotropic agents and in patients with low cardiac output in whom significant stimulation of the myocardium is required, a sympathetic agent such as dobutamine is usually preferred at least in the short term.

Adverse effects

> The foxglove when given in very large and quickly-repeated doses, occasions sickness, vomiting, purging, giddiness, confused vision, objects appearing green or yellow; increased secretion of urine, with frequent motions to part with it, and sometimes inability to retain it; slow pulse, even as low as 35 in a minute, cold sweats, convulsions, syncope, death.
>
> William Withering (1785)

Toxicity should be considered in any patient taking digoxin who presents with a new arrhythmia and/or a disturbance of atrioventricular conduction. Adverse effects can be classified according to the organ principally affected: heart, nervous system, eye and gut.

Dysrhythmias and heart block. Almost any dysrhythmia can occur in patients with digoxin toxicity. The most common are ventricular extra beats including bigeminal rhythm, atrioventricular junctional escape rhythms, atrial tachycardia with atrioventricular block, ventricular tachycardia, sino-atrial nodal block or sinus arrest and ventricular fibrillation. Fast atrial fibrillation is more likely to be due to inadequate treatment rather than toxicity. All degrees of heart block can occur, and the combination of junctional or ventricular arrhythmias with atrioventricular nodal block is very suggestive of digoxin toxicity.

Neurological effects. Headache, drowsiness, fatigue and general malaise are relatively common symptoms of digoxin toxicity. Mental symptoms including disorientation, confusion, delirium and visual hallucinations can occur, and are particularly common in elderly patients with cerebral atherosclerosis.

Visual disturbances are relatively common features of digoxin toxicity and minor abnormalities may go unnoticed. Vision may be blurred, white borders may appear around darker objects and images may acquire a frosted appearance. Colour vision is frequently affected, the typical disturbance being xanthopsia or disturbance of yellow–green vision, although other colours may sometimes be involved. Retrobulbar neuritis, amblyopia and diplopia have occasionally been described. Visual effects are dose related and are rare within the defined therapeutic range.

Gastrointestinal effects.   Anorexia, nausea and vomiting are often the earliest features of digoxin toxicity. Vomiting occasionally occurs as a single manifestation, but is usually preceded by nausea and anorexia and sometimes accompanied by abdominal pain. Vomiting occurs soon after intravenous administration, probably due to a direct effect on the medulla oblongata. Diarrhoea, on the other hand, is probably due to a local effect on the gastrointestinal tract.

Other effects

Other toxic effects are relatively uncommon; those reported include gynaecomastia, thrombocytopenia and urticarial rashes associated with eosinophilia. Intramuscular administration can cause muscle necrosis and should be avoided if possible. Severe hyperkalaemia has been reported with both accidental and deliberate overdoses of digoxin because of inhibition of the sodium/potassium pump and reduced movement of potassium into cells. A high plasma potassium concentration is associated with a poor prognosis, and a figure >5.5mmol/l is an important indication for treatment with anti-digoxin antibody fragments.

Factors which modify the action of digoxin

Several factors can increase the amount of digoxin in the body and hence the plasma digoxin concentration for a given dose: renal failure is the most important condition for which dosage should be reduced. A variety of drugs can increase plasma digoxin concentrations and increase the risk of toxicity, usually because of impaired renal and extra renal clearance of digoxin (Table 6.8). Other factors are important in modifying the sensitivity of the heart to a given concentration of digoxin (Table 6.9). Of these, hypokalaemia is the most important, and patients taking digoxin and a potassium-wasting diuretic should generally be given a potassium-sparing diuretic. A low serum magnesium concentration and a high serum calcium concentration may also contribute to digoxin toxicity. Patients with chronic

Table 6.8.   Some important cardiovascular drugs which increase the serum digoxin concentrations

Drug	Average increase in steady state (%)
Amiodarone	70–100
Propafenone	25–35
Quinidine	100
Spironolactone	20
Verapamil	50–100

Table 6.9. Factors increasing sensitivity to digoxin at therapeutic plasma
concentrations

Underlying pathology
  Corpulmonale
  Myxoedema
  Chronic hypoxaemia
  Acute rheumatic or viral carditis
  Acute myocardial infarction

Electrolyte disorders
  Hypokalaemia
  Hypomagnesaemia
  Hypercalcaemia

Other diseases
  Hypothyroidism

hypoxia and corpulmonale appear to be more sensitive to the effects of
digoxin. Hypothyroidism increases the risk of toxicity, partly because of
impaired renal elimination and partly because of increased myocardial
sensitivity.

Avoiding digoxin toxicity

Several factors contribute to the development of digoxin toxicity: over-
estimation of loading or maintenance doses, increased sensitivity to the
drug, deterioration in renal function, and the administration of other drugs.
Selection of doses based on renal function and lean body weight, awareness
of the numerous manifestations of digoxin toxicity, measurement of steady-
state plasma concentrations and a knowledge of the drugs and diseases that
can alter the effects of digoxin, are all important in avoiding toxicity. In
most patients a plasma digoxin concentration between 0.8 and 2.0 ng/ml
(1.0–2.6 nmol/l) is associated with therapeutic benefit and a low risk of
toxicity. In some patients higher plasma concentrations will be required for
adequate treatment, but the risk of toxicity rises sharply at concentrations
greater than 3 ng/ml.

Treating digoxin toxicity

Most patients who develop digoxin toxicity will respond to discontinuation
of the drug and potassium administration if there is associated hypokalaemia. The control of arrhythmias is problematical, but amiodarone,
lignocaine, and phenytoin are the preferred antiarrhythmic agents.
Ventricular pacing may be required for advanced heart block or severe
sinus bradycardia unresponsive to atropine. Patients with serum potassiums

>5.5 mmol/l and/or those with life-threatening dysrhythmias, should receive anti-digoxin antibody fragments (Digibind). The plasma digoxin concentration is not a good guide to the severity of toxicity but it can be used to estimate the dose of antibody required.

Other inotropic drugs

Sympathomimetic amines

A number of sympathetic amines are in clinical use most commonly to elevate blood pressure and to increase cardiac output. The rationale for their use relates to the well-described actions of catecholamines on the heart and blood vessels and activation of the alpha, beta and dopamine receptors.

Beta subtypes

The $beta_1$ and $beta_2$ receptors were originally classified by the relative activity of adrenaline and noradrenaline at these receptors. $Beta_1$ receptors have approximately equal affinity for adrenaline and noradrenaline, while $beta_2$ receptors have a higher affinity for adrenaline rather than noradrenaline (Table 6.10). A third subtype (β_3) has now been identified which has some properties of each of these receptor types (Table 6.11).

Alpha subtypes

The division of alpha receptor subtypes into $alpha_1$ and $alpha_2$ was also based on their affinity for different alpha agonists (Table 6.11). Further

Table 6.10. Relative selectivity of adrenoceptor agonists

Alpha agonists	Relative receptor affinities
Phenylephrine	$\alpha_1 > \alpha_2 \gg \beta$
Clonidine	
Methylnoradrenaline	$\alpha_2 > \alpha_1 \gg \beta$
Combined alpha and beta agonists	
Noradrenaline	$\alpha_1 = \alpha_2; \beta_1 > \beta_2$
Adrenaline	$\alpha_1 = \alpha_2; \beta_1 = \beta_2$
Beta agonists	
Dobutamine	$\beta_1 > \beta_2 \gg \alpha$
Isoprenaline	$\beta_1 = \beta_2 \gg \alpha$
Salbutamol	$\beta_2 \gg \beta_1 \gg \alpha$
Dopamine agonists	
Dopamine	$D_1 = D_2 \gg \beta \gg \alpha$

Table 6.11.   Cellular and cardiovascular actions of adrenoceptor agonists

Receptor	Agonist	Cellular effects	Actions on the cardiovascular system
Alpha$_1$-type	Phenylephrine Methoxamine	$\uparrow$IP$_3$ DAG	Vasoconstriction Elevated blood pressure. Positive inotropic activity
Alpha$_2$-type	Clonidine	$\downarrow$cAMP	Variable effect on vascular smooth muscle. Lowers blood pressure by central action
Beta$_1$-type	Isoprenaline Dobutamine	$\uparrow$cAMP	Increased rate and force of cardiac contraction
Beta$_2$-type	Salbutamol Terbutaline	$\uparrow$cAMP	Vasodilation especially muscle blood vessels Increased heart rate (reflex and/or β_1 effects)
Beta$_3$-type	BRL 37344	$\uparrow$cAMP	[Activates lipolysis]
Dopamine$_1$-type	Dopamine	$\uparrow$cAMP	Dilates renal blood vessels
Dopamine$_2$-type	Bromocriptine	$\downarrow$cAMP $\uparrow$K$^+$channels	[Modulates transmitter release at nerve endings]

IP$_3$ – inositol–1,45 triphosphate. DAG – diacylglycerol. cAMP – cyclic adenosine monophosphate.

subdivision of these receptors has been proposed. Based on radioligand binding, two subtypes of the alpha$_1$ receptor have been identified as α_{1A} and α_{1B}. Both occur in the heart, brain and kidney, but the spleen and liver contain mainly the $\alpha_{1\beta}$ receptor. Similarly, α_{2A} and α_{2B} receptors have been identified and compounds such as prazosin, chlorpromazine and yohimbine have different affinities for these receptors.

Dopamine receptors

Dopamine produces a variety of biological effects which are mediated by interactions with specific dopamine receptors. These are distinct from the alpha and beta receptors and are particularly important in the brain and in the splanchnic and renal vasculature. The terminology of the various subtypes has not been generally agreed but at present D$_1$, D$_2$, D$_3$, D$_4$ and D$_5$ subtypes are in general use (Figure 6.3).

Receptor selectivity

Selectivity implies that a drug may preferentially bind to one subgroup of receptors at concentrations which are too low to interact with other receptor subgroups. For example, noradrenaline preferentially activates the beta$_1$ receptors compared to the beta$_2$ receptors (Table 6.10). However, at higher concentrations this selectivity may be lost. For inotropic activity, selectivity at the beta$_1$ receptor is clearly an advantage.

Molecular mechanisms of sympathomimetic action

The effects of catecholamines are mediated by cell surface receptors (Figure 6.4). These receptors are coupled by G proteins to the various effector proteins whose activities are regulated by those receptors. G proteins of particular importance for adrenoceptor function include G$_s$ the stimulating G protein of adenylyl cyclase, G$_i$ the inhibitor G protein of adenylyl cyclase and G$_q$, the protein coupling alpha receptors to phospholipase C (Figure 6.4). Activation of all three beta receptor subtypes results in activation of adenylyl cyclase and increased conversion of ATP to cAMP (Figure 6.4). In the heart this results in increased calcium influx and sequestration inside the cell. The mechanism of beta receptor activation to relax vascular smooth muscle is uncertain, but may involve the phosphorylation of myosin light chain kinase to an inactive form. The most commonly observed effect of alpha$_1$ receptor stimulation is an increase in cytosolic calcium concentration which does not involve a change in adenylyl cyclase activity or cyclic AMP concentration within the cell. Alpha$_2$ receptors inhibit adenylyl cyclase activity and decrease intracellular cAMP levels. This is mediated by the

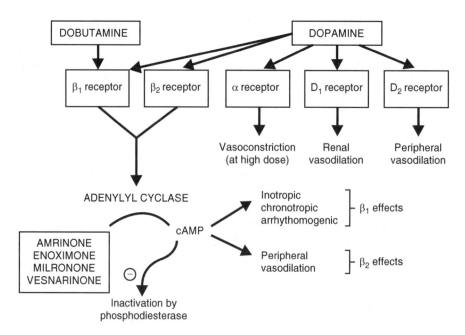

Figure 6.3. Modes of action of the inodilators.

inhibitory protein G_i which couples the alpha$_2$ receptor to the inhibition of adenylyl cyclase. Activation of potassium channels and closing of calcium channels has also been described. The dopamine$_1$ receptor typically produces increased concentrations of adenyl cyclase when activated, while the dopamine$_2$ receptors inhibit adenylyl cyclase activity, open potassium channels, and decrease calcium influx.

Receptor regulation

Responses mediated by adrenoceptors are not constant. The number and function of adrenoceptors on the cell surface and their responses can be altered by the concentration of catecholamines at the receptor, the presence of other hormones and drugs, age and a number of disease states. The best described example is desensitisation of adrenoceptors to catecholamines and other sympathomimetic drugs. After a tissue has been exposed for a period of time to an agonist, the tissue becomes less responsive to further stimulation by that substance. The process has significant clinical importance because it limits the long-term use of several sympathomimetic drugs in the management of heart failure.

Sympathomimetic drugs used in the treatment of heart failure

Dopamine and dobutamine are the beta agonists most commonly used in the treatment of heart failure. They are usually limited to short courses in patients with severe heart failure unresponsive to other measures, or in cardiogenic shock following an acute myocardial infarction. The use of

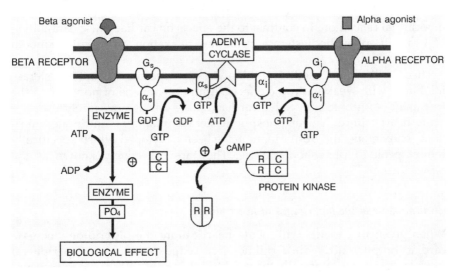

Figure 6.4. Proposed cellular modes of action for the adrenoceptor agonists.

dobutamine infusions lasting more than 72 hours is limited because tolerance often develops. Intermittent infusions of dobutamine have been administered to outpatients with severe refractory heart failure and improvements in haemodynamics and functional capacity have been described. However, in one controlled study the mortality was double that of patients in the control group.

Various orally administered beta agonists have been evaluated in the treatment of chronic heart failure such as pirbuterol, prenalterol, ibopamine and xamoterol. All produce short-term improvement in left ventricular performance which is not maintained long term, probably due to down-regulation of the beta receptors. In addition, a recently developed orally active $beta_1$ partial agonist, xamoterol, was associated with a higher mortality than placebo in the long-term treatment of heart failure. The value of these drugs in the long-term management of heart failure is extremely doubtful.

Phosphodiesterase inhibitors

Modes of action

Several distinct forms of phosphodiesterase isoenzymes, have been identified in mammalian cells. Peak III is the predominant form and a variety of inhibitors have been developed. Inhibition of peak III phosphodiesterase results in increased intracellular cyclic AMP in cardiac muscle and subsequent phosphorylation of cellular proteins by cyclic AMP dependent protein kinase (Figure 6.4). Increased cyclic AMP in cardiac muscle leads to increased contractility and to an enhanced rate of myocardial relaxation. In contrast to the effects on cardiac muscle inhibition of peak III, phosphodiesterase promotes relaxation of vascular smooth muscle.

Theophylline and methylxanthine are non-specific phosphodiesterase inhibitors with weak inotropic effects. Aminophylline is of no value in the treatment of chronic congestive cardiac failure and is now rarely used for acute heart failure. Newer phosphodiesterase inhibitors, amrinone, milrinone, enoximone and vesnarinone have been developed which specifically inhibit peak III phosphodiesterase. They are collectively known as the bipyridines.

Clinical value of the bipyridines in heart failure

When given to patients with acute heart failure the bipyridines increase cardiac output and reduce pulmonary wedge pressure and peripheral vascular resistance. Normally there is little change in arterial blood pressure or heart rate. Despite these beneficial effects, their long-term use is associated with a high incidence of toxicity. Amrinone frequently causes nausea and vomiting, thrombocytopenia, elevated liver transaminases and polyserositis, although these are substantially less common with milrinone, enoximone and vesnarinone.

Oral amrinone when administered chronically failed to improve symptoms and exercise capacity in patients with severe heart failure. Milrinone, although more potent and less toxic, was found to be no more effective than digoxin in most patients and was associated with a significantly higher mortality than placebo. Similar results have been described with enoximone. In contrast, vesnarinone when given over a 25-week period was associated with a significant decrease in cardiovascular morbidity and mortality. The latter study also showed that the therapeutic margin of safety was narrow with 60 mg daily causing a decrease in mortality and 120 mg a significant increase in deaths. A recent study did not confirm the beneficial effects of low dose vesnarinone on mortality. In a pooled analysis of mortality, the type III phosphodiesterase inhibitors were associated with a mortality rate approximately 40% higher than placebo. At present, therefore, this group of drugs has no place in the management of chronic heart failure. Milrinone and enoximone are available for intra-venous use in the United Kingdom for the short-term treatment of severe heart failure unresponsive to other therapies.

Other possible drug treatments

Beta adrenoceptor antagonists

Recent clinical trials suggest benefit from beta$_1$ selective adrenoceptor antagonists, metoprolol and bisoprolol, and a non-selective beta blocking drug with vasodilating properties, carvedilol. The Swedish metoprolol in dilated cardiomyopathy study randomised 383 patients with non-ischaemic cardiomyopathy with NYHA, classes III and IV and ejection fractions less than 40% to metoprolol or placebo. The reduction in combined primary endpoints of total mortality and need for cardiac transplantation almost achieved statistical significance at the 5% level. The cardiac insufficiency bisoprolol study (CIBIS) randomised a mixed population of 350 patients with ischaemic cardiomyopathy and 232 patients with non-ischaemic cardiomyopathy who had NYHA classes III and IV and ejection fractions less than 40% to bisoprolol or placebo. No significant differences were observed in mortality or incidence of sudden death, but subgroup analysis suggested improved survival in patients with non-ischaemic congestive cardiomyopathy. A larger study (CIBIS II) with greater statistical power was designed to test for differences in morbidity and mortality based on the results of the first study. This second study demonstrated a significant reduction in all-cause mortality, sudden death and hospitalisations due to worsening heart failure in patients with ischaemic and non-ischaemic cardiomyopathy.

Analysis of the United States carvedilol heart failure study programme which included four trials and involved more than 1000 patients, has recently been published. Carvedilol, a non-selective beta adrenoceptor antagonist with alpha$_1$ blocking activity demonstrated a reduction in all-cause mortality, and hospitalisations for cardiovascular events were significantly reduced. It has been suggested that non-selective beta adrenoceptor antagonists such as carvedilol and bucindolol may be more effective and better tolerated than beta$_1$ antagonists, metoprolol and bisoprolol because beta$_1$ receptors are down-regulated in heart failure and the cardiac beta$_2$ receptors are unprotected from increased sympathetic activity. This has not been formally tested in clinical trials. It is important to start with a very small dose and slowly titrate upwards otherwise dropout rates tend to be high.

Calcium channel antagonists

All the first-generation calcium channel antagonists, verapamil, diltiazem and nifedipine result in clinical and haemodynamic deterioration in a considerable number of patients and increase the incidence of cardiac events in patients with heart failure following a myocardial infarction. However, amlodipine, a second-generation dihydropyridine, has been shown to improve exercise time and reduce the symptoms of heart failure more than placebo. It seems possible that some of the newer generation calcium antagonists will have little detrimental effect on cardiac function, and amlodipine has been shown to improve morbidity in patients with non-ischaemic cardiomyopathy.

In general, first-generation calcium channel blockers should be avoided in patients with chronic heart failure. For those with symptoms of myocardial ischaemia, nitrates are the preferred agents. Amlodipine is at present the safest available calcium antagonist in patients with poor left ventricular function.

Amiodarone

Amiodarone has been shown to reduce mortality from sudden death and progressive pump failure in patients with severe heart failure. These studies were small, had untypical populations and the follow-up periods were relatively short. At present amiodarone should not be used in patients with heart failure without symptomatic arrhythmias, although it may restore and maintain sinus rhythm in patients with heart failure and atrial fibrillation, even in those with enlarged left atria. It is, however, the drug of first choice in patients with heart failure and symptomatic arrhythmias and it is certainly preferable to group 1 antiarrhythmic drugs which are proar-rhythmic and increase the incidence of sudden death.

Flosequinan

Flosequinan is an orally active fluoroquinolone compound with a long duration of action. It is principally a vasodilator but probably also has positive inotropic effects. Although it resembles the bipyridines in many ways, its mode of action is unclear. It has weak non-selective phospho-diesterase inhibitory effects and has no effect on sodium/potassium ATPase or cyclic AMP concentrations. Early clinical trials were promising, but a long-term study in heart failure found that the higher dose of 100 mg was associated with increased mortality. Although some patients seemed to benefit from the drug and the 50 mg was not associated with increased mortality, it has now been withdrawn in the United Kingdom.

Losartan

Losartan is the first of a group of drugs known as the angiotensin II receptor antagonists. To date there is only one outcome study published with this drug in congestive heart failure (ELITE (Evaluation of Losartan in The Elderly)). Although the primary endpoint was changes in renal function, which showed no difference between the two treatments, the study suggested a reduction in overall death rate and hospitalisations in the losartan-treated group compared with the captopril-treated group. Losartan also appeared to be better tolerated. A follow-up study with morbidity and mortality as the primary endpoints is now under way (ELITE II).

If losartan proves to be more effective than captopril, it could be due to the observation that ACE inhibitors do not completely reverse the abnormal vasoconstriction seen in heart failure as a result of conversion of angiotensin I to angiotensin II by other enzymes such as chymase.

Warfarin

Warfarin is of proven value in patients with heart failure accompanied by atrial fibrillation. Patients with a history of systemic or pulmonary embolism, or with an endocardial thrombus, should receive long-term oral anticoagulation. The evidence for long-term prophylaxis in those with enlarged hearts and sinus rhythm is inconclusive, but many physicians would recommend anticoagulation in selected patients with large hearts and low ejection fractions. It is also probably advisable in patients with large ventricular aneurysms.

7 Drug Treatment of Hyperlipidaemia

Introduction

Almost all lipids in human plasma are transported as protein complexes. With the exception of fatty acids which are bound to albumin, lipids are carried as specially developed macromolecular complexes known as lipoproteins. The hyperlipoproteinaemias refer to a number of metabolic disorders in which the plasma lipoprotein concentrations are elevated and the term 'hyperlipaemia' relates to those conditions where the triglycerides are elevated. The term 'hyperlipidaemia' embraces both groups of conditions.

The link between hyperlipidaemia and atherosclerosis

Epidemiological evidence has linked a variety of plasma lipoproteins to accelerated atherogenesis. The lipoproteins which contain apolipoprotein B-100 have been identified as the principal transporters of cholesterol into the arterial wall. These are low density (LDL), intermediate density (IDL), very low density (VLDL) and Lp(a) lipoproteins. Cholesteryl esters found in the foam cells in the process of atherogenesis also occur in the extracellular matrix and initiate collagen formation by fibroblasts. Macrophages have a major role in the development of atheroma. Oxidation of lipoproteins facilitates their uptake by specialised scavenger receptors, giving rise to the characteristic foam cells in which cholesteryl esters accumulate.

Total cholesterol and risk

The relationship between total serum cholesterol and risk is exponential (Figure 7.1). The problem is to decide at what point on the curve to intervene so that the benefits outweigh the risks of treatment. In the past, total cholesterol was used to assess the risk of coronary heart disease. Levels between 5.2 and 6.5 mmol/l were considered to represent 'moderate' risk,

Table 7.1. Guidelines of the European Atherosclerosis Society. Reproduced from the *Eur. Heart Journal* for distetes and diabetes 1994; 15: 1300–1331: Anderson, K. M. *et al.* Reproduced with permission from W.B. Saunders Company Ltd.

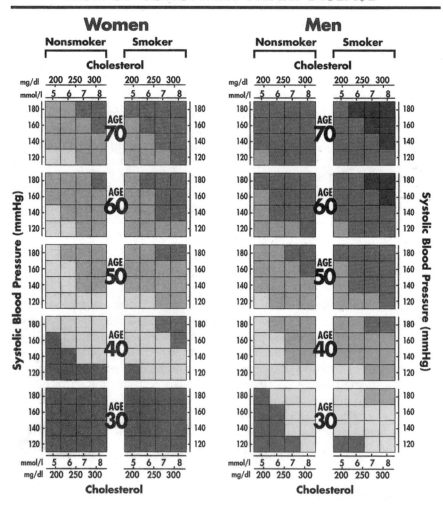

HOW TO USE THE RISK TABLES

1. To determine a person's absolute 10-year risk of a coronary event (heart attack), identify the table relating to the person's sex, smoking status, and age.

2. Within the table, find the cell nearest to the person's systolic blood pressure (mmHg) and cholesterol.

3. Compare cell colour with key and read the risk level.

4. The effect of lifetime exposure to risk factors cab be assessed by following the table upwards with increasing age.

5.
> **Notice – For patients with coronary heart disease, the level of risk should be increased by at least one category.**
> People with family history of coronary event at an early age, distetes, or a family history of hyperlipidaemia are also at increased risk.

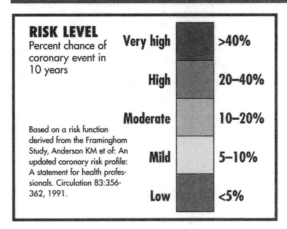

RISK LEVEL
Percent chance of coronary event in 10 years

Very high	>40%
High	20–40%
Moderate	10–20%
Mild	5–10%
Low	<5%

Based on a risk function derived from the Framingham Study, Anderson KM et of: An updated coronary risk profile: A statement for health professionals. Circulation 83:356-362, 1991.

The table assumes the HDL cholesterol to be 1.0 mmol/l (39 mg/dl) in men and 1.1 mmol/l (43 mg/dl) in women. People with lower levels and/or with triglycerides above 2.3 mmol/l (200 mg/dl) are at higher risk.

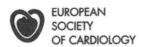

EUROPEAN
SOCIETY
OF CARDIOLOGY

EUROPEAN
ATHEROSCLEROSIS
SOCIETY

EUROPEAN
SOCIETY OF
HYPERTENSION

Prevention of Coronary Heart Disease in Clinical Practice
Adapted from rEcommendations of the Task Force of the European Society of Cardiology, European Atherosclerosis Society, and European Society of Hypertension, published in *Eur Heart J 1994; 15*:1300-1331 and *Atherosclerosis 1994; 110: 121-161.*

CHD MRFIT STUDY

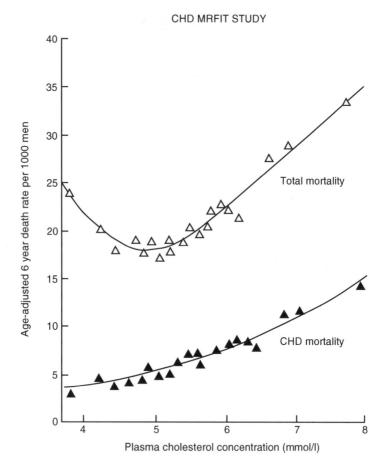

Figure 7.1.   After Martin, M. *et al.* (1986) *The Lancet*, 2: 933–6. © The Lancet Ltd, reproduced with permission.

values between 6.6 and 7.8 mmol/l, high risk and values greater than 7.8 mmol/l, very high risk. This was a gross oversimplification because it ignored the way in which cholesterol was transported in the plasma. If most of the cholesterol is transported as low density lipoproteins then the risk is increased, while if a large percentage is transported as high density lipoprotein, then the risk will be reduced. In addition, the impact of raised cholesterol on the risk of coronary heart disease is profoundly influenced by the presence of additional risk factors or existing heart disease. Hypertension, cigarette smoking, diabetes, a positive family history of heart disease and other lipid abnormalities should be taken into consideration when deciding to treat hyperlipidaemia. For example, data from the Framingham

Table 7.2. Major lipoproteins of human serum

Type of lipoprotein	Electrophoretic mobility in agarose gel	Density interval (g/cm³)	Core lipids	Diameter (nm)	Apolipoproteins
HDL	Alpha	1.063–1.21	Cholesteryl esters	7.5–10.5	A-I, A-II, C, E, D
LDL	Beta	1.019–1.063	Cholesteryl esters	21–22	B-100
IDL	Beta	1.006–1.019	Cholesteryl esters Triglycerides	25–30	B-100, E, C
VLDL	Pre-beta slow pre-beta	<1.006	Triglycerides Some cholesteryl esters	30–100	C species B-100 E
Chylomicrons	Remain at origin	<1.006	Triglycerides Some cholesteryl esters	80–500	B-48, C, E A-I, A-II
Lp(a) lipoproteins	Pre-beta	1.04–1.08	Cholesteryl esters	21–30	B-100, Lp(a)

study has demonstrated that taking into account the relative risk of coronary heart disease before the age of 55 for a patient of average risk (total cholesterol of 6 mmol/l and a systolic blood pressure of 120 mmHg), 50 individuals need to be treated to save one individual from death due to coronary heart disease. For those with cholesterols of 7 mmol/l and systolic blood pressures of 150 mmHg, only 25 individuals need to be treated to save one life.

Primary prevention

Primary prevention studies have shown that lowering total cholesterol in a population is associated with a reduction in morbidity and mortality due to coronary heart disease. Early studies, mainly involving bile acid-binding resins and fibric acid derivatives, failed to show a reduction in all-cause mortality probably due to the relatively small numbers studied and the short duration of these investigations. The *West of Scotland Coronary Prevention Study* published in 1995 was a landmark in the evaluation of the benefits of statin therapy. It showed that pravastatin produced a significant reduction in cardiovascular mortality and morbidity in asymptomatic men with hypercholesterolaemia and a decrease in all-cause mortality. Subgroup analyses demonstrated a relationship between multiple cardiovascular risk factors and absolute benefit from treatment with pravastatin. Using the information derived from this study it has been possible to draw up guidelines for primary prevention using the presence of additional risk factors (Table 7.1).

Secondary prevention

Secondary prevention studies have clearly shown that lowering the LDL cholesterol using drug therapy is associated with reductions in fatal and non-fatal myocardial infarction with no increase in non-cardiovascular deaths or events. A 25% reduction in LDL cholesterol is also associated with a similar reduction in arteriographically defined coronary artery lesions and a 20% increase in regression of atheromatous plaques. It is clear from the available evidence that patients with established coronary heart disease can benefit from aggressive lowering of the LDL cholesterol with regard to changes in the coronary lumen and clinical events. Data from the major secondary studies, CARE (cholesterol and recurrent events) trial and 4S (Scandinavian simvastatin survival study), demonstrate that all groups of patients with known coronary heart disease benefit from reductions in total cholesterol irrespective of their cholesterol when treatment is started. These benefits occur across the spectrum of total cholesterol levels in men and women and are additive to other commonly prescribed treatments including aspirin and beta adrenoceptor antagonists. Guidelines, based on these two major studies suggest that patients with angina, myocardial infarction or other evidence of atherosclerosis should have their cholesterol lowered with pravastatin or simvastatin if the total cholesterol is greater than 5.2 mmol/l. A reduction of 20–25% is achievable and effective.

Pathophysiology of hyperlipoproteinaemia

Normal lipoprotein metabolism

The major lipoproteins which occur in the plasma are spherical particles with hydrophobic core regions containing cholesteryl esters and triglycerides (Figure 7.2). A monolayer of unesterified cholesterol and phospholipids surrounds the core. Specific proteins called apolipoproteins are located on the surface of the particle. Some of these lipoproteins contain very high molecular weight apolipoproteins (B proteins) which do not migrate between particles and groups of smaller apolipoproteins which do. There are two principal forms of apolipoprotein B: B-48 which is formed in the intestine and found in chylomicrons and their remnants, and B-100 which is formed in the liver and found in VLDL, VLDL remnants, LDL and Lp (a) lipoproteins.

Smaller apolipoproteins distribute among the lipoproteins. ApoA-I is a co-factor for lecithin cholesterol acyltransferase (LCAT). ApoC-II is a co-factor for lipoprotein lipase, while several isoforms of ApoE are required for

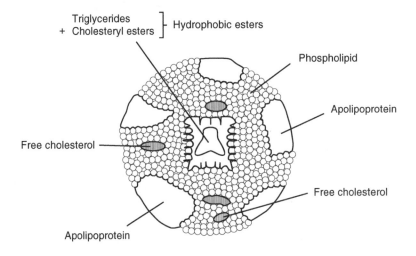

Figure 7.2. A generic lipoprotein particle or micelle.

the uptake of lipoprotein remnants by the liver. The properties of the major lipoproteins in human serum are listed in Table 7.2.

Synthesis and breakdown of the major lipoproteins

High density lipoproteins (HDL)

The apolipoproteins of HDL are secreted by the liver and intestine. Most of the lipid in HDL comes from the surface monolayers of chylomicrons and VLDL during lipolysis. HDL also acquire cholesterol from peripheral tissues in a pathway which protects the cholesterol homeostasis of cells. In this process, free cholesterol absorbed from cell membranes is acquired by a small particle termed pre-beta$_1$ HDL. The cholesterol is then esterified by L CAT, resulting in the formation of larger HDL species. The cholesteryl esters are transferred to VLDL, IDL, LDL and chylomicron remnants by cholesteryl ester transfer protein (CETP). As a result the cholesteryl ester is eventually delivered to the liver by endocytosis of the acceptor lipoproteins (Figure 7.3).

Low density lipoproteins (LDL)

Most low density lipoproteins are catabolised in the liver and other nucleated cells by high affinity receptor mediated endocytosis. Cholesteryl esters from the LDL core are then hydrolysed, producing free cholesterol for cell membrane synthesis. Cells also acquire cholesterol by a pathway involving the formation of mevalonic acid by HMG-CoA reductase. Production of this enzyme and the number of LDL receptors is regulated by the amount of cholesterol inside the cell.

Very low density lipoproteins (VLDL)

Very low density lipoproteins are secreted by the liver and assist in the transport of triglycerides to peripheral tissues. They contain apolipoproteins B-100 and C. The triglycerides are then hydrolysed by lipoprotein lipase after their exit from the liver to produce free fatty acids for storage in adipose tissue and for oxidation in metabolically active tissues such as cardiac and skeletal muscle. As the triglycerides are depleted, smaller particles or remnants are formed. These are referred to as intermediate density lipoproteins (IDL). Some of these particles undergo endocytosis by the liver while the remainder are converted to LDL by further removal of triglycerides.

173

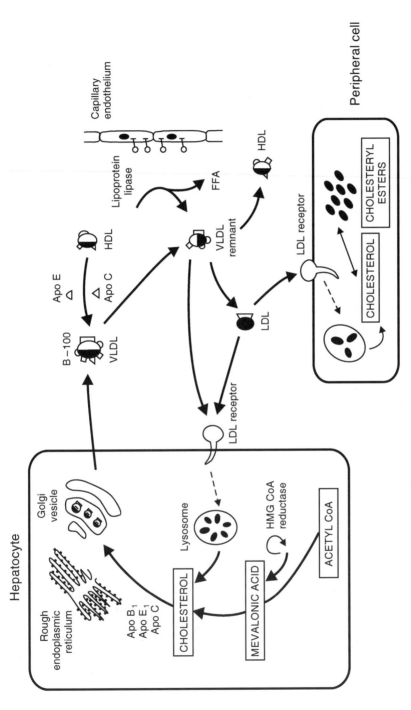

Figure 7.3. Metabolism of lipoproteins produced by the liver. After Kane and Malloy "Disorders of lipoproteins". In *The Molecular and Genetic Basis of Neurological Disease.* Rosenberg, R. N. *et al.* (editors), Butterworth–Heinemann, Woburn, MA, 1993. Reproduced with permission.

Chylomicrons

These are the largest of the lipoproteins and are synthesised in the small intestine to carry triglycerides of dietary origin. A small amount of esterified cholesterol is also present in the chylomicron core. The surface monolayer is composed of phospholipids, free cholesterol and newly synthesised lipoproteins such as ApoB-48, A-I and A-II. Triglycerides are removed from the chylomicrons in extrahepatic tissues by a pathway shared with VLDL. This involves hydrolysis by lipoprotein lipase with heparin and ApoC-II acting as co-factors for the reaction. As with VLDL, a progressive decrease in particle diameter occurs as the triglycerides in the core are depleted. Surface lipids, ApoA-I, ApoA-II and ApoC are transferred to HDL and the resulting chylomicron remnants are removed by the hepatocytes. The cholesteryl esters are hydrolysed in lysosomes, and cholesterol excreted in the bile, oxidised and excreted as bile acids or secreted into plasma in lipoproteins.

Lipids and atherosclerosis

The precise mechanism by which increased levels of cholesterol induce the lesions of atherosclerosis is unclear. Most current theories link low density lipoprotein (LDL) and beta-very low density lipoproteins (βVLDL) to the process of atherogenesis. LDL is a major carrier of cholesterol in plasma and is the molecule most strongly linked to the risk of coronary heart disease in epidemiological studies. Higher concentrations of LDL in the plasma probably increase the rate of penetration into the arterial wall and its subsequent uptake and degradation by vascular smooth muscle cells and infiltrating macrophages. However, the local conditions of the intima are probably more important for the accumulation of cholesterol esters and the formation of foam cells. For example, LDL complexes with intimal proteoglycans which facilitate the extracellular deposition of LDL choles-terol and the uptake of LDL proteoglycans – complexes by macrophages and the formation of foam cells. Peroxidation of lipoproteins is probably one of the most important mechanisms in causing endothelial damage and increasing the risk of atherosclerosis in patients with hyperlipidaemia. Oxidised LDL is more readily taken up by macrophages than native LDL, and the availability of naturally occurring antioxidants such as vitamin E, vitamin C and ubiquinol may therefore be important factors in the development of coronary artery disease. Likewise the use of antioxidant medications is of potential value in preventing or delaying the development of atheroma. Epidemiological evidence also suggests that the level of HDL cholesterol in plasma is inversely related to the risk of coronary artery

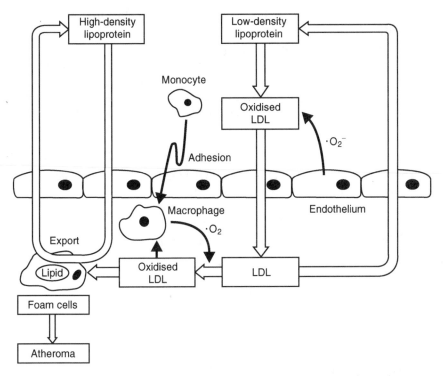

Figure 7.4. Proposed role of oxidised low density lipoproteins in the pathogenesis of atheroma.

disease, suggesting a protective effect of HDL against atherogenesis. HDL exerts an antioxidant effect on other lipoproteins and may protect the endothelium. The most likely beneficial role for HDL, however, involves the participation of HDL in the retrieval of cholesterol from peripheral tissues (Figure 7.4).

Although the function of Lp(a) is not established, the compound is associated with thrombotic and atherogenic properties. Its presence with ApoB100 in atherosclerotic plaques and its avid binding to fibrin has led to the suggestion that Lp(a) delivers cholesterol to proliferating cells by binding fibrin at sites of vascular injury. Excess local Lp(a) at injury sites may be oxidatively modified, taken up by macrophages and may contribute to foam cell formation within atheromatous plaques. Lp(a) also competes with plasminogen at the plasminogen receptor on the vascular endothelium. Therefore, Lp(a) could impede the access of plasminogen to endothelial cell tissue plasminogen activator and produce a prothrombotic state by suppressing local fibrinolysis. Standard lipid-lowering therapy is ineffective in reducing elevated levels of Lp(a). Nicotinic acid alone or in combination with neomycin has a small effect but flushing, hepatic and ototoxicity are major problems with long-term therapy. There is also preliminary evidence that fish oils may be beneficial.

The relationship between atherosclerosis and hypertriglyceridaemia is more difficult to assess. Severe elevation is a cause of acute pancreatitis and requires aggressive treatment by diet, abstinence from alcohol and drug therapy. In general, most authorities do not consider elevated triglycerides to be an independent risk factor. However, there is some experimental evidence to suggest that some triglyceride-rich lipoproteins such as intermediate density and very low density lipoproteins, play a role in atherogenesis and that patients with low levels of HDL cholesterol may benefit from reductions in total triglycerides.

Classification of hyperlipidaemia – primary

Hypertriglyceridaemia

Chylomicronaemia

Primary chylomicronaemia is an autosomal recessive condition which is due to lipoprotein lipase or lipoprotein lipase co-factor deficiency and often presents as acute pancreatitis. However, eruptive xanthomas, hepatosplenomegaly, hypersplenism and lipid-laden foam cells in the bone marrow, liver and spleen, are important associated features. Some patients have elevated VLDL proteins and a presumptive diagnosis can be made by demonstrating a pronounced decrease in plasma triglycerides a few days after a fat-free diet. The condition tends to be made worse by oestrogen therapy and during pregnancy. Treatment is with diet and drug therapy is not required.

Familial hypertriglyceridaemia

Mixed. This usually results from impaired removal of triglyceride-rich lipoproteins. Most patients demonstrate elevated VLDL cholesterol, central obesity and insulin resistance. Severe lipaemia results in eruptive xanthomas, lipaemia retinalis, epigastric pain and pancreatitis. Again treatment is largely dietary.

Endogenous lipaemia. The primary abnormality of increased VLDL is aggravated by several factors which increase secretion from the liver. These include diabetes, obesity, high alcohol intake and oestrogen therapy. Treatment involves weight reduction, restriction of dietary fat and avoidance of alcohol and oestrogen therapy. In patients with an established or strong family history of atherosclerosis, drug therapy with a fibric acid derivative or nicotinic acid is required.

Combined. In this type of hypertriglyceridaemia LDL, VLDL or both, are elevated and the pattern may change with time. Serum cholesterol and triglycerides are usually only moderately elevated and xanthomas are usually absent. A reductase inhibitor or combination therapy with a resin or fibric acid derivative may be required for elevated LDL–cholesterol levels.

Dysbetalipoproteinaemia. In familial dysbetalipoproteinaemia remnants of chylomicrons and VLDL accumulate. In contrast to most other forms of hyperlipidaemia, levels of LDL are usually decreased although total cholesterol is usually high. The diagnosis is confirmed by the absence of the E_3 and E_4 isoforms of apoE. Patients tend to be obese with impaired glucose tolerance and xanthomas. Reduction in weight, alcohol and total fat is often sufficient, but a fibric acid derivative sometimes combined with nicotinic acid may be required in some cases.

Hypercholesterolaemia

Familial

This disorder is transmitted as an autosomal dominant trait. Cholesterol levels are usually very high and are present at a very early age, triglycerides tend to be normal and the condition is associated with a very high incidence of premature coronary artery disease. The disease is related to defects in the high-affinity receptors for LDL. Non-functioning, malfunctioning and reduced numbers of LDL receptors have all been described and these abnormalities are most marked in the homozygous form of the disease. These patients respond best to reductase inhibitors and resins.

Familial ligand-defective apolipoprotein B

Defects in the ligand domain of ApoB-100, the region that binds to the LDL receptor, impair the endocytosis of LDL and elevate the serum cholesterol. Tendon xanthomas can occur.

Familial combined

In this condition LDL levels are markedly elevated but total cholesterol is usually less than 8.0 mmol/l.

Lp(a) hyperlipoproteinaemia

This is a familial disorder which is associated with premature athero-sclerosis. It is in part determined by genes which initiate increased production of the lipoprotein and by defects in the removal of LDL which tend to increase the levels of Lp(a).

HDL deficiency

Certain rare genetic disorders are associated with very low levels of serum HDL. These patients tend to develop premature atherosclerosis. Those with associated hypertriglyceridaemia may benefit from a reduction in triglycerides which usually reduces the HDL cholesterol levels to normal.

In contrast to this relatively complex classification, various specialist groups have defined lipid abnormalities on the basis of cholesterol and triglyceride levels. For example, the European Atherosclerosis Society has defined hypercholesterolaemia as a total cholesterol greater than 5.2 mmol/l with a fasting triglyceride level below 5.2 mmol/l. Mixed hyperlipidaemia consists of both fractions being above 5.2 mmol/l, while hypertriglyceridaemia is defined as a triglyceride level above 5.2 mmol/l with a normal cholesterol. This classification has its limitations, but is easy to remember and relates well to the guidelines on management outlined in Table 7.2.

Secondary

The more common conditions associated with secondary hyperlipidaemia are summarised in Table 7.3. These usually resolve when the underlying condition is successfully treated. Treatment of the hyperlipidaemia due to the nephrotic syndrome requires treatment since atherosclerosis is more

Table 7.3. Conditions which are associated with secondary hyperlipidaemia

Elevated triglycerides	Elevated cholesterol
Diabetes mellitus	Hypothyroidism
Excess alcohol	Nephrotic syndrome (early)
Nephrotic syndrome (late)	Anorexia nervosa
Oestrogens	Cholestatic jaundice
Uraemia	Hypopituitarism
Corticosteroids	Corticosteroids
Hypothyroidism	
Hypopituitarism	
Acromegaly	

common in these patients. Patients with chronic cholestasis and neuropathy caused by xanthomatous involvement of peripheral nerves also require treatment of hyperlipidaemia.

Dietary modification

Alteration of diet is always the first step in the management of hyperlipidaemia, and may be the only treatment necessary for patients with milder forms of hypercholesterolaemia and those with hypertriglyceridaemia. General guidelines of the American Heart Association diet include a daily cholesterol intake of 200 g or less and no more than 7% of the total calorie intake as saturated fat. Calories should be restricted to achieve and maintain ideal body weight. This is particularly important in patients with elevated triglycerides when small reductions in weight can reduce triglyceride levels substantially.

Alcohol should be restricted especially in patients with hypertriglyceridaemia to decrease VLDL secretion. Omega-3 fatty acids found in cold water marine fish are of some value in selected patients with severe hypertriglyceridaemia but tend to be of little value in other lipid disorders. However, they do have other beneficial properties on platelet and endothelial function. Conventional wisdom at present suggests that monounsaturated fats are preferable to polyunsaturated fats because they have a lower carcinogenicity potential and increase HDL cholesterol levels. Contemporary nutritional research also suggests that adequate intake of naturally occurring antioxidants such as ascorbic acid, beta carotene and tocopherol may be important in preventing free-radical mediated oxidative process, especially the oxidation of LDL cholesterol. The daily requirements of these supplements in the diet have not been accurately defined. Certain types of dietary fibre, notably the bran found in oats and other cereals, the soluble fibre found in certain types of pulses, and uncooked garlic have a limited ability to lower levels of LDL cholesterol.

Drug treatment

If diet, exercise and treatment of the underlying diseases are unsuccessful, then drug therapy is indicated. Diet has been relatively unsuccessful in most of the primary intervention studies probably due to poor compliance. Much better results have been achieved with dietary and drug intervention in the secondary prevention studies, in large part due to greater motivation by those who took part. These studies in particular illustrated the value of drug treatment combined with dietary modification. With the exception of chylomicronaemia, drug treatment should be started immediately in adult patients with severe genetic hyperlipidaemia and in patients with symptomatic coronary heart disease and hyperlipidaemia. Decisions to use drug therapy should be based on the specific metabolic defect, the condition's potential for causing atherosclerosis or pancreatitis, the patient's age and the nature and incidence of adverse effects. No drugs should be given to pregnant or lactating women, and the fibrates and HMG co-enzyme reductase inhibitors should be avoided in women who are likely to become pregnant. Children with heterozygous familial hypercholesterol-aemia may be treated with a bile acid-binding resin usually after 7 or 8 years when myelination of the central nervous system is largely complete. The decision to treat an individual child should be based on the level of plasma LDL, the family history and the child's age.

In the elderly there is a less clear relationship between elevated cholesterol and the incidence of coronary heart disease. On the other hand, the absolute risk of events due to atherosclerosis is much higher and treating hyperlipidaemia in this population remains a priority. Unfortunately, limited data are available in those patients over 65 years. In elderly Swedish men elevated triglyceride levels were stronger predictors of coronary heart disease than cholesterol levels.

Bile acid binding resins

Chemistry

Cholestyramine and colestipol are very large polymeric anionic exchange resins which are insoluble in water. They bind bile acids in the intestinal lumen and prevent their reabsorption. Chloride is released from the quaternary ammonium binding sites in exchange for bile acids, but the resin is not absorbed.

Mode of action

About 95% of bile acids and cholesterol metabolites are reabsorbed in the jejunum and ileum. This can be reduced up to tenfold by resin administration which interrupts the enterohepatic circulation of bile acids (Figure 7.5). The increased clearance results in enhanced conversion of cholesterol to bile acids in the liver via 7α hydroxylation which is normally controlled by a negative feedback due to the presence of bile acids. This results in a variety of compensatory mechanisms, particularly increased synthesis of cholesterol and an increase in the number of high affinity LDL receptors. LDL catabolism in the plasma is enhanced and the levels fall. Despite increased cholesterol production, plasma cholesterol and LDL

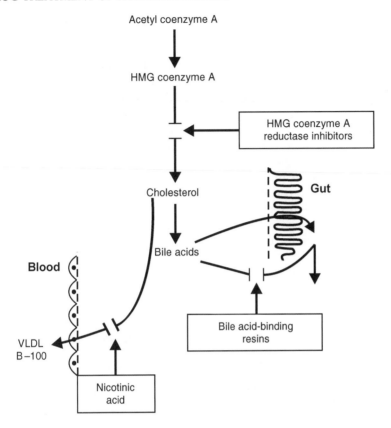

Figure 7.5. Main sites of action of HMG coenzyme A reductase inhibitors, bile acid-binding resins and nicotinic acid.

concentrations decrease in patients with type II hyperlipidaemia because of enhanced clearance of LDL from the plasma. They are ineffective, however, in patients with homozygous familial hypercholesterolaemia who have no functioning LDL receptors.

Therapeutic efficacy and use

Colestipol and cholestyramine are very effective in lowering LDL cholesterol (Table 7.6). They are given in daily doses up to 30 g and 24 g respectively, and can reduce levels by 15–30%. Starting daily doses are 5 g and 4 g and can be increased regularly by these amounts over a few weeks to increase tolerability. The patients should be instructed to mix the resin with water, dilute juice or soft food and take it with their meals. Although twice-daily dosage is preferred for convenience, they tend to be more effective when taken with each meal. These drugs have no place in the treatment of lipid disorders other than hypercholesterolaemia and are generally reserved for the treatment of type II hyperlipoproteinaemia. If they are used to treat elevated LDL levels in patients with combined hyperlipidaemia they can increase VLDL levels necessitating the use of another drug.

The use of bile acid sequestrants in patients at high risk of developing ischaemic heart disease has been shown to reduce morbidity and mortality. Administration of cholestyramine for up to 10 years reduces the risk of coronary heart disease in asymptomatic men with primary hypercholesterolaemia. Mean plasma concentration reductions of total and LDL cholesterol of 13.4% and 20.3% respectively, were associated with a 24% reduction in deaths attributed to coronary heart disease and a 19% reduction in non-fatal myocardial infarction. However, the two groups did not differ in terms of overall mortality.

Adverse effects and interactions

The most common complaints are constipation and a bloating sensation which can be relieved to some degree by increased dietary fibre or mixing psyllium seed with the resin. Heartburn and diarrhoea occasionally occur, while in patients with inflammatory bowel disease or cholestasis, steatorrhoea can occur. Malabsorption of vitamin K and folic acid rarely occur but minor changes in vitamin K absorption can cause difficulty in controlling warfarin therapy. Dry, flaking skin and gallstones occasionally complicate therapy with resins.

Colestipol and cholestyramine impair the absorption of a variety of drugs. These include the digitalis glycosides (especially digitoxin), thiazide diuretics, warfarin, tetracycline, vancomycin, thyroxine, iron salts, statins, folic acid, aspirin and vitamin C. In view of this, it is best to prescribe other medication 1 hour before or at least 2 hours after resin administration.

Fibric acid derivatives

Mode of action

The principal action of the fibric acid derivatives is to increase the activity of the enzyme lipoprotein lipase so increasing the catabolism of VLDL triglyceride and promoting the transfer of cholesterol to HDL. VLDL production may also be decreased. Their main clinical effects are reduction in triglycerides, modest increases in HDL and variable effects on LDL cholesterol. Gemfibrozil is a more effective inhibitor of VLDL synthesis than clofibrate. Bezafibrate, fenofibrate and ciprofibrate are more potent than clofibrate or gemfibrozil and are more effective in reducing LDL cholesterol levels.

Pharmacokinetics

The pharmacokinetic values of the principal fibric acid derivatives are summarised in Table 7.4.

Therapeutic efficacy and use

The fibrates differ mainly in terms of their duration of effect and potency. However, all presently available compounds are administered in divided doses. The newer drugs, bezafibrate, fenofibrate and ciprofibrate appear to be more effective than gemfibrozil and clofibrate in reducing LDL cholesterol levels. All three drugs have been shown to reduce LDL cholesterol by 15–30% as opposed to 5–20% with gemfibrozil. The effects on triglyceride levels are comparable for all five drugs (20–75% reduction) and with the exception of clofibrate an elevation in HDL cholesterol of about 20% is usually observed (Table 7.6).

Most outcome information with fibrates relates to clofibrate and gemfibrozil. In the Helsinki Heart Study which used gemfibrozil as the lipid-lowering agent, there was a 34% reduction in the incidence of coronary heart disease endpoints. The original World Health Organisation study using clofibrate also showed a reduction, but an excess of adverse effects, mainly gallbladder disease and gastrointestinal cancer, was observed. The impact of the more potent fibrates on cardiovascular events is limited and they have rarely been included in the lipid-lowering regimens employed in the secondary prevention studies.

Adverse effects and interactions

Common adverse effects of fibrate therapy include nausea, abdominal pain and flatulence. Skin rashes, myalgia or overt myositis, hypokalaemia, arrhythmias and derangement of liver function tests have also been reported. The risk of muscle damage including rhabomyolysis is greatest when these drugs are combined with HMG co-enzyme A reductase inhibitors. These agents are best avoided in patients with hepatic or renal dysfunction and should not be given to patients with a history of primary biliary cirrhosis or gall-bladder disease because of the increased risk of gallstones. With the exception of clofibrate, however, the risk is small. All five drugs should be avoided during pregnancy and in nursing mothers. Data from the Helsinki heart study extension suggested that gemfibrozil

184

Table 7.4. Pharmacokinetic values of the fibrates

	Bezafibrate	Ciprofibrate	Clofibrate	Fenofibrate	Gemfibrozil
Time to onset of action	2–5 days	2–5 days	2–5 days	Not known	2–5 days
Time to peak action	4–12 weeks	2–4 weeks	3 weeks	2 weeks	4–12 weeks
Plasma half-life	≈2 hours	25–90 hours	≈16 hours	≈22 hours	≈1.3 hours
Metabolism	Hepatic metabolism to several different metabolites	50–90% is metabolised to the glucuronide. Remainder is as unchanged drug or minor metabolites	De-esterified in the intestine to clofibric acid; glucuronide formed in the liver	De-esterified in plasma and liver to fenofibric acid	Liver metabolism to four metabolites
Oral bio-availability (%)	90	80	80	Not known	Almost 100
Excretion	40% excreted unchanged in the urine – 20% glucuronide, 20% other metabolites in urine, 2% faeces	Renal excretion of the metabolites and unchanged drug	Renal excretion 20% as clofibric acid, 60% as glucuronide	Renal excretion as metabolites, mostly conjugates	70% renal excretion as conjugates and metabolised drug – 5% unchanged 5% faecal

(and possibly other fibrates) should be used with caution in patients with combined hyperlipidaemia and symptoms of coronary heart disease.

The fibric acid derivatives tend to increase the anticoagulant effect of warfarin and other orally active anticoagulants, potentiate the hypogly-caemia action of sulphonylureas and increase the risk of rhabomyolysis associated with HMG co-enzyme reductase inhibitors. Oral contraceptives have been shown to reduce the effectiveness of clofibrate while probenecid may inhibit its clearance and potentiate its effect.

Competitive inhibitors of HMG-Co enzyme A reductase

These compounds are structural analogues of HMG-Co A (3-hydroxy-3-methylglutaryl co-enzyme A). Simvastatin, pravastatin, fluvastatin, ator-vastatin and cerivastatin are available for use in the United Kingdom. Lovastatin is used widely in the United States.

Mode of action

HMG-Co A reductase mediates the first important step in sterol biosynth-esis (Figure 7.5). The active forms of these compounds are structural analogues of the HMG-Co A intermediate which is formed by HMG Co A reductase in the synthesis of mevalonate (Figure 7.6). They also induce an increase in high affinity LDL receptors so increasing the fractional catabolic rate of LDL and the hepatic extraction of LDL precursors (VLDL remnants). The plasma pool of LDL is therefore reduced. Modest decreases in plasma triglycerides and small increases in HDL cholesterol concentrations also occur. However, atorvastatin has demonstrated reductions in triglycerides ranging from 25 to 45% over the dose range 10–80 mg in patients with mixed hyperlipidaemia.

Chemistry and pharmacokinetics

Lovastatin was the first inhibitor available for clinical use and was isolated from cultures of the fungus *Asperigillus terreus*. Simvastatin and pravastatin are chemical modifications of lovastatin while fluvastatin, atorvastatin and cerivastatin are entirely synthetic HMG-Co A reductase inhibitors (Figure 7.7). Those of fungal origin share a hydronaphthalene-ring structure with a hydroxy acid appendage (Figure 7.6). The hydroxy acid can form a six-member lactone ring, but it is the open ring which mimics the HMG-Co A reduced intermediate and acts as the inhibitor.

To maximise receptor-mediated reductions in LDL cholesterol while minimising the effects of cholesterol deprivation, these drugs should act only on the liver. With the exception of cerivastatin, all currently available

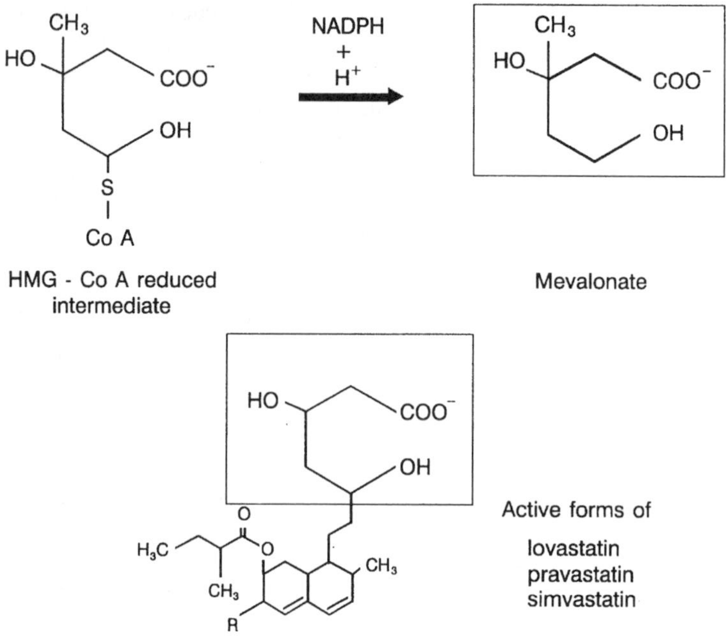

Figure 7.6. Conversion of the HMG Co A precursor to mevalonate, an essential compound in the synthesis of cholesterol and the structural similarity to HMG Co A reductase inhibitors.

statins demonstrate extensive first-pass metabolism so limiting systemic exposure and all except pravastatin are highly protein bound. Although much has been made by individual pharmaceutical companies about differences in lipophilicity and penetration of the blood–brain barrier, these seem to be unimportant in clinical practice. Lovastatin and simvastatin pass to some degree but pravastatin, atorvastatin, cerivastatin and fluvastatin do not. Further details of pharmacokinetic values are listed in Table 7.5.

Therapeutic efficacy and use

The HMG-Co A reductase inhibitors are useful lipid-lowering agents when used alone or in combination with a variety of other lipid-lowering drugs. They are particularly useful for reducing LDL cholesterol. Reductase inhibitors are best given in the evening because of the diurnal pattern of cholesterol biosynthesis. Moderately elevated LDL levels often respond to a single daily dose given in the evening. In patients with heterozygous familial hypercholesterolaemia standard doses reduce total cholesterol levels by 20–30%. At present they are the most effective and best tolerated

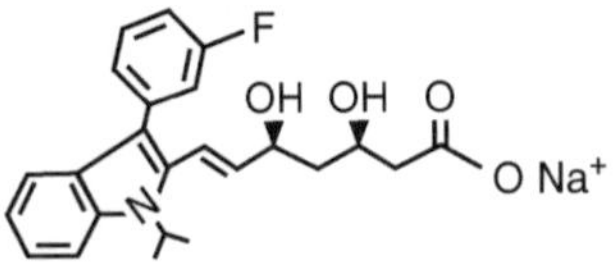

Fluvastatin

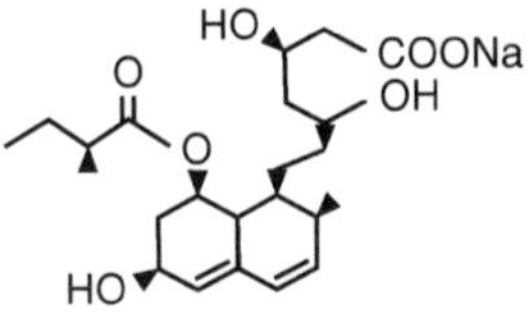

Pravastatin

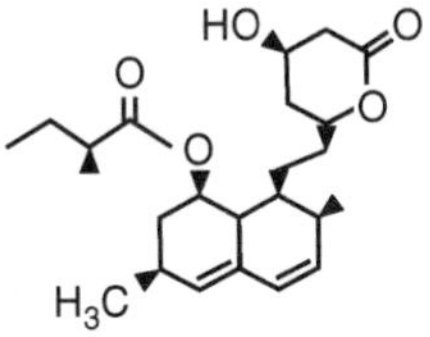

Lovastatin

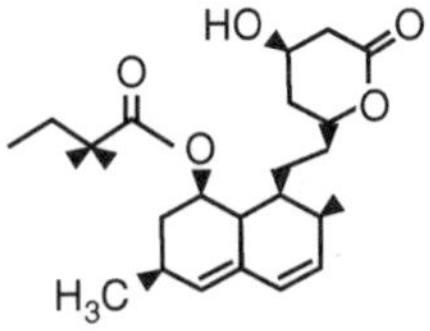

Simvastatin

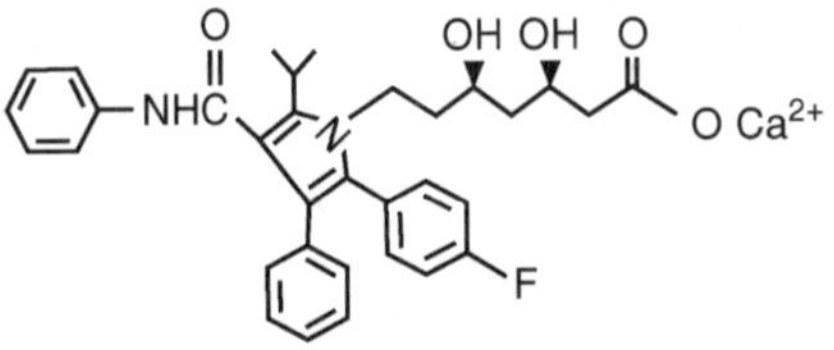

Atorvastatin

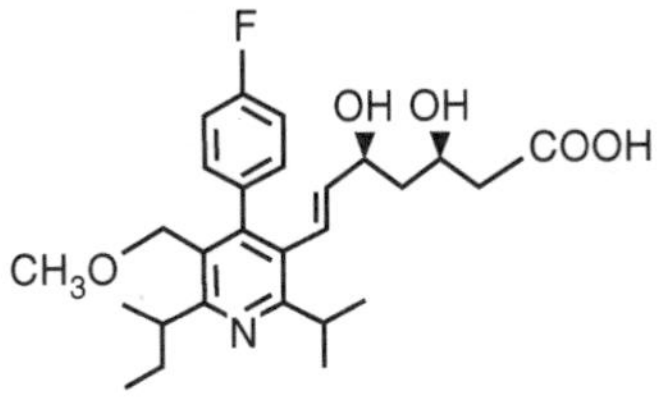

Cerivastatin

Figure 7.7. Molecular structures of 3-hydroxy-3 methyl glutaryl-coenzyme A reductase inhibitors, fluvastatin, pravastatin, lovastatin, simvastatin, atorvastatin and cerivastatin.

Table 7.5. Pharmacokinetic values of the statins

	Fluvastatin	Pravastatin	Simvastatin	Atorvastatin	Cerivastatin
Time to onset of action*	1–2 weeks	1–2 weeks	1–2 weeks	1–2 weeks	1–2 weeks
Time to peak activity*	4–6 weeks	4–6 weeks	4–6 weeks	4–6 weeks	4–6 weeks
Plasma half life	0.5–1.0 hours	≈1.5 hours	≈2 hours	≈14 hours	2–3 hours
Metabolism	Almost 100% metabolised to several metabolites	Metabolised in the liver to several metabolites	Hydolysis to several metabolites in the liver including active hydroxy metabolite	Oxidised to active metabolites which account for 70% of the drug's activity	Oxidised to active metabolites which have similar activity to parent compound
Oral bio-availability %	≈25	≈20	< 5	≈12	≈60
Excretion	Mainly biliary via faeces	40% in urine 60% in faeces	Mainly biliary via faeces	Parent compound and active metabolites are excreted in the bile	70% biliary 30% urinary excretion

*Based on short-term studies examining the lipid effects over 4-6 weeks.

Table 7.6. Effects of drugs (with diet) on plasma lipid profiles in patients with coronary heart disease or mild hypercholesterolaemia for one year

Drug/Diet	Total cholesterol	LDL cholesterol	HDL cholesterol	Tryglycerides
Diet	↓	↓	—	↓
Resins	⬇	⬇	—	↑
Fibrates	↓	↓	⬆	⬇
Statins	⬇	⬇	↑	↓ ⬇*
Nicotinic acid	↓	↓	↑	⬇
Probucol	↓	↓	⬇	—

*Atorvastatin ↓ → ⬇ 5–40% change.

drugs for lowering LDL cholesterol. Although they may induce modest reductions in VLDL with the possible exception of atorvastatin, they are presently not recommended for mixed lipid disorders or hypertriglyceridaemia (Table 7.6). Levels of HDL cholesterol may also be increased in some patients. Drug regimens which have included HMG co-enzyme A reductase inhibitors have achieved regression of atheroma in patients with coronary artery disease, and recently simvastatin and pravastatin have been shown to reduce morbidity and mortality in primary and secondary prevention trials.

Adverse effects and interactions

These drugs have no common important short-term adverse effects. Gastrointestinal symptoms, headache, insomnia, rashes and fatigue have been reported. Small increases in transaminases, skeletal muscle and creatinine kinase can occur in the absence of symptoms. The serious adverse effects of chemical hepatitis and a myopathic syndrome are rare. The myopathy may present with muscle pain, tenderness or weakness and can progress to rhabdomyolysis with myoglobinaemia and renal failure if the drug is not stopped. A syndrome resembling dermatomyositis has rarely been described. The risk of developing the myopathic syndrome is increased when other drugs are co-administered. These drugs include cyclosporin, fibric acid derivatives, nicotinic acid and erythromycin. The drugs should be avoided in patients with liver disease and are not recommended for pregnant or nursing mothers.

Nicotinic acid (Niacin)

Mode of action

The main action of nicotinic acid is probably inhibition of VLDL secretion and decreased production of LDL. Increased clearance of VLDL via the lipoprotein lipase pathway also reduces plasma triglyceride levels. The catabolic rate for HDL is decreased with an associated rise in the HDL_2 subfraction and the levels of HDL cholesterol and apolipoprotein A-1 increase in the plasma. The drug also reduces the circulating levels of fibrinogen and increases the concentrations of tissue plasminogen activator which may have an impact on the development of atherogenesis. In addition, nicotinic acid is a potent inhibitor of the intracellular lipase system in adipose tissue.

Chemistry and pharmacokinetics

Nicotinic acid is a water-soluble vitamin. It is converted to the amide and then incorporated into nicotinamide adenine dinucleotide. Nicotinic acid is rapidly absorbed reaching peak plasma levels 1 hour after oral administration. Its plasma elimination half-life is about 1 hour, metabolism is negligible and the drug is mostly excreted unchanged in the urine.

Therapeutic efficacy and use

In combination with bile acid-binding resins, nicotinic acid substantially reduces LDL cholesterol in patients with heterozygous familial hypercholesterolaemia. In severe mixed lipaemia, triglyceride levels in the plasma also decrease. One advantage over most other lipid-lowering agents is that the levels of HDL cholesterol increase substantially. When used as a single agent, nicotinic acid produces a reduction in LDL cholesterol with an associated rise in the plasma concentrations of HDL cholesterol (Table 7.6).

Monotherapy with nicotinic acid has been shown to reduce death due to coronary heart disease and to decrease overall mortality. Beneficial effects on mortality have also been demonstrated in combination with clofibrate and when combined with colestipol, regression of atheromatous lesions in the coronary arteries has been described.

Adverse effects and interactions

Most patients experience a warm flushing sensation when the drug is started and when the dose is increased. The effect can be reduced by taking aspirin or ibuprofen about 30 minutes before drug administration. Tolerance, however, usually develops within a few days at any dose level. Pruritis, rashes, dry skin and acanthosis nigricans have been reported. Some patients develop abdominal discomfort with nausea which usually responds to dosage reduction and/or antacid therapy. The drug is best avoided in patients with peptic ulcer disease. Moderate elevations in the levels of aminotransferases or alkaline phosphatase occur in a small percentage of patients, but severe liver toxicity, necessitating drug withdrawal, is rare. Carbohydrate tolerance may be moderately impaired but is usually reversible except in patients with latent diabetes. Hyperuricaemia occurs in about one-fifth of patients and it occasionally precipitates gout. Other reported symptoms include atrial dysrhythmias, hypotension, and a reversible toxic amblyopia.

Probucol

Mode of action

The mode of action of probucol is poorly defined. It probably inhibits sterol biosynthesis and improves the transport of cholesterol from the peripheral tissues to the liver. Recent evidence suggests that probucol may have an impact on atherogenesis by acting as a potent antioxidant. Reducing the concentrations of oxidised low density lipoproteins inhibits the formation of foam cells in the arterial intima.

Pharmacokinetics

Probucol is structurally unrelated to any other lipid-lowering agent. Its duration of effect and elimination half-life are very variable with low bioavailability and high urinary excretion. The drug is extensively protein bound.

Therapeutic efficacy and use

Probucol is generally regarded as a second-line agent for the treatment of primary hypercholesterolaemia because of its modest effects on atherogenic lipoproteins and its potentially adverse effects on HDL cholesterol. When used as a single agent plasma LDL levels decrease by 8–15% and HDL levels decrease by about 25%. The value of probucol as an antioxidant agent in the prevention and treatment of atheroma has not been clearly defined.

Adverse effects and interactions

Probucol is generally well tolerated but the drug causes prolongation of the *QT* interval and can induce ventricular tachycardia in patients with coronary heart disease. It is probably best avoided in patients with long *QT* intervals due to disease or drugs such as amiodarone, sotalol, quinidine, digoxin, erythromycin, and those agents causing hypokalaemia. Uncommon adverse effects of probucol include abnormal liver function tests, myopathies, hyperuricaemia, thrombocytopenia, hyperglycaemia, neuropathy and angioneurotic oedema.

Oestrogens

Post-menopausal women who take oestrogens have fewer cardiovascular deaths than those who have never received them. This may be related in part to lower levels of LDL cholesterol and higher levels of HDL cholesterol. Triglyceride levels tend to increase, however. It seems likely that oestrogens will prove to be effective in post-menopausal women with high LDL, low HDL and normal triglycerides, but studies to date have been observational and the results of randomised, controlled outcome studies are awaited.

Alcohol

Modest quantities of alcohol appear to offer protection against coronary heart disease. Beneficial effects include raised HDL cholesterol and the antioxidant activity of flavanoids in red wine. High alcohol intake is associated with increased triglyceride levels.

Other antioxidant agents

Based on the assumption that atherogenesis is linked to the oxidation of low density lipoprotein cholesterol, there would seem to be considerable potential for the clinical use of antioxidant agents to slow the progression or prevent the development of atherosclerosis. Drugs which lower LDL cholesterol and have antioxidant activity such as probucol, may slow the progression of atherosclerosis more than other lipid-lowering drugs which do not have this property. Epidemiological studies support the idea that an increased intake of monosaturated fats and beta carotene, both with antioxidant properties, can reduce the incidence of coronary heart disease. Vitamin C has been shown to prevent the oxidation of LDL and protect naturally occurring antioxidants such as vitamin E and beta carotene present in LDL cholesterol. In addition, an inverse relationship between the concentrations of vitamin E and mortality due to ischaemic heart disease has been described, and vitamin E reduces free radical-mediated myocardial dysfunction after coronary artery bypass surgery.

8 Drug Treatment of Cardiac Dysrhythmias

Introduction

Cardiac dysrhythmias are common in clinical practice. They vary greatly in their prognostic significance and an accurate diagnosis is essential before treatment is started. Treatment is required if the rhythm is too rapid, too slow or so irregular that cardiac function is significantly compromised. Other rhythm disturbances, notably ventricular tachycardia and fibrillation are life threatening while some can precipitate serious dysrhythmias. In these situations, drug therapy can be life saving. The wisdom of treating arrhythmias to prevent sudden death however has been severely questioned as a result of the CAST (cardiac arrhythmia suppression trial). This investigation demonstrated that class 1C antiarrhythmic agents used to suppress ventricular premature beats after an acute myocardial infarction produced a threefold increase in mortality. This effect may not be restricted to 1C agents but may occur with all class 1 agents (Table 8.1).

The general view at present would seem to be that asymptomatic or minimally symptomatic arrhythmias should not be treated with drug

Table 8.1. Odds ratios and 95% confidence intervals for mortality in patients receiving active antiarrhythmic therapy (classes I–IV) versus placebo control from the randomised clinical trials of antiarrhythmic drugs. Odds ratios greater than 1.0 suggest increased mortality

Antiarrhythmic class	Odds ratios	95% Confidence intervals	Probability value
I	1.13	1.01–1.27	$p = 0.04$ (61 trials)
II	0.81	0.78–0.87	$p < 0.00001$ (56 trials)
III	0.83	0.72–0.95	$p = 0.01$ (14 trials)
IV	1.03	0.94–1.13	NS (26 trials)

NS = non-significant.

therapy. Treatment of arrhythmias can be beneficial in patients with very rapid, slow or severely disordered rhythms which impair cardiac reserve. The management of prognostically important rhythm disturbances such as ventricular fibrillation and sustained ventricular tachycardias, is more difficult. At present antiarrhythmic agents are not routinely recommended for these patients for two reasons. First, for most rhythm disturbances of this type, the prognosis is determined more by the nature of the underlying condition than the type of arrhythmia. Second, non-drug therapies such as cardioversion, cardiac pacing, catheter ablation and surgery are often more effective in selective cases.

Electrophysiology of normal cardiac rhythm

The electrical impulse which initiates normal cardiac contraction originates in the sino-atrial node at a regular frequency of 60–100 beats/minute. The impulse then spreads rapidly through the atria and reaches the atrio-ventricular node. Conduction through this node is slow, providing time for atrial contraction to propel blood through the atrioventricular valves. The impulse then spreads through the His–Purkinje system to all parts of the ventricles (Figure 8.1). Delay at the atrioventricular node lasts 150 ms while ventricular activation is complete in less than 100 ms (Figure 8.1). Arrhythmias occur when cardiac depolarisation deviates from the normal in one or more aspects. This could be due to an abnormality at the site of origin of the impulse or in its rate, rhythm or conduction.

The role of ion transport in maintaining membrane electrical activity

The electrical potential across the membrane of cardiac cells is determined by the concentrations of several ions particularly sodium (Na^+), potassium (K^+) and calcium (Ca^{2+}) on each side of the membrane and the permeability to each ion. Ions diffuse across the membrane through ion-specific channels and the rate of movement is thought to be controlled by flexible peptide chains or energy barriers referred to as "gates". Each ion channel has its own gate or gates which open and close depending on specific transmembrane conditions (Figure 8.2). For example the sodium channel appears to have four activation gates and one inactivation gate which respond to changes in the membrane potential. Since sodium is more abundant outside the cell (140 mmol/l) than inside (10 mmol/l), sodium will rapidly enter down the concentration gradient if the membrane is permeable to sodium ions. Therefore at rest, most cells are not significantly permeable to sodium. However, at the start of each action potential, per-meability to sodium increases and later calcium and potassium move down their concentration gradients as the permeability to these ions increases during

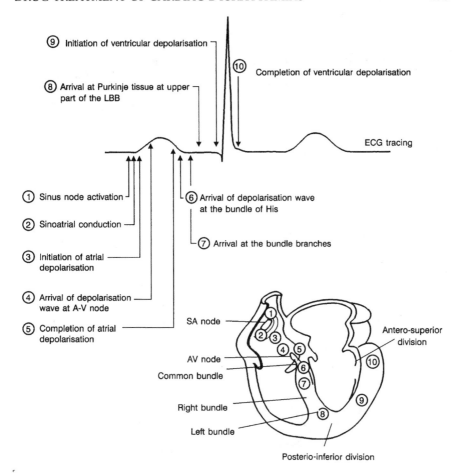

Figure 8.1.   The sequence of depolarisation within the heart.

the later stages of action potential (Figure 8.3). The myocardial cell must therefore have mechanisms to maintain stable transmembrane ionic conditions. The most important of these is the sodium pump $Na^+/K^+ATPase$ which together with other active ion carriers maintain the gradients necessary for diffusion to occur through the ion channels during activation. In addition, some pumps and exchangers produce a net current flow, for example by exchanging two K^+ ions for three Na^+ ions. These exchange systems are called electrogenic.

The cardiac action potential and the role of ion channels

The upstroke (phase 0) of the cardiac action potential is almost entirely dependent on the sodium current. Depolarisation to the threshold voltage

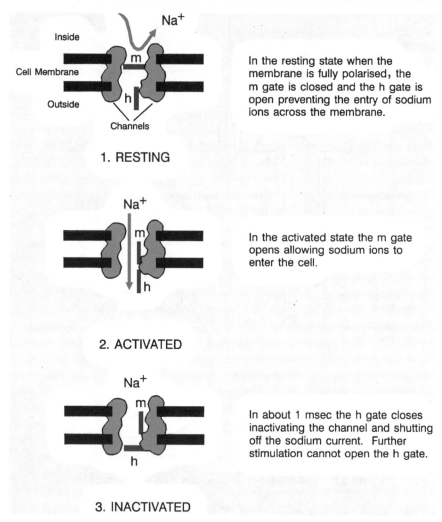

In the resting state when the membrane is fully polarised, the m gate is closed and the h gate is open preventing the entry of sodium ions across the membrane.

1. RESTING

In the activated state the m gate opens allowing sodium ions to enter the cell.

2. ACTIVATED

In about 1 msec the h gate closes inactivating the channel and shutting off the sodium current. Further stimulation cannot open the h gate.

3. INACTIVATED

Figure 8.2. Schematic diagrams of the cardiac sodium channel during (1) resting, (2) activated and (3) inactivated stages.

results in the opening of the (m) gates of the sodium channels. If the inactivation (h) gates of these channels have not already closed, the channels will be open and activated and sodium permeability will be markedly increased (Figure 8.2). Extracellular sodium will then diffuse down the electrochemical gradient into the cell and the membrane potential will move back to the equilibrium potential (about $+70\,mV$ when extracellular sodium is $140\,mmol/l$ and intracellular sodium is $10\,mmol/l$). This occurs over a

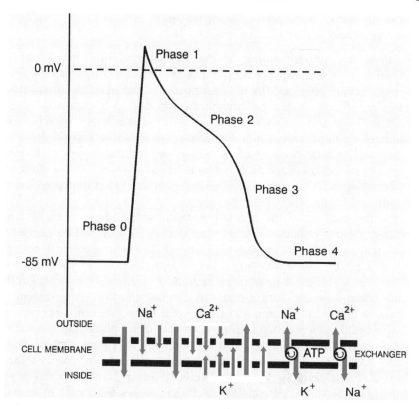

Figure 8.3. Schematic diagram of the changes in ion permeability and transport mechanisms which occur during the cardiac action potential and the following diastolic period.

very short period of time because the opening of the m gates is rapidly followed by closure of the h gates after depolarisation. A similar pattern of activation and inactivation affects the calcium channels but in this situation the principal channel is the L type. The movement of calcium occurs more slowly and at more positive potentials (Figure 8.3). The action potential plateau (phases 1 and 2) is associated with reduced sodium current, the activation and inactivation of the calcium current followed by the slow development of a repolarisation potassium current (Figure 8.3). Final repolarisation (phase 3) of the action potential occurs as a result of sodium and calcium channel inactivation and increased permeability to potassium so that the membrane potential approaches the potassium equilibrium potential. Ion concentrations on either side of the membrane are maintained in the resting state by a variety of ion pumps and exchangers, notably $Na^+K^+ATPase$ and the $Na^+ Ca^{2+}$ exchanger (Figure 8.3).

Relationship between the resting potential and the cardiac action potential

Essential to our understanding of the mechanisms of action of anti-arrhythmic agents is the relationship between the cell resting potential and its evoked action potential. In the resting state, the majority of sodium channels are closed in the cell membrane producing a potential range between $-75\,mV$ and $-55\,mV$. Therefore fewer channels are available for diffusion of sodium ions when the action potential is evoked from a potential within this range than from a lower value. Important consequences of a reduction in the peak permeability to sodium include reduced upstroke velocity (V_{max}), reduced action potential amplitude, reduced excitability and conduction velocity.

During the plateau of the action potential, most sodium channels are inactivated. When repolarisation takes place the h gates open and the channels are once again available for excitation. A less negative resting potential results in a prolongation of the recovery time and an increase in the effective refractory period, i.e. the time from the beginning of the action potential until the time when a second action potential can be initiated. Hyperkalaemia, inhibition of the sodium pump and myocardial ischaemia can decrease the resting potential by depressing sodium currents during phase 0 of the action potential. Depolarisation of the resting potential to values greater than $-55\,mV$ abolishes all sodium currents since all sodium channels are inactivated. These severely depolarised cells, however, have been shown to produce special action potentials which are associated with increased permeability to calcium or decreased permeability to potassium. These "slow" responses are features of the sino-atrial and atrioventricular nodes since these tissues have resting potentials in the range $-50\,mV$ to $-70\,mV$. They are also important in the generation of certain dysrhythmias.

Factors causing arrhythmias

There are several factors which can precipitate rhythm disturbances or increase the risk of arrhythmias occurring. These include myocardial ischaemia, scar tissue, hypoxia, various metabolic and biochemical disturbances, autonomic dysfunction, excessive catecholamine production and drug therapy (especially digoxin and type I antiarrhythmic drugs).

Problems with impulse formation

Decreasing the duration of the action potential and/or the diastolic interval increases the pacemaker rate. The diastolic interval, which is the more important of the two measurements is determined by three factors: the maximum diastolic potential, the slope of phase 4 depolarisation and the threshold potential (Figure 8.4). Increased pacemaker discharge is usually associated with increased phase 4 depolarisation slope which is caused by hypokalaemia, acidosis, fibre stretch, beta$_1$ adrenoceptor stimulation and certain types of myocardial injury. After-depolarisations interrupt phase 3 and phase 4 of the cardiac action potential (Figure 8.5) and occur when intracellular calcium is increased. They occur more often at high heart rates and may be responsible for the arrhythmias caused by digitalis overdose, myocardial ischaemia, catecholamines and arrhythmias associated with a long QT interval.

Problems with impulse conduction

Severely depressed conduction can result in atrioventricular nodal block or bundle branch block. One of the most common conduction abnormalities, however, is re-entry or circus movement in which an impulse re-enters and excites areas of the conducting tissue more than once. This circulating impulse often produces secondary impulses which spread to other areas of the myocardium. A few ectopic beats or a sustained tachycardia can result depending on the number of round trips of the pathway the impulse makes before eventually dying out. For re-entry to occur three conditions must coexist:

1. A physiological or anatomical obstruction to normal conduction so that a circuit is formed around which a wavefront can spread.
2. There must be unidirectional block at some point in the circuit so that the impulse continues in one direction and dies out in the opposite direction.

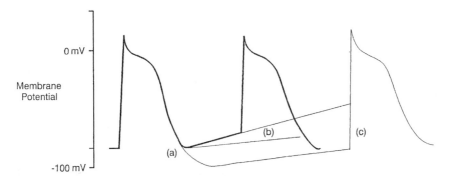

Figure 8.4. Three important mechanisms which determine the pacemaker rate: (a) more negative maximum diastolic potential; (b) reduced slope of the diastolic depolarisation; (c) more positive threshold potential.

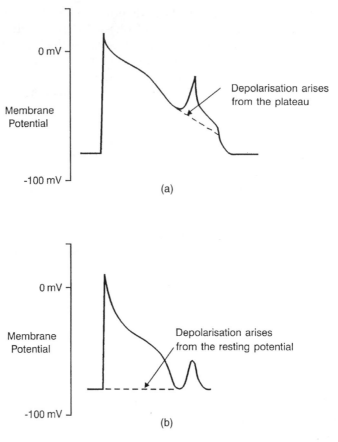

Figure 8.5. (a) Prolonged action potential plateau with early after depolarisation; (b) normal action potential with delayed after depolarisation.

3. Conduction time around the circuit must be sufficiently long to prevent the impulse entering refractory tissue as it travels around the obstacle. In other words the conduction time must exceed the effective refractory period.

Ischaemia and other types of damage to the conducting system depress conduction to a variable degree. If conduction velocity is excessively slow, bi-directional rather than unidirectional block tends to occur and the impulses tend to die. If conduction is too rapid, unidirectional block is more common, although if the impulses travel around the obstacle too rapidly they will reach tissue which is still refractory and the impulses will also die. Slowing of conduction occurs when sodium or calcium channels are depressed. Drugs which are effective in preventing re-entry either work by further depression of conduction by blocking the sodium or calcium current or occasionally by increasing conduction by enhancing sodium or calcium flux. Lengthening or shortening of the refractory period also makes re-entry less likely. The longer the refractory period in tissue near the site of block, the greater the likelihood that it will still be refractory when re-entry occurs. Alternatively, the shorter the refractory period in the depressed region, the less likely for unidirectional block to occur.

Mechanisms of action of antiarrhythmic drugs

Arrhythmias occur as a result of abnormal pacemaker activity or abnormal impulse conduction. The principal aim of antiarrhythmic therapy is therefore to reduce ectopic pacemaker activity and prevent circus movement in re-entrant circuits. Currently available antiarrhythmic drugs achieve this goal by blocking the sodium or calcium channels, prolonging the effective refractory period and by antagonising the effects of catecholamines at the cardiac beta$_1$ receptors. Antiarrhythmic agents decrease the automaticity of ectopic pacemakers more than nodal tissue. They also have a greater effect on depolarised tissue than normally polarised tissue. This is achieved mainly by selectively blocking sodium or calcium channels in depolarised cells. Antiarrhythmic drugs which affect the ion channels mainly block activated channels during phase 0 or inactivated channels during phase 2. They have little effect on resting channels. Therefore these drugs block electrical activity in the presence of rapid tachycardia which is characterised by several activations and inactivations per unit time. Channels in normal cells, which become blocked by drug therapy during normal activation–inactivation cycles, will rapidly lose the drug from the receptors during the resting period of the cycle.

Most antiarrhythmic drugs reduce the slope of phase 4 of the cardiac action potential in cells with normal automaticity by reducing the permeability of sodium or calcium channels relative to that of potassium. Other agents render the membrane threshold more positive. Beta adrenoceptor antagonists reduce the phase 4 slope by antagonising the chronotropic action of noradrenaline at the beta$_1$ receptors. In re-entrant arrhythmias which are usually related to depressed conduction, most antiarrhythmic drugs slow conduction further by reducing the number of available unblocked channels or by prolonging the recovery time of the channels and increasing the effective refractory period. As a result early extrasystoles are blocked and late ectopic beats spread more slowly and are subject to bi-directional conduction block.

When dosage is increased, however, antiarrhythmic drugs will also depress normal conducting tissue and eventually produce a drug-induced dysrhythmia. Even at "therapeutic" plasma concentrations, several anti-arrhythmic drugs can demonstrate this pro-arrhythmic effect in the presence of sinus tachycardia, acidosis and electrolyte abnormalities. The balance of antiarrhythmic and pro-arrhythmic activity is clearly important in the long-term management of cardiac disease. A recent meta analysis of the effect of antiarrhythmic drugs on prognosis of patients with persisting arrhythmias after myocardial infarction with congestive cardiomyopathy showed that class 1 agents have an adverse effect on mortality, calcium channel antagonists were of no benefit while patients treated with amiodarone or beta adrenoceptor antagonists had lower death rates. These observations are probably due to differences in pro-arrhythmic activity (Table 8.1).

Classification of antiarrhythmic drugs

The antiarrhythmic drugs have traditionally been classified into four or possibly five groups on the basis of their mode of action. Class 1 includes those drugs which inhibit the movement of sodium ions by blocking the sodium channels. This group is further divided into classes 1A, 1B and 1C according to their effects on the duration of the cardiac action potential. Drugs in class 1A increase, 1B reduce and 1C have none or minimal effect on the length of the action potential. Drugs which antagonise the $beta_1$ receptors are included in group II. Group III is composed of drugs which lengthen the effective refractory period by mechanisms which are not primarily due to inhibition of the sodium channel while class IV consists of the calcium channel antagonists. A fifth group is sometimes included containing adenosine, potassium and magnesium. This classification ignores several differences among drugs within the same class. For example several class 1 drugs have class III-like activity and a drug may have antagonistic effects on both the sodium and calcium channels. New classifications have been proposed but to date these have not received widespread acceptance.

Class I (sodium channel antagonists)

Subclass 1A

This group includes three orally active drugs: quinidine, procainamide and disopyramide. Two drugs, imipramine and amiodarone, have similar effects on the sodium channel and action potential but are usually not included because both drugs have other important pharmacological properties.

Quinidine

Mode of action. Quinidine lengthens the refractory period and depresses excitability and conduction in depolarised tissue more than normal tissue. To a large extent this is related to the ability of quinidine to block the activated sodium channels. Quinidine also lengthens the action potential duration and hence the *QT* interval on the electrocardiograph. Blockade of the potassium channels with a reduction in the repolarisation outward current is probably responsible for this effect. A class III effect produces additional lengthening of action potential and is usually seen at slow heart rates. The pro-arrhythmic effect of quinidine is largely related to prolongation of the *QT* interval. Quinidine inhibits peripheral and myocardial alpha adrenergic receptors which increase the risk of hypotension following intravenous administration. It also has anticholinergic activity which increases the heart rate in atrial fibrillation and flutter and can cause sinus tachycardia.

Pharmacokinetics and dosage. Quinidine is an orally active agent which is rapidly absorbed from the gastrointestinal tract. It is 70–80% protein bound; 80% is metabolised and the remainder is excreted unchanged in the urine. Its half-life is about 6 hours (Table 8.2). This is often increased in congestive cardiac failure, and sometimes in liver and renal disease. Acidification of the urine increases the urinary excretion. Quinidine is usually administered orally as the sulphate. An initial dose of 250 mg is given to detect hypersensitivity followed by a maintenance dose between 500 and 1250 mg twice daily. The commonly quoted plasma therapeutic range at steady state is 3–5 μg/ml. Intravenous preparations are available but are almost never used in clinical practice. Hypotension due to peripheral vasodilatation is common with this method of administration.

Clinical indications. Quinidine is now rarely used in the United Kingdom but continues to be widely prescribed in the United States and other countries. It is used most frequently in an attempt to convert atrial fibrillation or flutter to sinus rhythm sometimes combined with digoxin or verapamil before cardioversion is attempted. The drug can also be used prophylactically to reduce recurrences of paroxysmal atrial and ventricular tachycardias.

Adverse effects. The anticholinergic effects of quinidine increase the sinus rate and atrioventricular conduction, so overcoming some of the direct

Table 8.2. Pharmacokinetic values of type 1 antiarrhythmic drugs

	Disopyramide	Flecainide	Lignocaine	Mexiletine	Procainamide	Propafenone	Quinidine	Tocainide
Time to onset of action	½–3½ hours	1–2 hours	Intermediate (iv)	½–2 hours	1 hour	1 hour	1 hour	Unknown (iv) (immediate)
Time to peak action	½–3 hours	2–4 hours	Unknown	Unknown	1–2 hours	2–3 hours	1–4 hours	1–1½ hours
Plasma half-life	≈ 7 hours	13–19 hours	1–2 hours	10–12 hours (normal) 15–17 hours (MI) 25 hours (CHF)	2–5 hours	2–10 hours (normal)	≈ 6 hours	≈ 14 hours
Metabolism	50% to active and inactive metabolites	60% to inactive metabolites	90% to active metabolites	85% converted to inactive metabolites	25%–40% acetylated	Up to 90% 5-hydroxy N-desalkyl	Hepatic – some metabolites	Hepatic – all inactive metabolites
Oral bio-availability (%)	85–95	≈ 95	<5 (oral)	Unknown	75–95	10–50	Unknown	Almost 100
Excretion	50% unchanged	28% renal 5% faeces	Renal – unchanged and metabolites	Mainly biliary 10% renal	Renal – parent compound and metabolites	Renal and biliary excretion of metabolites	Renal – unchanged+ metabolites	Renal 40% unchanged
Protein binding	10–70% (dose dependent)	40%	60–80% (dose dependent)	60–75%	15–20%	75–90%	70–80%	10%

membrane effects. In atrial flutter and fibrillation this can be prevented to some degree by co-administering a drug which induces atrioventricular block such as verapamil, digoxin or a beta adrenoceptor antagonist. Up to 5% of patients develop a syndrome called "quinidine syncope" characterised by recurrent light-headedness and fainting episodes. The symptoms are mainly due to recurrent episodes of ventricular tachycardia which are associated with lengthening of the cardiac action potential and these usually terminate spontaneously. In patients with the sick sinus syndrome, a direct depressant effect of quinidine can occur, while in others nodal depression is overridden by the anticholinergic effects. Widening of the QRS by 30%, plasma concentrations $>5\,\mu g/ml$ and a serum potassium level $>5\,mmol/l$ are all associated with increased risk of cardiotoxicity.

Subjective adverse effects are high and a recent double blind study revealed diarrhoea in a third of patients, nausea in 18%, headache in 13% and dizziness in 8%. Tinnitus also occurs at high dose. More rarely quinidine can cause rashes, angioneurotic oedema, fever, hepatitis and thrombocytopenia. A syndrome resembling lupus erythematosis has also been reported. In patients with myasthenia gravis, quinidine may increase the severity of the muscle weakness.

Interactions. Quinidine increases the plasma concentrations of digoxin and therefore the risk of digoxin toxicity. Quinidine also enhances the effects of beta adrenoceptor antagonists, verapamil and diltiazem, on the sino-atrial and atrioventricular nodes. Enzyme inducers such as phenytoin, barbiturates and rifampicin, and enzyme inhibitors such as cimetidine alter the metabolism of quinidine. Quinidine increases the anticoagulant effects of warfarin. Hypokalaemia decreases quinidine efficacy and increases the length of the QT interval. Type III antiarrhythmic agents such as amiodarone or sotalol are also contraindicated in this situation. Quinidine has also been shown to reduce the effectiveness of anticholinesterases used in the treatment of myasthenia gravis.

Contraindications. The presence of a long QT interval, especially if accompanied by ventricular dysrhythmias, is a contraindication to the use of quinidine and related antiarrhythmic agents. Other relative contraindications include congestive cardiac failure, sick sinus syndrome, bundle branch block, myasthenia gravis and severe liver disease. Information in pregnancy is limited and therefore quinidine is best avoided.

Procainamide

Mode of action. The electrophysiological actions of procainamide are similar to those of quinidine. The drug appears to be more effective in blocking the sodium channels in depolarised cells but less effective in suppressing abnormal ectopic pacemaker activity. The most important difference, however, is that procainamide has less anticholinergic effects than quinidine so that the depressant actions of procainamide on the sino-atrial and atrioventricular nodes are preserved. Procainamide also tends to have fewer effects on the QT interval. Although the drug has ganglion blocking activity its vasodilator and hypotensive effects are less marked than quinidine. Hypotension is therefore usually only seen when the drug is administered as a rapid intravenous infusion.

Pharmacokinetics and dosage. Oral procainamide requires frequent administration because of rapid elimination, especially in fast acetylators. It has a high oral bioavailability and gives rise to an important longer acting metabolite, N-acetyl procainamide (NAPA). This substance has class III antiarrhythmic activity and acts as a weak sodium channel blocker. High levels of this metabolite have been implicated in causing ventricular dysrhythmias. The half-life of procainamide is 2–5 hours but the value for NAPA is considerably longer. Both parent compound and metabolite are excreted by the kidney and dosage needs to be reduced in patients with renal impairment (Table 8.2). Owing to the clinical activity of NAPA it is important to measure procainamide and the acetylated phenotype when adjusting dosage.

In order to achieve 24-hour antiarrhythmic activity a sustained release preparation should be administered every 6 hours in most patients. A total oral dose of 2–5 g/day is usually required, but lower doses will be necessary in those patients who accumulate NAPA. If a rapid effect is required an intravenous loading dose up to 12 mg/kg can be given over a 40-minute period followed by a maintenance of 2–5 mg/minute with careful monitoring of plasma concentrations. Toxicity is most likely to occur if plasma concentrations of procainamide exceed 8 μg/ml or NAPA concentrations are $>20\,\mu$g/ml.

Clinical indications. Long-term procainamide therapy is rarely used to prevent atrial and ventricular dysrhythmias because of the high incidence of serious adverse effects and the difficulties with dosage regimens. Procainamide is sometimes used as an alternative to lignocaine for sustained ventricular arrhythmias associated with an acute myocardial infarction.

Adverse effects. Procainamide's cardiotoxic effects are similar to those of quinidine. Hypotension after intravenous administration can occur especially at high dose and heart block and ventricular tachycardia have been reported. The most serious problem, however, is the high incidence of a syndrome resembling systemic lupus erythematosis with long-term oral therapy. The main differences from classical lupus include a higher male incidence, an older age group and a lower incidence of renal and central nervous system involvement. Approximately one-third of patients receiving long-term procainamide develop the syndrome. The main clinical features are arthralgia, fever, myalgia, pleuritis and pulmonary parenchymal disease. Anti-nuclear antibodies and other serological tests for lupus are present in most patients. Other adverse effects include nausea and vomiting, diarrhoea, hepatitis, agranulocytosis and allergic reactions. The weakness associated with myasthenia gravis may be increased.

Interactions. Cimetidine inhibits the clearance of procainamide and increases the risk of toxicity. Additive effects occur with antihypertensive agents, anticholinergic drugs and compounds which impair impulse formation at the sino-atrial and atrioventricular nodes.

Contraindications. Procainamide should be avoided in patients with congestive cardiac failure, digoxin overdosage, left bundle branch block and myasthenia gravis. Patients with autoimmune disease and those with positive antinuclear antibodies should not be started on procainamide. There are no useful safety data in children or pregnant women.

Disopyramide

Mode of action. The pharmacological effects of disopyramide are similar to quinidine, but the drug has substantially more anticholinergic and negative inotropic effects. In the treatment of atrial fibrillation and flutter it is therefore even more important to co-prescribe a drug which slows atrioventricular conduction. It should be used with great care in patients with left ventricular dysfunction or congestive cardiac failure. In rare instances it can cause heart failure in patients with apparently normal cardiac function. At high doses disopyramide can cause all the electrophysiological disturbances described with quinidine. Non-cardiac anticholinergic effects are relatively common. These include urinary retention especially in elderly males, dry mouth, blurred vision, constipation and worsening of pre-existing glaucoma.

Pharmacokinetics and dosage. Disopyramide has a high oral bioavailability. About 50% are metabolised in extra hepatic sites by N-dealkylation and the remainder excreted unchanged in the urine (Table 8.2). One metabolite has very marked anticholinergic effects. Protein binding varies with the plasma concentration – the higher the concentration in the plasma the lower the amount bound to plasma proteins. The defined therapeutic range is 3–8 μg/ ml, but variation in the degree of protein binding makes interpretation difficult. The elimination half-life is approximately 6–8 hours. The usual oral dose is 150 mg three times daily but daily doses of 1 g may be necessary in some patients. Lower doses are required in patients with renal impairment. Disopyramide has been given intravenously either as an initial dose of 2 mg/kg (but not exceeding 150 mg) given slowly over 5–10 minutes and followed by oral therapy or as an intravenous infusion of 0.4 mg/kg per hour.

Clinical indications. Disopyramide is probably as effective as other class 1A agents in treating ventricular dysrhythmias. It is also effective in the treatment of atrial tachycardias and fibrillation except when heart failure is present. The negative inotropic effect of disopyramide combined with its antiarrhythmic activity make it an ideal choice in hypertropic obstructive cardiomyopathy and there is some evidence that it is more effective than beta adrenoceptor antagonists in this condition. In the United States disopyramide is only approved for ventricular arrhythmias and it is at best a third-line antiarrhythmic drug in the United Kingdom.

Adverse effects. The main adverse effects of disopyramide are negative inotropic activity, anticholinergic effects and a pro-arrhythmic effect related to lengthening of the *QT* interval. The drug can therefore produce congestive cardiac failure in patients with poor left ventricular function and occasionally in those with apparently normal cardiac reserve. Anticholinergic effects are a particular problem especially in elderly patients, causing urinary retention, glaucoma and constipation. Disopyramide is the most likely type I agent to mask the direct depressant effects on nodal and conducting tissue and like other agents which prolong the *QT* interval can induce serious ventricular dysrhythmias. Other reported adverse effects include cholestatic jaundice, hypolgycaemia, sweating and acute psychotic reactions.

Interactions. Intravenous disopyramide can substantially reduce cardiac output in patients receiving drugs which also have negative inotropic effects such as beta adrenoceptor antagonists and calcium channel blockers. Similarly, problems are likely to arise if it is co-prescribed with drugs which cause depression of nodal or other conducting tissue, e.g. quinidine, digoxin, beta adrenoceptor blockers, verapamil and diltiazem. The risk of ventricular dysrhythmias is higher if disopyramide is prescribed with type III antiarrhythmic drugs such as amiodarone. Drugs with anticholinergic activity will clearly cause additional problems if prescribed with disopyramide. Enzyme inducers such as phenytoin have been reported to reduce plasma concentrations.

Contraindications. Uncompensated heart failure, glaucoma, hypotension, urinary retention and prolongation of the *QT* interval are absolute contraindications to the use of disopyramide. Milder degrees of heart failure, prostatic hypertrophy, a family history of glaucoma, severe constipation and "sick sinus" syndromes are relative contraindications. In pregnancy, disopyramide can stimulate uterine contraction and is excreted in breast milk. Hypoglycaemia has been reported in diabetic patients.

Subclass 1B

Class 1B drugs inhibit the fast sodium current, while shortening the duration of the action potential. Unlike class 1A drugs the *QT* interval is not prolonged. They act selectively on diseased or ischaemic tissue where they interrupt re-entry circuits and promote conduction block.

Lignocaine

Mode of action. Lignocaine acts exclusively on the sodium channel. Unlike quinidine, which mostly blocks sodium channels in the activated state, lignocaine rapidly blocks both activated and inactivated sodium channels. As a result, a large number of the unblocked sodium channels become blocked during each action potential. During diastole most of the sodium channels rapidly become free in normally polarised cells. Diastole is usually prolonged as the action potential shortens and the time available for recovery is prolonged. As a result, lignocaine suppresses the electrical activity of depolarised, arrhythmogenic tissues while having little effect on normal tissues. These actions relate to the drugs' well-described clinical properties, showing beneficial therapeutic effects in ischaemic (depolarised) tissue and little effect in atrial fibrillation or flutter (polarised).

Pharmacokinetics and dosage. Less than 5% of an orally administered dose of lignocaine reaches the plasma due to extensive first-pass metabolism. Therefore lignocaine has to be given parenterally. The elimination half-life in patients with normal hepatic function is about 2 hours (Table 8.2). Protein binding is variable probably due to the presence of α-acid glycoprotein which binds lignocaine. Larger doses are required in patients with high levels of the glycoprotein.

In patients with congestive cardiac failure the apparent volume of distribution and total body clearance are reduced. If both are reduced to a similar degree then the elimination half-life will not change significantly. Accumulation can, however, occur in some patients. In patients with chronic liver disease, plasma clearance is usually reduced while the apparent volume of distribution is often increased. The elimination half-life is therefore markedly prolonged, and the time taken to reach steady state may be as long as 36 hours as opposed to 8 hours in patients with normal liver function.

In adults a loading dose of 50–100 mg given intravenously over 15 minutes followed by a maintenance infusion of 2–4 mg/minute is commonly prescribed. In patients with normal liver function this should produce steady-state plasma concentrations between 2 and 6 μg/ml.

Clinical indications. Lignocaine is effective in suppressing ventricular tachycardia and fibrillation after cardioversion, cardiac surgery and anaesthesia. Early studies suggested that lignocaine reduced the incidence of serious ventricular dysrhythmias in the first few days after an acute myocardial infarction. The popularity of this treatment after a myocardial infarction has declined substantially over the last 20 years for two principal reasons: the growth of more effective therapies such as thrombolytic drugs, aspirin and beta adrenoceptor antagonists, and the finding in later studies that mortality may be increased or unaffected when lignocaine is routinely used in patients after a myocardial infarction.

Despite the controversy, there is probably a place for lignocaine therapy during the first 6 hours after a myocardial infarction if intravenous beta adrenoceptors are contraindicated and ventricular premature beats are present. Routine prophylactic lignocaine after a myocardial infarction is probably not cost effective because the incidence of primary ventricular fibrillation is now less than 5%. Lignocaine should not be given when there is bradycardia or bradycardia with ventricular tachyarrhythmias. Lignocaine is largely ineffective in the treatment of supraventricular arrhythmias except when associated with the Wolff–Parkinson–White syndrome or digoxin toxicity.

Adverse effects. At "therapeutic" doses lignocaine is the least cardiotoxic of currently available type 1 antiarrhythmic agents. It has a low incidence of pro-arrhythmic activity, but in a small number of patients it can precipitate sino-atrial arrest and heart block following an acute myocardial infarction. At "toxic" concentrations lignocaine can depress myocardial contractility in patients with congestive cardiac failure.

The most commonly described adverse effects of lignocaine relate to its activity on the central nervous system usually occurring at high dose. These include paraesthesias, tremor, nausea, light-headedness, slurred speech, hearing disturbances and convulsions. Convulsions most often occur in elderly patients who receive high doses and in those with reduced drug clearance. They are usually short-lived and respond to discontinuation of the drug and intravenous diazepam.

Interactions. The hepatic clearance of lignocaine is impaired by cimetidine, propranolol and halothane so that the dose needs to be reduced to prevent toxicity. On the other hand the efficacy can be decreased by drugs which induce oxidative metabolism such as barbiturates, phenytoin and rifampicin. Problems can arise when lignocaine is administered with other antiarrhythmic drugs, but in general the risk of ventricular dysrhythmias and heart failure is much less than with type 1A antiarrhythmic agents.

Contraindications. It is best to avoid lignocaine in patients with bradycardia complicated by ventricular arrhythmias and to use with caution when congestive heart failure, reduced hepatic or renal function, hypokalaemia, hypertension or sinus bradycardia are present. The safety of lignocaine in children has not been established and it is best avoided during pregnancy and lactation.

Tocainide

Mode of action. Tocainide is an orally active analogue of lignocaine which does not undergo hepatic first-pass metabolism. Like lignocaine it has little negative inotropic activity and shortens or has little effect on the *QT* interval. At therapeutic concentrations tocainide has no effect on the effective refractory period, the duration of the action potential or sinus node recovery in healthy subjects.

Pharmacokinetics and dosage. The oral bioavailability of tocainide is almost 100% because of the absence of first-pass metabolism. Peak plasma concentrations occur about 2 hours after oral administration and almost 50% is recovered unchanged in the urine. The plasma elimination is about 14 hours with no active metabolites and is prolonged in patients with renal impairment (Table 8.2).

   The usual initial dose is 400 mg, three times daily adjusted according to the response and tolerability. The maintenance dose is normally 1200 mg given in three divided doses and increased to a total daily dose of 1800–2400 mg daily if necessary.

Clinical actions. Like lignocaine, tocainide is effective in suppressing ventricular arrhythmias but has little activity against atrial rhythm disturbances. Its main indication is when class 1A drugs have failed or as a follow-up treatment to successful lignocaine therapy.

Adverse effects. Tocainide frequently causes dose-dependent effects on the nervous and gastrointestinal systems. These include lightheadedness, paraesthesia, tremor, nausea, vomiting and diarrhoea. Tremor is a useful clinical indication that the maximum dose has been exceeded. Serious adverse immune effects such as pulmonary fibrosis, polyarthritis, leucopenia and thrombocytopenia occur in about 0.2%. Pro-arrhythmic effects and heart failure may also occur. In view of the high incidence of adverse effects, tocainide should be used only in severe life-threatening arrhythmias.

Interactions. Tocainide appears to be relatively safe when combined with other antiarrhythmic agents but there is a paucity of good clinical information. Care must be exercised, especially when combinations with beta adrenoceptor antagonists and type 1 antiarrhythmics are used.

Contraindications. Tocainide is contraindicated in patients with second and third degree heart block. A known hypersensitivity or a history of previous immune reactions are definite contraindications.

Mexiletine

Mode of action. The actions of mexiletine are similar to those of lignocaine and tocainide. It reduces the rate of depolarisation by blockade of the sodium channel, reduces conduction velocity in the His–Purkinje system and decreases the effective refractory period and action potential duration to a small degree.

Pharmacokinetics and dosage. Mexiletine is well absorbed with a high oral bioavailability and reaches peak levels in 2–4 hours. Almost 90% is metabolised in the liver to inactive metabolites and the remainder excreted unchanged in the urine. The elimination half-life is recorded between 10 and 25 hours depending on liver function (Table 8.2). Mexiletine is very lipid soluble with high central nervous system penetration and frequent adverse effects.

The oral loading dose is quoted at 400 mg followed by 300–1200 mg daily in three divided doses given with food 2–6 hours after the loading dose. The intravenous dose is usually between 100 and 250 mg at 12.5 mg/minute then 2.0 mg/kg per hour for $3\frac{1}{2}$ hours and 0.5 mg/kg per hour thereafter. The dose should be reduced in elderly patients and those with congestive cardiac failure and liver disease.

Clinical indications. The major indication for mexiletine is the treatment of symptomatic ventricular arrhythmias. Like several other agents, however, it may increase mortality when the drug is used for the chronic oral prophylaxis of ventricular arrhythmias following a myocardial infarction.

Adverse effects. A very high percentage of patients experience important adverse effects. During chronic oral therapy almost half the patients experience some gastrointestinal adverse effects. About 20% experience tremor, nystagmus and confusion. Other adverse effects include bradycardia, hypotension and hepatic damage. Pro-arrhythmic effects are rare. Adverse effects are clearly dose related with a quoted incidence of serious adverse effects in 35% of patients receiving more than 1 g daily.

Interactions. The oral absorption of mexiletine is delayed by co-administration of narcotic analgesics and accelerated by metoclopramide. Enzyme-inducing agents including cigarette smoking reduce plasma concentrations and mexiletine elevates plasma theophylline levels. Beta adrenoceptor antagonists and type 1A antiarrhythmic agents produce additional negative inotropic effects when combined with mexiletine.

Contraindications. The main contraindications to the use of mexiletine include complete heart block, severe bradycardia and previous drug hypersensitivity. Relative contraindications include hypotension, hepatic failure, epilepsy and severe renal failure.

Phenytoin

Mode of action. Phenytoin has similar electrophysiological effects to lignocaine. Its effects on the electrocardiograph are minimal apart from slight shortening of the *QT* interval. Variable effects on the atrioventricular node occur. Acceleration and slowing of AV (atrioventricular) nodal conduction have been described. As well as blocking the sodium channel, phenytoin inhibits the calcium channel and it is one of the antiarrhythmic drugs of first choice in the treatment of digoxin overdose.

Pharmacokinetics and dosage. Absorption of phenytoin from the gastrointestinal tract is almost complete although the time to peak plasma concentration varies from 3 to 12 hours. Phenytoin is highly bound to albumin. It is metabolised primarily by parahydroxylation and glucuronidation. The metabolites are clinically inactive and are excreted in the urine. The drug exhibits dose-dependent elimination kinetics. At low plasma levels phenytoin metabolism is proportional to the rate of delivery to the liver, i.e. first-order elimination kinetics. However, at high levels the capacity of the liver to metabolise phenytoin is maximal and small increases in dosage will produce marked increases in plasma levels. The elimination half-life at normal concentrations varies from 12 to 36 hours, but at high dose the plasma levels can remain elevated for much longer periods. The intravenous dose is usually 10–15 mg/kg over 1 hour followed by an oral maintenance of 400–600 mg/day (2–4 mg/kg per day in children). Phenytoin is an enzyme inducer and the dose may have to be increased during chronic oral therapy.

Clinical indications. Phenytoin is not a first-line antiarrhythmic drug, but there are three clinical situations in which it may have a specific role. First, in arrhythmias related to digitalis overdose, phenytoin maintains conduction and inhibits delayed after-depolarisations especially when the potassium is low. Second, it has been shown to be effective in treating ventricular dysrhythmias occurring after surgery for congenital heart disease. Finally, it appears to be useful in the treatment of congenital prolonged *QT* syndrome when beta adrenoceptor antagonists are ineffective.

Adverse effects. Most adverse reactions to phenytoin affect the central nervous system and are dose related. Nystagmus occurs early and does not usually require dose reduction. Diplopia, ataxia and sedation suggest overdose. Gum hyperplasia and hirsutism occur in most patients to a lesser or greater degree. Other adverse effects include peripheral neuropathy, osteomalacia, folate deficiency, fever, skin rashes, lymphadenopathy and agranulocytosis.

Interactions. Drug interactions involving phenytoin mainly relate to changes in metabolism and protein binding. Highly protein bound drugs can displace phenytoin from its protein binding sites and can cause short-lived increased toxicity. Phenytoin induces microsomal enzymes and can increase the metabolism of several other drugs such as quinidine, lignocaine and mexiletine. Other enzyme inducing drugs, notably phenobarbitone and carbamazepine, can decrease steady-state plasma concentrations.

Moracizine

Moracizine is a phenothiazine derivative which has electrophysiological effects similar to lignocaine but also prolongs the *PR* and *QRS* intervals. It has therefore properties of a class 1B and class 1C antiarrhythmic agent. A mechanism involving an effect on the central nervous system has also been suggested.

Clinical use. Moracizine is effective in the treatment of ventricular ectopy and in the suppression of non-sustained ventricular tachycardia. Unfortunately the drug has recently been shown to increase mortality in patients treated for symptomatic or minimally symptomatic ventricular ectopy following an acute myocardial infarction. However, it may have a continued role in the long-term management of arrhythmias in patients who have not sustained an acute myocardial infarction since long-term treatment is not associated with increased risk of sudden death. The usual adult dose is 600–900 mg in three divided doses.

Adverse effects and interactions. Oral therapy with moracizine appears to be better tolerated than most currently available antiarrhythmic agents. Apart from the important pro-arrhythmic effects following acute myocardial infarction, only dizziness, paraesthesia, headache and nausea have been consistently described. A low incidence of adverse effects, however, could reflect a paucity of clinical data and significant interactions have not been described.

Subclass 1C

Class 1C antiarrhythmic drugs have three major electrophysiological effects. They inhibit the fast sodium channel, delay conduction in the His–Purkinje system with widening of the *QRS* complex and shorten the action potential of Purkinje fibres while leaving the adjacent myocardial cells unaffected. A ventricular and more recently an atrial pro-arrhythmic effect have been described.

Flecainide

Mode of action. Flecainide is a potent sodium channel blocker used mainly to treat ventricular dysrhythmias. It also blocks some potassium channels which may account for its efficacy in treating atrial arrhythmias. It prolongs the *PR* interval and *QRS* complex and has negative inotropic effects which limit its usefulness in ischaemic heart disease and congestive heart failure. Like other members of the group it has important pro-arrhythmic effects.

Pharmacokinetics and dosage. Flecainide is well absorbed when given orally with a high systemic bioavailability and peak plasma concentration between 2 and 4 hours. The plasma elimination half-life is between 13 and 19 hours and 60% is metabolised by the liver to inactive metabolites and most of the remainder excreted unchanged in the urine (Table 8.2).

The oral dose of flecainide is 100–400 mg twice daily and the intravenous dose 1–2 mg/kg over 10 minutes followed by a continuous infusion of 0.15–0.25 mg/kg per hour. The dose needs to be reduced in patients with poor left ventricular function and renal disease to maintain plasma concentrations below 1.0 μg/ml.

Clinical indications. Flecainide should only be used to treat symptomatic, life-threatening ventricular tachycardia, Wolff–Parkinson–White syndrome and atrioventricular nodal re-entrant arrhythmias.

Adverse effects. Cardiac adverse effects include aggravation of ventricular arrhythmias and sudden death in about 10% of patients, especially in the presence of poor left ventricular function and conduction problems. Intravenous flecainide can sometimes precipitate heart failure in "at risk" patients. Although flecainide can be used to treat supraventricular tachycardia, a late atrial pro-arrhythmic effect has been described which can be prevented by the co-administration of digoxin, a beta adrenoceptor antagonist or verapamil to avoid accelerated atrioventricular conduction. Central nervous system effects of dizziness, headache, nausea, paraesthesia, fatigue and tremor are relatively uncommon. Other reported adverse effects include pneumonitis, pulmonary fibrosis, hepatic impairment, chest pain and sensory neuropathy.

Interactions. Additive effects on sinus or atrioventricular conduction occur with beta adrenoceptor antagonists, verapamil, diltiazem and digoxin, while beta adrenoceptor antagonists, verapamil and type 1A antiarrhythmic agents have additive negative inotropic effects with flecainide. Amiodarone increases steady-state plasma concentrations of flecainide by about 30%. Enzyme inducers and inhibitors can also affect plasma concentrations.

Contraindications. Flecainide should not be used where there is significant conduction delay, sick sinus syndrome, poor left ventricular function and following an acute myocardial infarction. Care is required in the elderly and in patients with poor renal function. The drug cannot be considered safe in pregnancy, during lactation or in children under the age of 12.

Encainide

Mode of action. The electrophysiological effects of encainide are similar to those of flecainide. The negative inotropic effects are probably less, although care must be exercised when administering this drug to patients with congestive cardiac failure.

Pharmacokinetics and dosage. Encainide can be administered intravenously or orally. After oral administration peak plasma concentrations occur 1–2 hours after dosing and about 75% of the drug is protein bound; 90% of the population are fast metabolisers and in these patients steady-state levels of the parent compound are low while the active metabolites are high (O-demethyl-encainide and 3-methoxy-O-demethylencainide). The remainder are slow metabolisers and have high levels of the parent compound. The mean elimination half-life in fast metabolisers is about 4 hours and 8 hours in the slow metabolisers.

The usual oral dose is 25–75 mg three times daily and this should be reduced in patients with renal failure and possibly congestive cardiac failure.

Clinical indications. Encainide is effective in suppressing a variety of ventricular and supra-ventricular arrhythmias. A significant pro-arrhythmic effect severely limits its long-term use.

Adverse effects. Adverse effects include vertigo, visual disturbances and headache. Encainide lengthens the *PR* interval and *QRS* complex and has pro-arrhythmic effects similar to other type 1C agents.

Interactions. Drugs with additive effects on atrioventricular conduction and negative inotropic activity should be avoided. Cimetidine increases plasma concentrations and enzyme inducers should decrease the levels.

Contraindications. Contraindications are the same as those for flecainide.

Propafenone

Mode of action. As a class IC drug, propafenone blocks the fast inward sodium channel producing membrane stabilising activity. The *PR* interval and width of the *QRS* complex increase but the *QT* interval remains unaffected. Propafenone has additional calcium channel and beta adrenoceptor antagonist activity.

Pharmacokinetics and dosage. Oral propafenone is rapidly absorbed, reaching peak plasma concentrations within 2 hours of administration. Oral bioavailability varies from 10% to 50% and metabolism to the 5-hydroxypropafenone and *N*-desalkyl propafenone is also variable (Table 8.2). As a result the elimination half-life is also variable being 2–10 hours in "normal" metabolisers and 12–32 hours in poor metabolisers. The usual oral dose is 150–300 mg three times daily. A loading dose of 2 mg/kg intravenously followed by an infusion of 2 mg/minute is occasionally used.

Clinical indications. Propafenone is limited for use in life-threatening ventricular arrhythmias, paroxysmal atrial flutter, fibrillation and re-entrant tachycardias involving the atrioventricular node or accessory pathway when standard therapy has been ineffective.

Adverse effects and interactions. Dose-dependent cardiac adverse effects include lengthening of the *PR* interval and *QRS* complex, conduction block and adverse effects on the sino-atrial node. A modest negative inotropic effect can induce heart failure in susceptible individuals. Pro-arrhythmic activity is probably less common than with flecainide and encainide. Disorders of taste and smell, dry mouth, blurred vision, diarrhoea and abdominal discomfort occur in more than 10% of patients. Skin rashes, cholestasis, lupus syndrome and seizures have also been reported occasionally.

As with other class 1C drugs, propafenone can have an additive effect when combined with drugs which depress nodal function, atrioventricular conduction or inotropic activity. Propafenone increases steady-state plasma digoxin concentrations and the anticoagulant effects of warfarin. Cimetidine has been shown to inhibit the drug's oxidative metabolism, while rifampicin and probably other enzyme-inducing drugs can induce the metabolism of propafenone and therefore reduce its clinical effect.

Contraindications. Pre-existing bradycardia, heart block or depressed left ventricular function are relative contraindications. The drug should be avoided especially at high dose in patients with obstructive airways disease because of the beta adrenoceptor activity. In patients with a cardiac pacemaker, reduced dosing may be required because pacing thresholds are altered. Safety and effectiveness have not been established in children or during pregnancy.

Class II (beta adrenoceptor antagonists)

Although beta adrenoceptor antagonists are used principally to treat hypertension and angina pectoris they have an important role in the management of arrhythmias, especially if they are precipitated by exercise and/or emotion. Rhythm disturbances which respond to beta blocker therapy include sinus tachycardia, paroxysmal atrial tachycardia, exercise-induced ventricular arrhythmias and those occurring in the hereditary prolonged *QT* syndrome. They are also useful in the treatment of arrhythmias associated with mitral valve prolapse and in phaeochromocytoma when combined with an alpha adrenoceptor antagonist.

The beneficial effects of beta adrenoceptor antagonists following acute myocardial infarction are probably in part due to the drugs' antiarrhythmic activity. The negative inotropic effects of this group of compounds can cause problems in overt congestive cardiac failure, but in patients with reasonable left ventricular function they can be used to prevent and control atrial nodal and ventricular arrhythmias, especially if sympathetic activity is high and other conditions such as angina and hypertension are present.

Additional properties of beta blockers are mostly unimportant. However, drugs with high partial agonist activity tend to be less effective in treating sinus tachycardia and atrial tachyarrhythmias. Sotalol which has additional class III antiarrhythmic activity will be considered later as a special case.

Class III Agents

Class III antiarrhythmic drugs act by lengthening the cardiac action potential duration and hence the effective refractory period and QT interval on the electrocardiograph. All three drugs discussed in this group block potassium channels in cardiac muscle and all three have distinctive additional properties. Amiodarone has significant sodium channel blocking activity, sotalol is a beta adrenoceptor antagonist and bretylium is an adrenergic neurone inhibitor which initially causes release of noradrenaline from the sympathetic nerve endings. Amiodarone and bretylium have little or no negative inotropic activity.

Amiodarone

Mode of action. Amiodarone has a large number of electrophysiological actions. It effectively blocks the sodium channels mainly when they are in the inactivated state. As a result, amiodarone has the greatest effect in tissues which have long action potentials, frequent action potentials or less negative diastolic potentials. At therapeutic concentrations, amiodarone lengthens the cardiac action potential duration probably by blocking the potassium channels. This effect is preserved even at rapid heart rates. Amiodarone also has weak type II and type IV effects and is a powerful inhibitor of abnormal automaticity. In keeping with these elctrophysiological effects, amiodarone slows the sinus rate and atrioventricular conduction and lengthens the QT interval and QRS complex. Atrial, atrioventricular nodal and ventricular refractory periods are increased. The pro-arrhythmic effects of amiodarone appear to be less than with most other orally active antiarrhythmic agents. The adrenoceptor antagonist and calcium channel blocking activity may account for amiodarone's antianginal activity. The drug also dilates resistance and coronary arteries and occasionally causes hypotension at high dose.

Pharmacokinetics and dosage. Amiodarone is slowly and irregularly absorbed from the gastrointestinal tract and is widely distributed throughout the body. Owing to the large apparent volume of distribution and relatively low clearance, the drug has a long elimination half-life which varies from 26 to 107 days during chronic oral administration. As a result the onset of action after oral administration is delayed (Table 8.3) and steady-state concentrations are not achieved for several months. To achieve earlier therapeutic plasma concentrations a large loading dose is required. The large apparent volume of distribution is due to high lipid solubility and extensive distribution into body tissues, especially the liver and lungs. Amiodarone undergoes extensive metabolism in the liver to desethylamiodarone which has similar antiarrhythmic properties to the parent compound. There is a poor correlation between steady-state plasma concentrations and effect and the therapeutic range is therefore poorly defined. Excretion is mostly in the bile although elimination through the skin and tears also occur. Dosage adjustment is required in patients with hepatic impairment but not in those with renal disease.

To achieve reasonably rapid control of an arrhythmia, the initial loading is usually 1200–1600 mg in two divided doses for 1–2 weeks. This is then reduced to 400–800 mg/day for a further 1–3 weeks and thereafter to 200–400 mg daily given as a single dose. If treatment is less urgent, a maintenance dose of 200–400 mg can be given from the beginning of therapy. In prolonged treatment, especially for atrial dysrhythmias, maintenance doses less than 200 mg daily may be sufficient. Intravenous administration is sometimes used for intractable arrhythmias or for atrial fibrillation following an acute myocardial infarction. The usually recommended doses

Table 8.3. Pharmacokinetic values of type III antiarrhythmic drugs

	Amiodarone	Bretylium	Sotalol
Time to onset of action	Hours to weeks	10–120 minutes	$\approx$ 60 minutes
Time to peak action	Several days to weeks	6–9 hours	2–3 hours
Plasma half-life	Acute $\approx$ 15 hours Chronic 26–107 days	5–10 hours	7–15 hours
Oral bio-availability %	20–90	—	$\approx$ 90
Metabolism	Extensive hepatic	<5%	<5%
Excretion	Biliary mostly	Renal as unchanged drug	Renal as unchanged drug
Protein binding	$\approx$ 96%	<5%	<5%

are 5 mg/kg over 20 minutes and 1000 mg over 24 hours followed by oral therapy. The advantages of intravenous therapy over oral therapy have not been clearly defined.

Clinical indications. Amiodarone is one of the drugs of first choice in preventing life-threatening ventricular arrhythmias and recurrent cardiac arrest. Unlike several class I antiarrhythmic drugs, the risk of sudden death in this situation not increased and may even show a slight reduction. Amiodarone is reported to be effective in more than 60% of patients who have not responded to other antiarrhythmic drugs. It is also effective in the treatment of atrial fibrillation, flutter and paroxysmal supraventricular tachycardia. Occasionally amiodarone is beneficial in patients with unstable angina accompanied by severe ventricular arrhythmias.

In patients with heart failure, ventricular arrhythmias are an important cause of death. This is related more to the nature of the underlying heart disease than the presence of heart failure although both are contributory. The results of the larger studies are summarised in Table 8.4. Although the results are not entirely consistent, a number of important conclusions can be drawn from the data. In contrast to class I and class III antiarrhythmic drugs, amiodarone appears to reduce the incidence of ventricular arrhythmias in patients with heart failure following a myocardial infarction. Since overall mortality is not affected, prophylactic use of amiodarone cannot be recommended in patients suffering from non-sustained ventricular arrhythmias. Amiodarone is more effective in patients with non-ischaemic heart disease and with more severe degrees of heart failure. In patients with symptomatic or sustained ventricular arrhythmias in the presence of heart failure, amiodarone is the drug of first choice and combines effectively with beta adrenoceptor antagonists. Although the pro-arrhythmic effect of amiodarone is very low, the long-term use of the drug is limited by a large number of frequent and serious extra cardiac effects.

Adverse effects. Amiodarone is reported to have an incidence of adverse effects ranging from 34% to 93% and 26% of patients discontinue the drug because of drug intolerance. The long elimination half-life leads to persistence of the adverse effects for extended periods after the drug is stopped. Apart from abnormalities in thyroid function tests, the commonest adverse effects involve the gastrointestinal tract and neurological system. Pulmonary toxicity is, however, the most serious complication of amiodarone therapy.

Effects on thyroid function. Amiodarone has complex effects on thyroid hormones and function probably because it is structurally related to

Table 8.4. Summary of the results of trials investigating the antiarrhythmic effect of amiodarone

Study	Medication	Ejection fraction	Percentage post-myocardial infarction	Severity of ventricular arrhythmias	Follow-up period	Results		
						Frequency of ventricular arrhythmias	Sudden deaths	Total deaths
EMIAT	200 mg/day (n = 743)	<40%	100%	>10/hour (40%)	1.7 years	—	↓ $p = 0.05$	—
	Placebo (n = 743)							
CAMIAT	200 mg/day (n = 606)	—	100%	>10/hour ≥ run of ventricular tachycardia	1.8 years	—	↓ $p = 0.02$	—
	Placebo (n = 596)							
GESICA	300 mg/day (n = 260)	<35%	40% (coronary heart disease)	>10/hour (70%)	2 years	—	—	↓ $p = 0.02$
	Standard (n = 256)							
CHF-STAT	300 mg/day (n = 336)	<40%	70% (coronary heart disease)	≥10/hour	3.8 years	↓ $p < 0.001$	—	—
	Placebo (n = 338)							
CASCADE	100–400 mg/day (n = 113)	14–35%	80%	Ventricular tachycardia or fibrillation	2.6 years	↓ $p = 0.05$	↓ $p = 0.01$	—
	Conventional (n = 115)							

EMIAT—European myocardial infarction amiodarone trial.
CAMIAT—Canadian amiodarone infarction arrhythmia trial.
GESICA—Gruppo de Esdo de la Sobrevida en la Insuficienaa Cardiaca en Argentina.
CHF-STAT—Congestive heart failure survival trial of antiarrhythmic therapy.
CASCADE—Cardiac Arrest in Seattle: conventional vs amiodarone drug evaluation.

thyroxine and contains high concentrations of iodine. The principal action of amiodarone appears to be the inhibition of the peripheral conversion of T_4 to T_3. This results in a rise in the level of T_4 and a small decrease in the levels of T_3. Serum reverse T_3 is increased in relation to the cumulative dose prescribed. In the majority of patients thyroid function remains unaltered in the dose range 100–200 mg despite biochemical alterations. About 5% develop hyperthyroidism or hypothyroidism. Younger patients are more likely to present with hyperthyroidism while older patients more frequently develop hypothyroidism.

Effects on the gastrointestinal tract. Nausea and vomiting have been reported in almost half the patients receiving amiodarone with congestive cardiac failure, even if low doses of 200 mg daily are used. Constipation and abnormal liver function tests occur in about 20% of patients. Taste disturbances rarely occur.

Neurologial effects. Adverse neurological effects are common and include proximal muscle weakness, peripheral neuropathy, tremor, ataxia, headache, insomnia and impaired memory. Optic neuritis and impotence have also been reported.

Effects on the lung. A spectrum of pulmonary adverse effects occur in 1–10% of patients ranging from pneumonitis to pulmonary fibrosis. These effects are probably dose related, and although a few fatalities have been reported most pulmonary complications regress when amiodarone is discontinued provided extensive fibrosis has not occurred.

Cardiac effects. In patients with sinus or atrioventricular nodal disease, amiodarone can cause symptomatic bradycardia or heart block. *Torsades de pointes* occasionally occurs if the QT interval is excessively prolonged. Heart failure may occur in susceptible patients.

Other adverse effects. Corneal micro deposits develop in the great majority of patients receiving amiodarone therapy. These rarely cause visual disturbances except for occasional halos and loss of peripheral vision especially in the dark. Impaired visual acuity is rare and responds to dose reduction or discontinuation. After prolonged high dose therapy a photosensitive slate-grey or bluish skin discoloration occurs which slowly improves on drug withdrawal. A photo dermatitis also occurs and patients must avoid exposure to the sun. Other uncommon adverse effects include bronchospasm, anaphylaxis, flushing and sweating after intravenous therapy, thrombocytopenia, and non-infectious epididymitis.

Interactions. A variety of important interactions occur with amiodarone. The potentially most serious is the combination with other drugs which lengthen the *QT* interval. These include class 1A and III antiarrhythmic drugs as well as tricyclic antidepressants, phenothiazines and large doses of thiazide diuretics. Amiodarone increases the anticoagulant effect of warfarin probably by an effect on the liver and elevates steady-state plasma digoxin concentrations by as much as 100%, increasing its non-arrhythmogenic adverse effects. When adding amiodarone to digoxin therapy it is therefore advisable to reduce the maintenance digoxin dose by half. Amiodarone inhibits nodal activity and additive effects may be seen with beta adrenoceptor antagonists and calcium channel blockers. Amiodarone also reduces the clearance and increases the risk of toxicity of theophylline, quinidine, procainamide, flecainide and phenytoin.

Contraindications. Treatment should always be started in hospital where monitoring facilities are available. Care is needed in patients with congestive cardiac failure and when the drug is added to other antiarrhythmic agents. Hypokalaemia can render the drug ineffective and predisposes to ventricular arrhythmias. Relative contraindications include a history of thyroid disease, liver disease, pulmonary fibrosis and asthma. Care should be exercised in patients allergic to iodine. Amiodarone should not be used during pregnancy as it is teratogenic and should be avoided during lactation since significant amounts are excreted in breast milk.

Sotalol

Mode of action. Sotalol is a non-selective beta adrenoceptor agent with class III antiarrhythmic properties. The beta blocking activity resides on the L-enantiomer while the class III antiarrhythmic activity resides on the D-enantiomer. The cardiac action potential duration is prolonged resulting in a long *QT* interval on the electrocardiograph. This property can occasionally predispose to life-threatening arrhythmias including ventricular fibrillation.

Pharmacokinetics and dosage. Sotalol has low lipid solubility with an oral bioavailability of about 90%. Its onset of action is relatively rapid, reaching peak plasma concentrations within 1 to 2 hours. Its plasma half-life of 7–15 hours is longer than most other commonly used beta adrenoceptor antagonists and the drug can be effectively administered once daily. Sotalol is not metabolised and is largely excreted unchanged in the urine (Table 8.3). The drug tends to accumulate in the elderly and in patients with poor renal function.

The dual mode of action of sotalol makes dose adjustment difficult and higher doses may be required to achieve the type III antiarrhythmic activity. The usual initial and maintenance dose for arrhythmias is 120–240 mg/day in single or divided doses with a recommended maximum dose of 320 mg/day.

Clinical indications. Sotalol has been shown to be efficacious in the suppression of ventricular arrhythmias, even in patients refractory to treatment with other antiarrhythmic agents. However, the pro-arrhythmic potential is of concern. This severe adverse effect is probably dose related and is usually reported with doses greater than 320 mg/day. Studies which have demonstrated a reduction in mortality have used the racemic mixture of d- and l-sotalol and it seems likely that the beneficial effects are due to the beta adrenoceptor antagonist component (l-sotalol). In support of this, d-sotalol treatment resulted in increased mortality in patients with poor left ventricular function following an acute myocardial function. Further studies are required to clearly define the role of sotalol in the treatment of symptomatic or asymptomatic arrhythmias.

Adverse effects and interactions. Sotalol shares all the commonly reported adverse effects of beta adrenoceptor antagonists. Drowsiness and fatigue are probably more common than with beta$_1$ selective antagonists such as metoprolol, atenolol and bisoprolol. Sotalol also has a significant pro-arrhythmic effect and increases the risk of *torsade de pointes* in about 5% of patients treated. This is more likely to occur if hypokalaemia is present. When used primarily as an antiarrhythmic agent, bradycardia and heart failure are important adverse effects.

As with amiodarone, combinations with other agents which lengthen the *QT* interval or decrease the serum potassium increase the risk of serious ventricular arrhythmias. Sotalol is one of the agents most commonly associated with hypoglycaemic unawareness and conduction problems can arise when the drug is combined with non-dihydropyridine calcium antagonists.

Contraindications. Important contraindications to the use of beta blockers – heart failure, peripheral vascular disease and asthma clearly apply to sotalol. The drug is best avoided in patients with second and third degree heart block and "brittle" diabetics. Pregnancy and lactation are relative contraindications.

Bretylium tosylate

Mode of action. Bretylium was first introduced as an adrenergic neurone blocker for use in patients with hypertension. It interferes with the neuronal release of noradrenaline at the post-ganglionic adrenergic nerve endings and blood pressure tends to fall. Bretylium also lengthens the ventricular action potential duration and effective refractory period, an effect which is more pronounced in ischaemic cells where the action potential duration is reduced. Since bretylium facilitates the release of catecholamines, a positive inotropic effect can occur after the first dose. This can also induce ventricular arrhythmias and limits the use of the drug in emergencies. There is little inhibitory effect on nodal or conduction tissue.

Pharmacokinetics and dosage. Following intravenous administration, bretylium is widely distributed with no liver metabolism. Excretion is via the kidneys by active tubular secretion. The commonly quoted elimination half-life is 5–10 hours which is significantly prolonged in patients with renal impairment (Table 8.3).

In adults an intravenous bolus of bretylium tosylate 5 mg/kg is usually administered over a 10-minute period and repeated after 30 minutes. Maintenance therapy can be achieved by similar bolus or intramuscular injections every 4–6 hours, or by constant infusion of 0.5–2.0 mg/minute.

Clinical indications. The main indication for bretylium is in the treatment of ventricular fibrillation unresponsive to cardioversion and lignocaine.

Adverse effects and interactions. The most important adverse effect of bretylium is hypotension which can be largely reversed by tricyclic antidepressants. This blocks the reuptake of noradrenaline at the post-ganglionic adrenergic nerve endings. Release of noradrenaline following the first dose can induce arrhythmias and increase blood pressure. Nausea and vomiting have been reported after intravenous bolus administration. Other reported adverse effects include tissue necrosis following intramuscular injection, angina, hyperthermia and respiratory depression. Bretylium may increase the risk of adverse effects caused by digoxin and sympathomimetics by increasing noradrenaline release.

Contraindications. Care should be exercised in patients receiving drugs which lower blood pressure, lengthen the *QT* interval or whose effects are increased in the presence of high circulating levels of catecholamines. The drug is best avoided in patients with congestive cardiac failure, and during pregnancy and lactation.

Class IV (calcium channel antagonists)

Verapamil and diltiazem inhibit slow calcium channel dependent conduction through the atrioventricular node. Both are effective in the acute and long-term management of supraventricular arrhythmias. In rapid atrial fibrillation, intravenous verapamil reduces the ventricular rate and converts a small percentage to sinus rhythm. In atrial flutter the degree of atrioventricular blockade is increased and some may convert to atrial fibrillation. Neither drug is effective in treating ventricular tachycardia and can be lethal in wide complex ventricular tachycardia. However, some patients with exercise induced ventricular tachycardia may respond well.

Class V (adenosine, digitalis, magnesium and potassium)

Some antiarrhythmic drugs do not fit the conventional class I–IV classification. These include digoxin which has previously been discussed, adenosine, magnesium and potassium.

Adenosine

Mode of action

Adenosine is a naturally occurring nucleotide primarily formed as a degradation product of adenosine triphosphate. Its mechanism of action is complex but involves increased potassium conductance and inhibition of cyclic adenosine monophosphate-induced calcium influx. The overall effect is marked hyperpolarisation and suppression of calcium-dependent action potentials. When given as an intravenous bolus, adenosine directly inhibits atrioventricular nodal conduction and increases the atrioventricular nodal refractory period but has little effect on sino-atrial nodal function.

Pharmacokinetics and dosage. Adenosine is rapidly metabolised to inactive metabolites and has a short duration of action after intravenous administration. Its peak action is seen after about 10 seconds and the effect normally lasts about 10 seconds. The elimination life is less than 10 seconds and the metabolites are cleared by the kidney.

The drug is administered as a rapid intravenous bolus; 3 mg over 2 seconds followed by 6 mg and 12 mg given over 2 seconds if the arrhythmia does not respond to the lower doses.

Clinical indications. The main indication for adenosine is in the treatment of paroxysmal atrial and nodal tachycardias including those associated with Wolff–Parkinson–White syndrome. It can be given safely to patients with broad complex tachycardia, poor left ventricular function and severe hypotension because of its short duration of effect. It is also useful in helping to distinguish between broad complex tachycardias of ventricular or supraventricular origin. In general, ventricular tachycardias do not respond except those related to exercise. Adenosine is of no value in atrial fibrillation or flutter.

Adverse effects and interactions. Adenosine causes flushing, shortness of breath, bronchospasm and chest burning in 10–20% of patients receiving the drug. Induction of high grade atrioventricular block can occur but is usually brief. Transient new arrhythmias at the time of chemical conversion commonly occur and may include *torsade de pointes*. Less common adverse effects include headache, hypotension, nausea, paraesthesias, neck pain, blurred vision, hyperventilation and a metallic taste in the mouth.

Dipyridamole inhibits the breakdown of adenosine and the dose should be reduced in patients on this drug treatment. Methylxanthines such as theophylline and caffeine competitively antagonise adenosine, reducing its effectiveness as an antiarrhythmic agent. Additive effects occur with other drugs which impair atrioventricular conduction, but in general these are rarely serious because of the short duration of drug action.

Contraindications. Patients with atrial fibrillation or flutter should not receive adenosine as it is ineffective and in the presence of an accessory bypass tract, it may exacerbate the arrhythmia. Care is necessary in patients receiving dipyridamole when smaller doses should be used. In general, it is best to avoid the drug in patients with sick sinus syndrome or high grade atrioventricular block. The drug is probably safe to administer during pregnancy.

Magnesium

Magnesium was originally used to treat digitalis-induced arrhythmias in patients with low levels of magnesium. Magnesium, however, has antiarrhythmic properties in patients with normal magnesium concentrations. Magnesium has various cellular actions. It affects Na^+/K^+ ATPase, sodium, calcium and potassium channels. Apart from treating arrhythmias due to digoxin overdosage, magnesium has been shown to be useful in the management of *torsades de pointes* and the arrhythmias associated with an early myocardial infarction.

Potassium

Hypokalaemia predisposes to serious ventricular arrhythmias especially following an acute myocardial infarction by increasing the risk of early and delayed after-depolarisations and ectopic pacemaker activity. This is further increased if the patient is receiving a cardiac glycoside. Since hyperkalaemia is also arrhythmogenic, potassium has no place in the routine management of arrhythmias in patients with normal body potassium, but the aim should be to normalise potassium serum concentrations in patients at risk of developing arrhythmias.

Pro-arrhythmic effects of antiarrhythmiac agents and the risk of sudden death

Following the CAST (cardiac arrhythmia suppression trial) report, it was clearly demonstrated that a variety of class 1 antiarrhythmic agents increase the risk of sudden death. The idea that antiarrhythmic agents are also pro-arrhythmic, however, is not new. Soon after the introduction of quinidine in the 1920s syncope and sudden death were reported in a significant number of patients receiving the drug. All antiarrhythmic agents are capable of precipitating ventricular arrhythmias, but there is considerable variation between different drugs. In general the concept of pro-arrhythmia is used to define an increase or the appearance of a ventricular arrhythmia as a consequence of drug administration. However, syncope and sudden death can on occasions be due to severe bradyarrhythmias. The mechanisms involved can be direct or indirect and related to depressed left ventricular function, the development of bradycardia with a long QT interval, alteration in autonomic nervous system function and myocardial ischaemia.

The basic manifestations of the pro-arrhythmic effect are prolongation of the cardiac action potential and lengthening of the QT interval and wide complex tachycardias terminating in ventricular fibrillation. Class 1A and III lengthen the QT interval and predispose to *torsade de pointes* while class 1C drugs tend to produce wide complex tachycardias. In addition, ventricular arrhythmias can complicate therapy with any class 1 drug if conduction is markedly depressed. The present advice would be to avoid class 1 drugs if possible, to treat only where overall benefit has been defined and to avoid antiarrhythmic drugs altogether in subjects at high risk.

Treatment of arrhythmias in congestive heart failure

Prophylactic antiarrhythmic drugs should not be used in patients with congestive cardiac failure. When the arrhythmia is contributing to poor left ventricular function, amiodarone has been shown to have beneficial effects on ejection fraction, although there is no favourable effect on mortality.

Conclusions

Symptomatic supraventricular arrhythmias require therapy with digoxin, calcium channel antagonists, and adenosine, etc. The treatment for ventricular arrhythmias remains controversial and a clear distinction needs to be made between suppression of premature ventricular complexes and the treatment of ventricular tachycardia and fibrillation. Lignocaine is still probably the drug of first choice for ventricular arrhythmias following an acute myocardial infarction and beta adrenoceptor antagonists, the drugs of choice for long-term prophylaxis. All seriously symptomatic arrhythmias need therapy and in this country amiodarone is probably the preferred agent. Until clear evidence is available that certain anti-arrhythmic agents have beneficial effects on prognosis, routine treatment of asymptomatic arrhythmias is not indicated.

9 Drug Treatment of Hypertension

Hypertension is the level of blood pressure at which the benefits of action exceed those of inaction.   G. Rose (1980)

Introduction

Elevated blood pressure is a major risk factor for the development of stroke and is an important risk factor for the development of coronary heart disease. It is an essentially treatable condition and drug treatment has been shown to reverse the hypertension attributable risk of stroke and substantially reduce the risk of myocardial infarction and other major cardiovascular events, at least in the short term. Effective management of hypertension would therefore have a major impact on public health.

Relationship between blood pressure and risk

The overall results of several epidemiological studies demonstrate a direct, continuous and independent association between the level of blood pressure and the risk of coronary heart disease and stroke (Figure 9.1). From this data it has been estimated that an increase in diastolic blood pressure of 5 mmHg results in a 34% increase in the risk of stroke and a 21% increase in the risk of coronary heart disease. Although there is no clear evidence of a threshold below which treatment is unlikely to reduce risk, maintaining diastolic blood pressure below 90 mmHg will reduce the relative risk below 1. A cut-off point between 90 and 100 mmHg therefore has been used in most of the large intervention studies with target blood pressure below 90 mmHg. In the recently published HOT[†] (Hypertension Optimal Treatment) trial the optimal blood pressure for reduction of cardiovascular events was 139/83 mmHg, but maintaining the blood pressure below 150/90 produced almost equally good results.

[†]Hansson, L., Zanchetti, A., Carruthers, S. G. *et al.* Effects of intensive blood pressure lowering and low-dose aspirin in patients with hypertension: principal results of the Hypertension Optimal Treatment (HOT) randomised trial. *Lancet*, 1998; 315: 1755–1762.

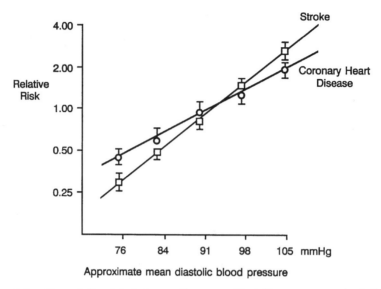

Figure 9.1. The relationship between the mean diastolic pressure and relative risk of developing a stroke or coronary heart disease. Reproduced from MacMahon, S., Peto, R., Cutler, J. *et al. Lancet,* 1990; 335: 765–774. Blood pressure, stroke and coronary heart disease. © by The Lancet Ltd, reproduced with permission.

Risks in different populations

Women tolerate elevated blood pressure better than men, demonstrating lower mortality and morbidity rates at all levels of blood pressure. This is equally true for systolic and diastolic blood pressure and the differences are even more marked in women aged 65 years and above. Racial differences have been described between North American blacks, whites and Hispanics. Blacks tend to have higher levels of blood pressure than whites and overall mortality rates are greater, mainly due to a higher incidence of stroke. In contrast, Hispanic men have lower rates than non-Hispanic whites despite higher risk scores and poorer control of blood pressure.

Age and blood pressure

Blood pressure, particularly systolic blood pressure, increases progressively with age, and elderly hypertensives have a greater risk of developing cardiovascular disease than younger hypertensive patients. Isolated systolic hypertension defined as a systolic blood pressure greater than 160 mmHg and a diastolic blood pressure less than 90 mmHg is present in about one-quarter of patients over the age of 80 years. In the Framingham study, systolic blood pressure was a better predictor of risk than diastolic blood pressure and this relationship held in patients over the age of 65 years. However, in patients over 75 years, the risk declines and those aged 85–88 years old with mildly elevated blood pressure have lower mortality rates than patients with lower blood pressures. The reason may be that low blood pressures in this population are an indication of impending cardiovascular events.

Benefits of lowering blood pressure

The benefits of drug therapy in malignant hypertension were easy to demonstrate because the condition had a predictable, relatively brief and almost uniformly fatal course in untreated patients. A small number of studies confirmed the value of treatment in reducing mortality in this condition. Demonstrating the value of drug therapy in non-malignant severe hypertension took longer to demonstrate, but in the 1960s a series of controlled studies were published which suggested that reducing blood pressure over a period of several years reduced most of the major complications. However, the first adequately designed placebo controlled study which provided convincing evidence of protection by drug treatment in non-malignant hypertension was the Veterans Administration Co-operative study started in 1963. Although patient selection and definition of endpoints was less than ideal, major complications occurred in 29% of the placebo group and 12% in the treated group. The benefits were greater for patients with initial diastolic blood pressures between 105 and 114 mmHg than for those with values between 90 and 104 mmHg.

Trials in mild hypertension

The promising results of the Veterans Administration study prompted the initiation of a number of studies in hypertensive patients with diastolic blood pressures below 115 mmHg. Demography and drug therapy in these studies are listed in Table 9.1. Although earlier meta analyses of these studies showed the expected reduction in the incidence of stroke and vascular death, the reduction in mortality from coronary heart disease was only 11%, less than expected, and not statistically different from the untreated group. The most recent meta analysis which included studies in elderly patients again confirmed the complete reversal of the risk of stroke (−38%) and a larger and significant impact on coronary events (−16%) when diastolic blood pressure was lowered by 5–6 mmHg (Figure 9.2). In all but two of these studies, a diuretic was the initial drug treatment and a beta adrenoceptor antagonist was the most commonly used additional agent. More recently studies based on dihydropyridine calcium antagonists have demonstrated a similar impact on cardiovascular events. The disappointing

Table 9.1. Demography and drug therapy in the early outcome studies in hypertensive patients

Trial	No. of patients	Mean age (years)	% Male	Mean follow-up years	Principal drugs	Decrease in DBP (mmHg)
Veterans Administration (1978)	1 012	38	81	1.5	Chlorthalidone	7
Hypertension Detection and Follow-up Programme (1979) (Stratum I)	7 825	51	55	5.0	Chlorthalidone	5
Medical Research Council (1985)	17 354	52	52	5.0	Bendrofluazide Propranolol	6
Veterans Administration (1970)	380	51	100	3.3	Hydrochlorothiazide Reserpine Hydralazine	19
Hypertension Detection and Follow-up Programme (1979) (Stratum II)	2 052	51	55	5.0	Chlorthalidone	7

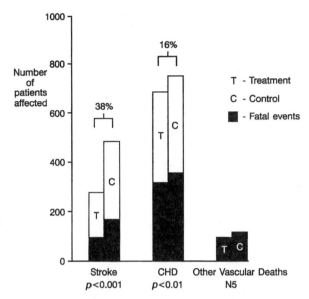

Figure 9.2. Reduction in stroke and coronary heart disease in treated hypertensive populations. Reproduced from "Blood Pressure, Antihypertensive Drug Treatment and the Risks of Stroke and of Coronary Heart Disease", Collins, R. and MacMahon, S. *British Medical Bulletin* 1994: 50; 272–298. Reproduced with permission from The British Council.

effect on coronary heart disease could therefore represent a type II statistical error, and the 95% confidence intervals for coronary mortality included either no effect or the expected reduction in mortality. Alternatively, the differences could reflect other aspects of the disease or its treatment since less impressive protection against coronary heart disease with antihypertensive therapy has been observed in free living populations. Higher mortality rates are observed in adequately treated hypertensive patients compared with age and sex-matched normotensive controls.

There are a number of possibilities to help explain why the excess risks associated with raised blood pressure are not reduced to levels seen in normotensive subjects. These include failure to address additional risk factors such as hypercholesterolaemia, smoking and diabetes, the short duration of intervention, inclusion of normotensive patients in the control group, metabolic effects of high dose diuretics and beta blocker therapy, under-treatment or possibly over-treatment of some patients.

Value of treatment in the elderly

A recent overview of seven major hypertensive trials in the elderly (Table 9.2) concluded that there is now clear evidence that active lowering of blood

Table 9.2. Effects of drug treatment in elderly hypertensive patients (odds ratios)

Complication	Australian Trial (1981)	EWPHE Amery (1985)	Coope and Warrender (1986)	SHEP (1991)	STOP-HT Dahlof (1991)	MRCE (1992)	SYST-EUR Trial (1997)
Coronary heart disease	0.82	0.80	1.03	0.73*	0.87†	0.81	0.72*
Stroke	0.67	0.64*	0.58*	0.67*	0.53*	0.75*	0.68*
Congestive cardiac failure	–	0.78	0.68	0.45*	0.49*	–	0.86*
All cardiovascular events	0.69	0.71*	0.76*	0.68*	0.60*	0.83*	0.73*

*Statistically significant.
†Statistically significant for myocardial infarction only.
EWPHE—European Working Party on high blood pressure in the elderly.
SHEP—Systolic hypertension in the elderly programme.
STOP-HT—Swedish trial in old patients with hypertension.
MRCE—Medical Research Council study in elderly hypertensives.

pressure in patients over the age of 65 years is associated with significant improvements in cardiovascular morbidity and mortality. In fact, the benefits appear to be more impressive in older than younger patients.

Other evidence for the benefit of antihypertensive therapy

In addition to the evidence on stroke and coronary heart disease in the large hypertensive studies, several smaller studies have examined the effects of lowering blood pressure on other endpoints. These have included total mortality and the distribution of specific causes of death as well as mortality and morbidity from end organ disease on the heart, brain, kidney and large arteries.

Total mortality rates have declined for hypertensive and normotensive populations in most Western industrial countries mostly due to a reduction in stroke. Analysis of the Framingham study also confirmed that control of hypertension significantly contributed to the decline in mortality from cardiovascular disease over the last 30 years. Before 1950, congestive cardiac failure was responsible for over one-half of the deaths in hypertensive patients. Although deaths related to coronary heart disease have increased since then, deaths from hypertensive cardiac failure have decreased significantly. This important benefit of antihypertensive therapy is often neglected.

There is also accumulating evidence that long-term reduction in blood pressure results in decreases in left ventricular mass, improves myocardial structure and function and increases coronary vasodilator reserve.

Two recent meta analyses suggested that ACE inhibitors are more effective than most other antihypertensive agents in reducing left ventricular hypertrophy, but because of the low frequency and poor quality of the studies involving older drugs both analyses were strongly biased towards newer agents. Three long-term comparative studies with examples of all the major antihypertensive agents were unable to confirm any benefits of ACE inhibitors over other forms of antihypertensive drugs and thiazide diuretics and beta adrenoceptor antagonists were at least as effective as other agents in reducing left ventricular mass.

The potential for better cardioprotection with angiotensin converting enzyme inhibitors cannot be totally dismissed, however, since this group of drugs reduces the progression of left ventricular dysfunction independent of their antihypertensive effects. In addition, although the degree of albuminuria in hypertensive patients with impaired renal function can be reduced by any drug which lowers blood pressure, the clinical benefit of lowering blood pressure on other measures of renal function is difficult to demonstrate except in diabetic patients. In this group of patients ACE inhibitors appear to produce benefit beyond their effect on blood pressure although this was not confirmed by the recent UK Prospective Diabetes

Table 9.3. Factors influencing the decision to treat with antihypertensive drug therapy

---

Presence of additional risk factors
- Cigarette smoking
- Hyperlipidaemia
- Obesity
- Family history of premature cardiovascular disease
- Diabetes

Evidence of end organ disease
- Angina, myocardial ischaemia or infarction
- Previous coronary artery surgery
- Congestive cardiac failure
- Left ventricular hypertrophy
- Transient cerebral ischaemia and strokes
- Renal disease
- Retinopathy

Study Group which demonstrated that lowering blood pressure with captopril or atenolol was equally effective in reducing blood pressure and the incidence of diabetic complications in type II diabetics. ACE inhibitors remain the drugs of first choice in type I diabetes especially if albuminuria is present. In type II diabetes ACE inhibitors have no clear advantages.

What level of blood pressure should be treated?

Although different opinions do exist, the consensus view is that blood pressure consistently greater than 150/95 mmHg should be treated. Those with persistent pressures between 140/90 and 150/95 should be treated if additional risk factors are present. Lower thresholds are recommended for type I diabetes ($\geqslant 140/90$) and type I diabetes with albuminuria ($\geqslant 120/75$) (Table 9.3).

Treatment targets

The general view, based on the experience of early hypertensive studies and extrapolation from epidemiological data, has been that the lower the blood pressure the greater the likely benefit. However, analyses of several clinical trials suggested that as the blood pressure was reduced below 85 mmHg little or no additional benefit occurred and the risk appeared to be increased. (Figure 9.3). The HOT trial demonstrated that the optimal blood pressure for reduction in cardiovascular events was 139/83. Reduction of blood pressure below the optimal level caused no harm and there was no evidence of J phenomenon. In

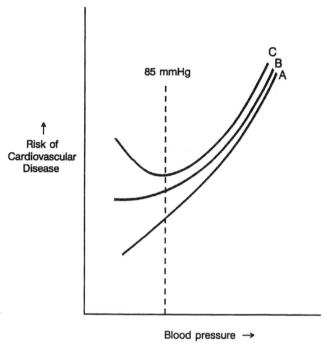

Blood pressure →

Figure 9.3. Three hypothetical models of the relationship between blood pressure and risk of cardiovascular disease. Lowering blood pressure below 85 mmHg results in (A) a reduction in cardiovascular disease, or (B) no additional benefit, or (C) increased cardiovascular disease (J curve).

hypertensive patients with diabetes there appeared to be a significant advantage in lowering diastolic blood pressure below 80 mmHg. Further evidence against the so-called 'J' curve was the finding that the expected reductions in cardiovascular morbidity and mortality occurred in elderly patients while the mean treated diastolic blood pressure was less than 80 mmHg.

Non-drug therapy

Although this chapter is mainly concerned with the drug treatment of hypertension it is essential that non-drug therapy should be considered first since all patients require lifestyle modification whether or not they receive drug therapy. There is as yet no evidence of the value of non-drug therapy alone in reducing morbidity and mortality in hypertensive patients. However, a number of studies in patients with mild hypertension have demonstrated that combinations of non-drug therapy will lower blood pressure to a small degree and reduce the number of antihypertensive drugs required to reduce blood pressure to the required value. The value of individual interventions will now be discussed.

Stopping smoking

Until recently it was widely stated that cigarette smoking had little effect on blood pressure and the main reason for recommending that the patient should stop smoking was that it represented a powerful independent risk factor for the development of coronary heart disease and stroke. However, recent evidence suggests that cigarette smoking is associated with an elevation in blood pressure following smoking a cigarette and this lasts 15–30 minutes on each occasion. These pressor effects have been described during 24-hour blood pressure monitoring and, although not proven, it is possible that the rises in blood pressure contribute to the increased incidence of vascular events in smokers and their apparent resistance to the effects of antihypertensive medication. Other adverse cardiovascular effects of cigarette smoking include lipid abnormalities, central obesity, insulin resistance and direct toxic effects on the vascular endothelium.

Reduced alcohol intake

Several population studies have confirmed a positive association between blood pressure and regular alcohol consumption. Blood pressure is higher in patients who consume more than three units daily and the risk of developing hypertension is two to three times more common in heavy drinkers. In men who consume more than 50 drinks per week the prevalence of hypertension rises to 13% and in hypertensive men who take alcohol regularly 36% of cases can be, in large part, attributed to alcohol. Reducing the intake of alcohol lowers blood pressure. A mean decrease in alcohol consumption from 452 to 64 ml per week resulted in a mean decrease of 5 mmHg in systolic pressure and a mean decrease of 3 mmHg in diastolic blood pressure in treated hypertensive patients and this occurred independent of changes in body weight. These patients were well controlled with a mean treated blood pressure of 142/85 mmHg. Larger reductions would be expected in patients with higher levels of blood pressure.

Weight reduction

Obesity, especially the type distributed in the upper part of the body, is associated with increased blood pressure. On average a decrease of 1 kg body weight is associated with a decrease of approximately 1% in systolic and diastolic blood pressures, and this decrease is independent of changes in salt and alcohol intake.

Salt restriction

Modest reduction of salt intake by about one-third has been shown to reduce systolic blood pressure by 4.9 ± 1.3 mmHg and diastolic blood pressure by 2.6 ± 0.8 mmHg. Elderly patients and those with the highest initial blood pressures seem to respond best to salt restriction. Few problems arise as a result of moderate salt restriction. Although, in general, the greater the degree of salt restriction the greater the effect on blood pressure, there is little to recommend severe sodium restriction. Reduction of daily sodium intake to 10 and 20 mmol/day can lead to increased lipids, insulin, reduced renal blood flow and salt-losing nephropathy. Similar or greater reductions can usually be achieved with small doses of thiazide diuretics and other antihypertensive agents. Given the real potential for benefit and the absence of important adverse effects moderate sodium restriction is a desirable goal for individual hypertensives and for the population at large.

Increased potassium intake

Some of the benefits observed with salt restriction are probably related to increased potassium intake in the diet and epidemiological evidence suggests an inverse relationship between potassium intake and blood pressure. Oral potassium supplements have been shown to lower systolic blood pressure by 8.2 mmHg and diastolic blood pressure by 4.5 mmHg, and high potassium intake is associated with a lower incidence of stroke than in populations receiving less dietary potassium. A high intake of potassium is potentially dangerous, however, especially in elderly patients with impaired renal function. Maintaining normal serum potassium with potassium supplements or potassium sparing diuretics in patients on diuretic therapy for hypertension is clearly of value. Recent evidence suggests that those on lower doses of diuretics, on potassium supplements and potassium-sparing diuretics have a lower incidence of sudden death than those receiving larger doses of thiazide diuretics without supplements or potassium-sparing agents.

Physical activity

Several intervention studies have observed the effects of physical activity on blood pressure. The majority of these were not randomised, were uncontrolled and did not consider confounding variables such as changes in weight and alterations in salt intake. In the best of these studies physical training resulted in a blood pressure reduction of 4/4 mmHg in normotensive subjects and 11/6 mmHg in hypertensive patients. The decrease in blood pressure was related to the initial systolic blood pressure and the increase in working capacity. In a follow-up study in 6000 patients lasting 1–12 years, those with low levels of physical activity were 50% more likely to develop clinical hypertension than those with high levels of physical activity.

Other non-pharmacological interventions

Several other non-pharmacological measures have been investigated in hypertensive populations, but most are of no proven value in reducing blood pressure long term. These include reduced intake of dietary calcium, increased magnesium, bio feedback and relaxation. There is limited evidence that a vegetarian diet may prevent increases in blood pressure with small but significant decreases in normotensive and hypertensive populations. It seems likely that these changes relate to alterations in the dietary intake of sodium and potassium. Diets rich in fish oils may also have a small impact.

In conclusion there is sound evidence that weight reduction, moderate salt restriction and alcohol reduction will lower blood pressure at least in the short term. It could be argued that other unproven interventions will do no harm, but there is a danger that useful measures could be overwhelmed by treatments of dubious value. Two recent long-term studies examining the combined effects of weight, salt and alcohol reduction produced rather disappointing results. The overall reductions achieved in both studies were too small for patients to avoid antihypertensive drug treatment. Although all patients should receive advice on lifestyle modification, there remains the danger that prolonged non-pharmacological treatment will result in sub-optimal treatment. This form of therapy should be regarded in most cases as a useful supplement to antihypertensive drug treatment and not an alternative to it.

The choice of antihypertensive agent

New antihypertensive drugs are being continually introduced into clinical practice. There is little evidence that these newer drugs have advantages over diuretics and beta adrenoceptors in terms of efficacy and adverse effects, and therapeutic choices are often based on promotional activities by pharmaceutical companies rather than the results of outcome of clinical studies. Almost all orally active drugs lower blood pressure by about 10% in patients with mild to moderate hypertension. When comparisons between various drugs are made, they almost always demonstrate similar efficacy and tolerability for periods of up to 5 years. With the exception of the Syst-Eur trial in isolated systolic hypertension in which patients received a dihydropyridine calcium antagonist followed by an ACE as initial therapy, most evidence comes from trials based on treatment with thiazide diuretics and beta adrenoceptor antagonists. To date we have no clear evidence that ACE inhibitor based regimens have the same or greater impact on stroke and coronary events as diuretic/beta blocker based regimens. Evidence of superiority of one group over another will only be answered when the results of large comparative trials such as ASCOT (Anglo–Scandinavian Cardiac Outcomes Trial) and ALLHAT (Antihypertensive and Lipid-Lowering Heart Attack Trial) are published.

There has recently been a major debate as to whether dihydropyridine calcium antagonists are associated with increased risk of coronary events, cancer, bleeding, depression and suicide. These observations were based on case control studies which often provide biased information. Clinical trials in heart failure and hypertension have failed to confirm these adverse effects but capsular nifedipine should no longer be prescribed to patients with ischaemic heart disease. Overall there is no convincing evidence to revise the current recommendations that diuretics and beta blockers should remain as first-line antihypertensive agents. Dihydropyridine calcium antagonists are probably preferable to beta blockers in elderly patients with systolic hypertension. The major indications and contraindications for the different agents are listed in Table 9.4. It is important, however, to remember that less than half of all patients with hypertension are controlled by monotherapy with any class of drug and a substantial proportion require three or more drugs.

Dose–response relationships

Over the last 30 years a variety of antihypertensive drugs have been introduced to clinical practice at an excessively high dose. For example, propranolol was introduced at doses up to 5000 mg, atenolol up to 2000 mg and captopril up to 1000 mg. Commonly used maintenance doses of 80 mg propranolol, 25 mg atenolol and 50 mg captopril have been shown to be effective in a significant number of patients. Doses of 200 mg hydrochlorothiazide were originally used and 12.5 mg has been shown to reduce blood pressure in many patients. Most doses used clinically are near or beyond the desirable dose range (Figure 9.4) and patients receiving these higher doses are at greater risk of developing adverse effects. The obvious solution is to start patients at doses which are less than the maximum and to titrate the dose until the desired effect is achieved. In many cases, especially with thiazide diuretics, these smaller doses are not always available.

Table 9.4. Indications and contraindications for the principal groups of antihypertensive agents

Drug class	Indications	Contraindications
Diuretics	First-line agents unless clear contraindications Good for elderly patients and those with heart failure	Gout Renal failure
Beta adrenoceptor antagonists	First-line agents unless clear contraindications Good for patients with angina and post-MI	Asthma, heart block, obstructive lung disease, peripheral vascular disease
Calcium channel antagonists	Useful in the elderly, especially those with isolated systolic hypertension	Heart block ⎫ especially verapamil and diltiazem Heart failure ⎭
ACE inhibitors	Diabetes Heart failure Left ventricular dysfunction	Pregnancy. Renovascular disease
Angiotensin II receptor antagonists	Those with ACE inhibitor-induced cough	Pregnancy. Renovascular disease
Alpha adrenoceptor antagonists	Prostatic hypertrophy ? Dyslipidaemia	Urinary incontinence
Centrally acting agents	Pregnancy (methyldopa)	Non-compliant patients. Those working in dangerous occupations and with machinery Diabetes (diazoxide).
Direct-acting vasodilators	Severe resistant hypertension Pregnancy (hydralazine)	Autoimmune disease (hydralazine)

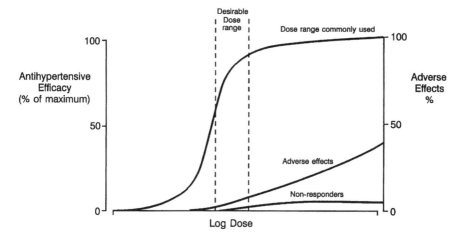

Figure 9.4. Schematic representation of the relationship between the dose, antihypertensive effect and adverse effects. Reprinted from G. D. Johnston. Dose response relationships with antihypertensive drugs. *Pharmacology and Therapeutics*, Vol. 55, pp. 53–93 (80), 1992 with permission from Elsevier Science.

Significance of trough : peak ratios

In 1988 the Cardiovascular and Renal Drug Advisory Committee of the United States Food and Drug Administration (FDA) and leading experts in the area of hypertension drew up a series of guidelines for the clinical evaluation of antihypertensive agents. One of the most important of these guidelines was that antihypertensive therapy should be assessed on the relationship between trough and peak responses rather than relying on a single 24-h value after dosing. For some drugs, especially the shorter acting calcium channel antagonists, doses titrated to the response at trough produced significant periods of hypotension throughout the dosage interval and doses based on peak responses resulted in long periods of inadequate therapeutic response. In an attempt to produce a better index of therapeutic efficacy, the guidelines proposed a value based on a peak blood pressure to trough ratio. In addition to maintaining a "useful" antihypertensive effect at the end of the dosage interval, it was agreed by the Advisory Committee that the trough effect should be at least half the peak effect once appropriate adjustments had been made for placebo effects. Fortunately or unfortunately the committee failed to define a useful antihypertensive effect. In addition, it was suggested that if the peak effect were modest then a trough to peak ratio of two-thirds would be necessary. In other words, the FDA guidelines offered an arithmetic index which helped to define the duration of action of an antihypertensive agent and hence the selection of the appropriate dosage interval, but did not provide measures of antihypertensive efficacy. It may be usefully combined with an assessment of the magnitude of the antihypertensive response.

The calculation of peak to trough ratio for an antihypertensive agent critically depends on the quality of the study design and the analysis of the results. The most important factors are the placebo and/or circadian effects. Ignoring the placebo effects can completely alter the interpretation of a study designed to calculate peak trough ratios and tends to exaggerate the response. For the same reasons, circadian change in blood pressure can reduce or increase the magnitude of the index depending on the timing of peak and trough responses.

To accurately define trough to peak ratios it is essential to have multiple measures of blood pressure made under controlled conditions in well-designed placebo controlled studies. As a result, the numbers of patients studied tend to be small and unrepresentative of hypertensive populations in general. If clinic blood pressures are used, the number of measurements will be small and the times of peak and trough arbitrarily defined. Ambulatory blood pressure is being more frequently used to define trough to peak ratios and should more accurately define trough peak ratios because of multiple measurements and recordings made during everyday activity. At present this seems to be the most useful way forward, but data to date are limited. Absolute values for trough to peak ratios depend on the methods used, and comparisons of the values obtained in independent studies should be viewed with considerable caution.

The major reason for the FDA guidelines was to prevent the licensing of antihypertensive agents at excessively high dose so that they could be marketed as once daily agents. Drugs with large trough peak ratios will be more likely to maintain adequate antihypertensive activity and therefore more likely to be safely administered once daily. In addition, omission of a single dose is less likely to have a major effect on blood pressure control.

Rationale for drug combinations of antihypertensive therapy

During chronic therapy, two or more antihypertensive drugs are often combined. This is based on the observation that a large number of antihypertensive drugs when combined have an additive or even synergistic effect on blood pressure. In addition, there is no blood pressure lowering drug which controls blood pressure in all patients, and for most agents a response between 50% and 70% is usually seen. The combination of two or more antihypertensive agents increases considerably the percentage of patients who achieve a therapeutic target. Commonly used drugs are listed in Table 9.5.

Table 9.5.   Useful combinations of antihypertensive drugs

Beta adrenoceptor antagonist and a diuretic
ACE inhibitor and a diuretic
Calcium channel antagonist and a diuretic
Beta adrenoceptor antagonist and a calcium channel antagonist
ACE inhibitor and a calcium antagonist
Beta adrenoceptor antagonist, a diuretic and a vasodilator drug (calcium antagonist,
    ACE inhibitor or selective alpha$_1$ antagonist)
ACE inhibitor, diuretic and calcium antagonist

Several antihypertensive agents cause salt and water retention during chronic therapy, especially those with powerful vasodilator activity. As a result the antihypertensive effect declines with time and may disappear altogether. These agents are more effective when a diuretic is added. In addition there are several antihypertensive drugs which induce reflex activation of the sympathetic nervous system. Increases in cardiac output antagonise the antihypertensive activity of minoxidil, hydralazine and other vasodilator drugs. This can be reversed by co-administering a beta adrenoceptor antagonist.

Long-term use of high dose diuretic therapy activates the sympathetic nervous system and renin angiotensin aldosterone system. Antagonism of reflex sympathetic activation of beta adrenoceptor antagonists and reduction of angiotensin II concentrations with ACE inhibitors probably contribute to the efficacy of these drug combinations.

Since low doses of individual agents can be used in combination to lower blood pressure it seems likely that combination therapy would be better tolerated than larger doses of individual agents. There is some evidence that the adverse metabolic effects of high dose diuretic therapy can largely be prevented by using lower doses combined with potassium-sparing diuretics or ACE inhibitors.

Individual antihypertensive agents

Diuretics

Despite mounting criticism from protagonists of new antihypertensive drugs, thiazide diuretics remain the cornerstone of antihypertensive drug therapy. They are inexpensive and have been used in the treatment of hypertension for almost 40 years. More importantly they have been the pivotal agents in most large therapeutic outcome studies including the recent STOP-hypertension and SHEP studies where positive benefits have been shown for cardiovascular and cerebrovascular disease. They are effective as monotherapy or in combination and appear to be particularly efficacious in elderly patients, black patients and those with renal insufficiency. When used as single agents, loop diuretics are less effective antihypertensive drugs than similar diuretic doses of thiazides but can be usefully combined with vasodilator drugs in more severe hypertension. There is recent evidence that combining thiazide diuretics with potassium-sparing diuretics is more effective in reducing the incidence of acute myocardial infarction than thiazides given at higher dose.

Classification

Diuretics differ in structure and major sites of action within the nephron. These differences influence the relative efficacy of the different agents as diuretic agents. Thiazide diuretics principally act on the cortical diluting segment of the distal tubule, the loop diuretics on the thick ascending part of the loop of Henle and the potassium-sparing diuretics on the distal tubule and collecting ducts (Figure 9.5).

Thiazide diuretics

Mode of action. Thiazide diuretics act by inhibiting sodium and chloride co-transport across the luminal membrane in the cortical diluting segment of the distal convoluted tubule where 5–10% of the filtered sodium load is reabsorbed (Figure 9.5). The precise mechanisms underlying the

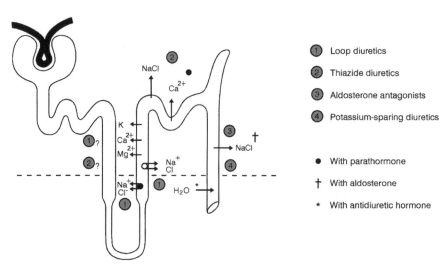

Figure 9.5. Sites of action of diuretics used in the treatment of hypertension.

antihypertensive effects of thiazide diuretics have not been clearly defined. The blood pressure lowering effects are probably in part related to producing a negative sodium balance although the recent observation that low doses of thiazide diuretics lower blood pressure without stimulating plasma renin activity is contrary to this view. Thiazide diuretics may also have weak potassium-channel opening activity and some of the antihypertensive activity could be related to peripheral vasodilatation and reduced peripheral vascular resistance and/or reduced vascular sensitivity to circulating pressor hormones. Alternatively, vasodilatation could be related to increased levels of vasodilator hormones such as prostacyclin and kallikrein.

With larger doses of diuretics, plasma and extracellular fluid volumes decrease initially, but return to normal within a few weeks as a result of humoral and intra-renal counter-regulatory mechanisms. Sodium intake and excretion are balanced within 3–9 days and peripheral resistance increases. Within 4–8 weeks, peripheral resistance declines and the blood pressure lowering effect is maximum. It is doubtful whether all these changes occur with the newly recommended lower dosages.

Dosage. The recommended daily doses of thiazide diuretics have been steadily decreasing over the last 30 years. Original doses of hydrochlorothiazide of 200 mg have been reduced to as little as 6.25 and 12.5 mg today. In hypertensive patients with good renal function these small doses significantly reduce blood pressure and have fewer biochemical adverse effects. Low doses which have been shown to be effective include 1.25 mg bendrofluazide, 125 µg cyclopenthiazide, 12.5 mg chlorthalidone and 500 µg metolazone. Some patients may respond better to larger doses, but it is worth remembering that the maximum antihypertensive may not be seen for 4 weeks or more so that upward dosage titration at shorter intervals can give the impression of a steep dose–response relationship.

Pharmacokinetics. The differences between the thiazide diuretics and related compounds indapamide, metolazone and chlorthalidone relate to differences in their pharmacokinetic behaviour. This affects the time to the onset of action and the duration of effect. Those that are highly substituted have greater lipid solubility, larger apparent volumes of distribution, lower renal clearances and greater tissue binding. Most thiazide diuretics are not significantly metabolised (Table 9.6).

Adverse effects. The disadvantages of diuretics relate mainly to their adverse biochemical effects. Almost all these adverse reactions are dose dependent and can be avoided or minimised by keeping the dose low. Adverse metabolic

Table 9.6. Pharmacokinetic values of the thiazide and thiazide-related diuretics

Drug	Bendrofluazide	Chlorthalidone*	Cyclopenthiazide	Hydrochlorothiazide	Indapamide[†]	Metolazone[‡]
Duration of action	12–18 h	6–36 hours	6–12 hours	6–12 hours	12–24 hours	24–48 hours
Time to peak action	2 hours	4 hours	2 hours	2 hours	<2 hours	2–4 hours
Plasma half-life	3–4 hours	≈54 hours	8 hours	6 hours	10–22 hours	8 hours
Metabolism	Extensive	Not metabolised	Not metabolised	Not metabolised	Extensive	5% metabolised
Oral bio-availability (%)	–	–	100	60	80	40–65
Excretion	30% renal	Unchanged 100% renal	Renal 100%	Renal 100%	60–70% in urine	70% renal 30% biliary
Protein binding	90%	90%	–	60%	70%	95%

*Structurally not a thiazide but similar activity.
[†]Indole derivative which may have additional vasodilator activity.
[‡]Works in patients with poor renal function.

effects which have caused concern include hypokalaemia, hypomagnesaemia, hyperuricaemia, hyperlipidaemia and glucose intolerance.

Hypokalaemia. Hypokalaemia mainly results from the loss of potassium in the urine secondary to diuretic activity and activation of the renin–angiotensin–aldosterone system due to volume contraction. Increased levels of aldosterone further increase potassium loss. Potassium loss is partially compensated with time by the kidney despite continued use of the drugs. Reduced tubular secretion of potassium and depression of distal nephron potassium excretion probably contribute. An incidence of up to 40% has been described in some studies. The frequency and severity relate to the dose, the duration of the diuretic activity, the dietary intake of potassium and sodium and the age of the patient. The importance of diuretic-induced hypokalaemia has caused considerable debate over the last decade. Interest has centred on the association between hypokalaemia, ventricular dysrhythmias and sudden death. The general view is that small reductions in the serum potassium do not constitute a risk in treated hypertensive patients but that larger decreases do represent a significant risk of sudden death. In addition, hypokalaemia increases the risk of toxicity in patients receiving digitalis glycosides and can induce ventricular dysrhythmias in patients with an acute myocardial infarction and those receiving drugs which prolong the *QT* interval on the electrocardiograph. A relationship between dose and the severity of hypokalaemia has been demonstrated for most thiazide diuretics which is not paralleled by effects on blood pressure. Diuretics should be prescribed at the lowest possible doses that effectively reduce blood pressure. The addition of a potassium-sparing diuretic may also be effective in reducing sudden death.

Hyperlipidaemia. There is a large body of literature detailing the adverse effects of thiazide diuretics on plasma lipids. These effects include an elevation of total cholesterol, triglycerides, LDL cholesterol with little effect on HDL cholesterol. Overall, however, these changes are difficult to identify in studies lasting more than 1 year and are dose related. The mechanism is unknown although the changes have been correlated with hypokalaemia and impairment of glucose tolerance. It has been suggested that these changes could negate the beneficial effects of lowering blood pressure produced by diuretics. Recent studies in the elderly are contrary to this hypothesis and when lower doses are used these effects are negligible and transient.

Hyperglycaemia and diabetes. Insulin resistance, diabetes, worsening of diabetic control and rarely hyperosmolar non-ketotic diabetic coma have all been described in patients receiving high doses of thiazide diuretics. Most evidence has been obtained in hypertensive patients who develop impaired glucose tolerance or overt diabetes mellitus. Not all studies have reported a worsening with chronic therapy. Although long-term impairment of glucose tolerance has been described with 10 mg bendrofluazide this has not been demonstrated with the 2.5 mg dose, and a relationship between dose and fasting blood glucose has been shown for bendrofluazide, chlorthalidone and hydrochlorothiazide in hypertensive patients. In addition, although conventional doses of thiazide diuretics increase insulin resistance, 1.25 mg bendrofluazide, a dose which was equally effective in lowering blood pressure had no effect on insulin resistance.

Hyperinsulinaemia seems to represent a cardiovascular risk factor and is associated with upper body obesity and hypertension. High dose thiazide diuretics have also been associated with an increased incidence of diabetic nephropathy and higher mortality than in those diabetic patients not receiving these drugs. Despite these reservations, low dose diuretics remain a useful option in diabetic patients with hypertension and recent evidence suggests favourable effects on outcome in this group of patients.

Hypomagnesaemia. Many of the problems related to hypokalaemia could in part be due to reduced levels of magnesium. Hypomagnesaemia is, however, rare with doses of hydrochlorothiazide below 100 mg. In general if low doses are used and/or potassium-sparing diuretics are co-administered, hypomagnesaemia should not be a problem.

Hyperuricaemia. Elevations of the serum urate concentrations commonly occur with thiazide diuretics and may precipitate gout in up to 5% of treated patients. Although an elevated uric acid is a marker that often coexists with other cardiovascular risk factors, there is no evidence that it represents an independent risk factor for ischaemic heart disease or stroke. In the short term, increases are dose-related for chlorthalidone, hydrochlorothiazide and cyclopenthiazide. After 1 year of treatment the urate levels tend to be lower.

Hyponatraemia. This occurs much less commonly in hypertensive patients than in those patients with congestive cardiac failure. Severe hyponatraemia is particularly likely to occur in elderly patients with increased water intake or hypothyroidism.

Other adverse effects. Impotence, lethargy, photosensitivity and dizziness have also been described at higher doses. Fever, chills, blood dyscrasias, pancreatitis, necrotising vasculitis, acute interstitial nephritis and non-cardiogenic pulmonary oedema have rarely been seen.

Loop diuretics. Loop diuretics block chloride reabsorption by inhibiting the $Na^+K^+2Cl^-$ co-transport system of the luminal membrane in the thick ascending limb of the loop of Henle (Figure 9.5) where 35–45% of the filtered sodium load is reabsorbed. They have a more rapid onset of action in terms of their diuretic activity than the thiazides and increasing the dose produces increasing diuresis. However, they have no clear advantages over low dose thiazide diuretics in terms of efficacy or adverse effects in the management of hypertension. Their major role is in patients with renal insufficiency or in combination with vasodilator drugs in resistant hypertension.

Adverse effects. Loop diuretics in general cause fewer metabolic problems than longer acting thiazide diuretics and related compounds. In addition to the well-described electrolyte changes, hyperlipidaemia, pancreatitis and allergic reactions have also been described. The risk of eighth nerve damage most commonly occurs with ethacrynic acid and least with bumetanide and is seen mainly in patients with renal impairment who receive high doses.

Potassium-sparing diuretics

These drugs act on the distal tubule to prevent potassium loss and facilitate the excretion of sodium. They either work by directly inhibiting sodium/

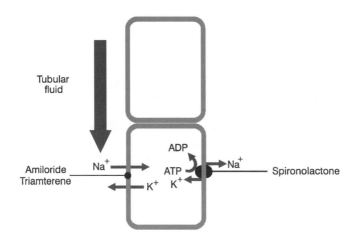

Figure 9.6. Mechanism of action of potassium-sparing diuretics on the distal tubules and collecting ducts. Spironolactone antagonises the effect of aldosterone at the basolateral surface. Amiloride and triamterene interact with lumenal membrane transporter systems. The net effect of both groups of drugs is to decrease sodium absorption and potassium secretion.

potassium exchange mechanisms (triamterene and amiloride) or antag-onising the effects of aldosterone (spironolactone) on the movement of sodium and potassium within the tubule (Figure 9.6). All three are weak diuretics and they are mainly used to reduce the hypokalaemia induced by thiazide and loop diuretics.

Amiloride. Amiloride inhibits a number of transport proteins which are involved in the movement of sodium ions alone or linked with hydrogen and calcium exchange systems. By preventing the entry of sodium into the distal convoluted tubular cells, potassium loss through the potassium channels is reduced.

Use in hypertension. Amiloride has some antihypertensive activity so that as well as reducing potassium loss it may potentiate the effect of thiazide diuretics on blood pressure. It is mainly used with thiazide diuretics and the combination may have some advantages over larger doses of thiazide diuretics in terms of hypokalaemia, arrhythmias and sudden death. Adverse effects include nausea, flatulence and skin rashes. Hyperkal-aemia is, however, the most common and most potentially dangerous adverse effect. Hyponatraemia is also relatively common in elderly patients especially in those with hypothyroidism and poor diet.

Triamterene. Triamterene has similar actions to amiloride. It inhibits potassium loss without hormonal adverse effects. It enhances the natriuretic effect of thiazides while minimising their kaliuretic activity. The drug is generally well tolerated with hyperkalaemia and hyponatraemia being the main adverse effects.

Spironolactone. Spironolactone is a synthetic steroid which binds to a cytoplasmic mineralocorticoid receptor and competitively antagonises the actions of aldosterone on the distal tubule (Figure 9.6). Although the drug is a more effective antihypertensive agent than other potassium-sparing diuretics and is useful in primary and secondary aldosteronism, its role in the treatment of hypertension is severely limited because of the high incidence of impotence and gynaecomastia in men.

Beta adrenoceptor antagonists

Proposed modes of action in hypertension

The precise modes of action of beta adrenoceptor antagonists in lowering blood pressure have been the subject of controversy since their introduction for the treatment of hypertension almost 30 years ago. All currently available beta blockers which lower blood pressure act on the $beta_1$ receptor and those agents which are selective for the $beta_2$ receptor have no significant antihypertensive activity. However, $beta_1$ selective agents are no more effective than non-selective drugs.

Three principal sites of action have been proposed – the nervous, cardiovascular and renin angiotensin systems. The majority of evidence is now against the central or peripheral nervous systems being major sites of action since most beta receptors involved with blood pressure control are of the $beta_2$ subtype. Most evidence now suggests renal and cardiac mechanisms. It is well documented that beta adrenoceptor antagonists lower plasma renin activity and it has been suggested that the fall in blood pressure is related to reduced renin release by the kidney. Although renin activity in the plasma decreases before there is a fall in blood pressure, renin involvement is still possible since the peripheral arterioles contain renin and have a slower turnover than that of the plasma. Subjects with very low renin activity show small reductions in blood pressure while those with very high renin activity show marked blood pressure reductions. However, these extremes form a small proportion of the hypertensive population and for the majority there is no useful relationship between the decrease in renin activity and the fall in blood pressure. In addition, higher plasma levels of beta adrenoceptor antagonists are associated with greater decreases in blood pressure than lower doses but have no additional effects on plasma renin activity, suggesting that if suppression of renin is involved it is not the only factor. The decrease in blood pressure is probably related mostly to decreases in heart rate and cardiac output although there is not a direct relationship between these two measures and blood pressure. Total peripheral resistance increases initially to compensate for the fall in cardiac output but returns to normal or near normal levels as baroreceptor activity declines. With time, cardiac output also tends to increase to near pre-treatment levels. The antihypertensive action of beta adrenoceptor antagonists therefore depends on at least two mechanisms: reduced renin release and a cardiovascular mechanism triggered by reductions in heart rate and cardiac output.

Choice of therapy

Most clinicians now use $beta_1$ selective adrenoceptor antagonists in the management of hypertension because of the lower incidence of adverse effects resulting from blockade of the $beta_2$ receptor. In this country atenolol is the most commonly used agent. The drug is cardioselective, lowers blood pressure throughout the 24-hour period and is eliminated unchanged by the kidney. Metoprolol is also widely used especially in Scandinavia despite variable metabolism and relatively short duration of effect. There are no clear advantages from using drugs with partial agonist activity in the management of hypertension.

Celiprolol is a recently introduced $beta_1$ selective adrenoceptor antagonist with mild $beta_2$ agonist and weak peripheral vasodilator activity. It has comparable antihypertensive efficacy to other beta adrenoceptor antagonists. Although theoretically this drug should be safer than most other beta blockers in asthma, it is generally better to choose a different group of antihypertensive agents. Celiprolol also has more favourable effects on plasma lipids but the importance of this property is unknown in the long-term management of hypertension. The claimed benefits of drugs with additional vasodilator activity such as carvedilol needs to be established in clinical practice and there is little advantage in choosing labetalol, a drug with alpha and beta blocking properties, except in pre-eclampsia and in resistant hypertension.

As with other antihypertensive therapy about 50% of patients demonstrate an adequate response to antihypertensive therapy. Overall, the response to treatment with beta blockers is poorer in Afro-Caribbean groups, but there is little evidence that other groups with low plasma renin levels respond less well to these drugs than to diuretics. Their efficacy in elderly patients with systolic hypertension has been disappointing. They are well tolerated in pregnancy with little evidence of foetal toxicity although delayed intrauterine growth has sometimes been identified.

Advantages

Beta adrenoceptor antagonists have additional beneficial effects which make them suitable for use in certain groups of hypertensive patients. They are particularly useful in patients with anxiety and related symptoms, especially those drugs which are highly lipid soluble and penetrate the central nervous system, such as propranolol. Patients with angina pectoris and arrhythmias as well as hypertension are particularly likely to benefit. In addition beta adrenoceptor antagonists reduce the incidence of reinfarction after an acute myocardial infarction although their role in primary prevention has still to be determined.

The value of beta blockers in reducing stroke and cardiovascular disease compared with diuretics is difficult to assess from the large intervention studies. In the Medical Research Council studies on the middle-aged and elderly, the beta adrenoceptor antagonists were less effective than the diuretics. Propranolol also had no impact on coronary events in smokers. However, in the MAPHY study (Metoprolol Atherosclerosis Prevention in Hypertensives Study, *Am. J. Hypertens.*, 1991; **4**: 151–8) metoprolol was more effective in reducing total mortality than the diuretic. In general beta blockers and diuretics are equally effective in lowering blood pressure but there may be a slight advantage in favour of diuretics, especially in preventing stroke. As previously stated these two groups of antihypertensive agents have been shown to reduce stroke and cardiovascular events, although there is preliminary evidence that dihydropyridine calcium antagonists may also be effective.

Combinations

In combination the antihypertensive effects of beta adrenoceptor antagonists are additive with most other agents. The combination with thiazide diuretic controls moderate to severe hypertension in about 60% of patients. They also reduce the adverse effects of the dihydropyridine calcium channel antagonists related to peripheral vasodilatation. This combination is particularly valuable in patients with hypertension and angina pectoris.

Calcium channel antagonists

The first reports documenting the antihypertensive effects of calcium channel antagonists appeared in the late 1960s, but there was little interest in their role as antihypertensive agents for almost a decade. All members of the group lower blood pressure by dilating the peripheral resistance arterioles. The decreases in blood pressure have been shown to be proportional to the pre-treatment blood pressure and plasma noradrenaline levels. An increase in sympathetic tone occurs as a result of increased baroreceptor activity, particularly with the dihydropyridine group of calcium antagonists. All calcium antagonists have direct negative inotropic and chronotropic effects although for the new dihydropyridines these effects are small. However, the haemodynamic profiles of the individual calcium antagonists differ substantially depending on their relative activity in different parts of the cardiovascular system and the balance between their various direct or indirect cardiac and vascular actions.

Verapamil

Verapamil produces a dose-dependent reduction in systolic and diastolic blood pressure in doses of 80–160 mg given three times daily. Its antihypertensive activity is similar to beta adrenoceptor antagonists and although it reduces heart rate particularly after exercise, this tends to be less than with beta blocking drugs. Verapamil in contrast to nifedipine and other dihydropyridines slows atrioventricular conduction and lengthens the PR interval. To avoid the inconvenience of multiple dosing, sustained release preparations are now available with comparable antihypertensive efficacy. Clinical evidence suggests that 120 mg twice daily of slow release verapamil is equivalent to 80 mg three times daily with conventional formulation. In general, verapamil combines well with other antihypertensive agents such as diuretics and ACE inhibitors. When given as an intravenous bolus injection to patients with conduction abnormalities caused by disease or beta blockers, sudden death has been reported. Few problems have been clearly documented in hypertensive patients. Although substantial decreases in heart rate and prolongation of the *PR* interval have been described, only one or two episodes of second degree heart block have been recorded in this group of patients. Until more data are available, however, the combination of verapamil and a beta blocker should be used with caution and only in patients with normal atrioventricular conduction, satisfactory left ventricular function and with no previous history of the sick sinus syndrome. Adverse vasodilator effects are less common than with the dihydropyridines but constipation is more common.

Diltiazem

In several comparative clinical studies, conventional diltiazem given in divided doses four times daily or as a sustained release preparation given twice daily has comparable antihypertensive activity to most other antihypertensive agents, and in a recent comparative study involving a diuretic, an ACE inhibitor, a beta adrenoceptor antagonist and a selective alpha adrenoceptor antagonist, diltiazem was the most effective antihypertensive agent. Like verapamil, resting heart rate is reduced but to a lesser degree than with most beta blockers. As with verapamil, diltiazem should not be administered in the presence of atrioventricular block, sino-atrial block or sick sinus syndrome. Adverse effects are uncommon and are mainly ankle swelling, abdominal discomfort and constipation, all of which are dose related. The more severe adverse effects are similar to verapamil, i.e. impaired atrioventricular conduction especially in patients with conduction abnormalities. Myocardial depression, however, is less of a problem. Care is necessary when diltiazem is combined with beta adrenoceptor antagonists, antiarrhythmic drugs and anaesthetic agents due to increased cardiodepressant effects on conduction and contractility. Plasma digoxin levels are increased by diltiazem.

Nifedipine

Daily treatment of mild to moderate hypertension with 10–20 mg of nifedipine given four times daily results in sustained reductions of blood pressure over a 24-hour period without evidence of postural hypotension. Unlike earlier vasodilator antihypertensive drugs, long-term therapy does not result in tolerance, sodium retention, plasma volume expansion or angina pectoris. The direct depressant effect on the myocardium is usually balanced by reflex tachycardia and a reduction in afterload. It therefore rarely causes heart failure. Longer acting preparations which can be administered once or twice daily are now available for the treatment of hypertension. Nifedipine combines very well with beta adrenoceptor antagonists and does not produce the problems with conduction seen with verapamil and diltiazem. The adverse peripheral vasodilator effects are reduced when the drug is combined with beta adrenoceptor antagonists and less impairment of physical performance has been found with the combination than with a beta blocker alone. Severe adverse effects – hypotension and depressed cardiac function – are rare and occur only in patients with severe underlying cardiac disease. Nifedipine also appears to be a useful agent in lowering blood pressure in acute hypertensive emergencies and in patients undergoing dialysis for acute and chronic renal failure. There have been recent worries that short-acting nifedipine may increase the incidence of myocardial infarction. For this reason capsular nifedipine is not recommended for the long-term treatment of hypertension and angina pectoris.

Other dihydropyridine calcium channel antagonists

The large majority of new calcium channel antagonists are structurally related to nifedipine and are referred to as the dihydropyridines. They are widely used in the treatment of hypertension and have similar effects to nifedipine. They have been developed because they appear to have greater affinity for peripheral vascular smooth muscle than cardiac muscle. Although experimental evidence suggests that several of these agents have less depressant effects on cardiac function, clear advantages over nifedipine have rarely been demonstrated in patients with poor cardiac reserve. Amlodipine, however, has recently been shown to produce favourable effects in congestive cardiomyopathy and no detrimental effects in patients with heart failure due to ischaemic heart disease.

Nicardipine

Nicardipine is well absorbed from the gastrointestinal tract, but like nifedipine has a low bioavailability due to extensive first-pass metabolism in the liver. The duration of effect is short so that the drug needs to be given three times daily and twice daily therapy has been shown to be ineffective. Animal studies suggest that nicardipine depresses myocardial function less than nifedipine, but it seems unlikely that the drug has any major advantages over nifedipine and the drug is contraindicated in patients with congestive cardiac failure and/or impaired left ventricular function. Early clinical studies suggested a lower incidence of flushing, headache and peripheral oedema than with nifedipine, but this has still to be confirmed in large population studies.

Amlodipine

Amlodipine's pharmacokinetic profile appears more favourable than other members of the dihydropyridine group for the treatment of hypertension. The time to peak concentration is relatively long, first-pass metabolism is minimal and the elimination half-life is about 35 hours. As a result the drug can be administered once daily. The drug's antihypertensive activity is comparable to atenolol, hydrochlorothiazide and other calcium channel antagonists. Unlike nifedipine, the blood pressure lowering effect is not accompanied by significant increases in heart rate and the drug appears to have fewer "vasodilator" adverse effects. Its safety in heart failure is now established.

Isradipine

Isradipine is readily absorbed from the gut with peak concentrations occurring after 2 hours. The duration of the drug's antihypertensive action varies from 12 to 21 hours and isradipine is therefore administered twice daily. Adverse effects are dose related and when doses >10 mg are used, their incidence is the same as nifedipine.

Felodipine

Felodipine is another vascular-selective dihydropyridine calcium antagonist which is available as an extended release formulation suitable for once daily administration. As monotherapy in mild to moderate hypertension it is as effective as other calcium antagonists, beta blockers, diuretics and ACE inhibitors. Adverse effects are comparable to other vascular selective dihydropyridines. Preliminary data indicate that felodipine may also be clinically useful in patients with congestive heart failure and the drug is currently under investigation for this condition.

ACE inhibitors

All currently available ACE inhibitors reduce blood pressure in patients with essential and renal hypertension. Patients with high plasma renin activity show the greatest decreases in blood pressure but reductions also occur in those with low plasma renin activity and in anephric subjects. ACE inhibitors offer an important option in the treatment of hypertension either as first-line treatment in diabetic patients or when other established drugs are contraindicated, poorly tolerated or when they do not have the desired

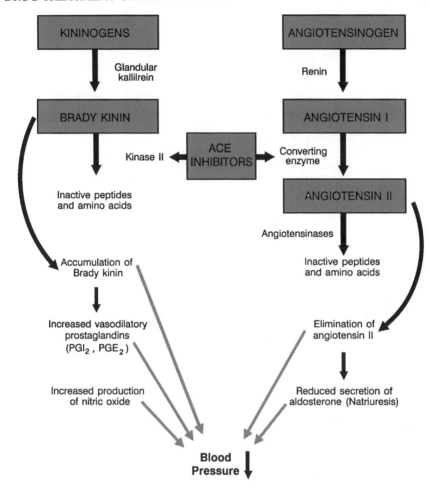

Figure 9.7. Mechanisms by which ACE inhibitors lower blood pressure.

therapeutic effect. Repeated clinical studies have demonstrated the efficacy of ACE inhibitors in lowering blood pressure and their ability to reduce left ventricular hypertrophy.

As monotherapy, these drugs have comparable efficacy to beta adrenoceptor antagonists and diuretics, although some large-scale studies have shown greater reductions in systolic blood pressure probably related to greater effects on arterial compliance. There is some evidence that longer-acting ACE inhibitors provide better control of blood pressure than short-acting drugs.

Table 9.7. Distribution of angiotensin converting enzyme inhibitors in different tissues and the possible role of enzyme inhibition

Tissue	Possible role of ACE inhibition
Lung	Contains very high concentrations of converting enzyme. Inhibition in the lung may be the cause of cough
Central nervous system	Reduced central sympathetic outflow may be due to ACE inhibition in the central nervous system
Kidney	Dilatation of the efferent arteriole decreases intraglomerular pressure, reducing microalbuminuria, delaying the development of diabetic nephropathy and predisposing to acute renal failure in conditions associated with low renal perfusion
Heart	Reduction of ventricular hypertrophy by direct effect on cardiac ACE. Reduction in arrhythmias
Arterial wall	Increased arterial compliance and myointimal proliferation

Mode of action

ACE inhibitors block the conversion of the inactive decapeptide angiotensin I to the active vasoconstrictor octapeptide angiotensin II (Figure 9.7). Reductions in angiotensin II levels produce a relative decrease in circulating aldosterone concentrations facilitating sodium loss and potassium retention. Plasma renin activity and angiotensin I levels tend to rise with chronic therapy and angiotensin II levels may increase as a result. ACE inhibitors prevent the breakdown of kinins, locally formed vasodilator peptides which not only have a vasodilatory action but also stimulate the synthesis of vasodilatory prostaglandins. Captopril may also produce vasodilatory prostaglandins by direct stimulation of cell membrane phospholipase. Kinins and prostaglandins may be involved in the antihypertensive effect of ACE inhibitors and the newly developed receptor antagonists, which do not affect these systems, should provide us with an answer. Endothelium-dependent vasodilatation is also improved by captopril. A central mechanism has also been postulated since naloxone blunts the antihypertensive effect of ACE inhibitors, but it is unlikely that this is of clinical importance.

ACE is found in most body tissues. ACE inhibitors appear to inhibit the enzyme in all these tissues but to a varying degree, depending on the amount of enzyme and the relative tissue penetration. Inhibition of ACE in different tissues could account for some of the effects seen with these drugs (Table 9.7). Unlike most other peripheral vasodilator drugs, ACE inhibitors do not cause reflex increases in heart rate. The reasons are unclear but may be related to reduced sympathetic tone or increased parasympathetic activity. In uncomplicated hypertension, renal perfusion is unaffected or slightly improved by ACE inhibition. In patients with congestive cardiac failure renal perfusion may decline to critical levels, especially in the more severe forms of this disease.

Pharmacokinetics

Most differences between ACE inhibitors relate to different rates of absorption, metabolism and renal excretion. Captopril and lisinopril are active as the parent compound but the majority require conversion to the active form in the liver. All are eliminated by the kidney as the parent compound or active metabolite, although fosinopril is significantly metabolised to the inactive form by the liver. These differences alter the speed of onset and the duration of effect in hypertension.

Captopril is rapidly absorbed following oral administration. A large proportion binds to tissue and plasma proteins or other sulphydryl-containing molecules by forming S–S bonds. This "reservoir effect" means that the antihypertensive effect lasts longer than would be predicted from its short elimination half-life, especially with long-term treatment. It has a rapid onset of action and plasma concentrations can be detected within 15 minutes of oral administration in fasting healthy volunteers. The presence of food appears to have little effect on absorption. Captopril is partially oxidised at the sulphydryl group to several metabolites such as the disulphide dimer of captopril, and other mixed disulphides with endogenous thiol compounds. Captopril and its metabolites are primarily excreted in the urine with minor elimination in the faeces (Table 9.8).

Most currently available ACE inhibitors are pro drugs, i.e. they are converted to their active form in the liver. Compounds converted to the active di-acid metabolite include, cilazapril, enalapril, fosinopril, perindopril, quinapril and ramapril (Table 9.8). The pharmacokinetics of pro-drug ACE inhibitors is exemplified by enalapril, the second drug to be available clinically for the treatment of hypertension. The parent drug is well absorbed after oral administration and reaches a peak about 1 hour later, decreasing rapidly as the active metabolite, enalaprilat, is formed in the liver. This means that the onset of action is relatively slow. Enalapril is slowly removed from the plasma through the kidney without further metabolism. The plasma elimination half-life is about 11 hours. Other pro-drugs show similar behaviour although quinapril and ramipril may undergo further metabolism (Table 9.8). Fosinopril, on the other hand, is conjugated in the liver to a significant degree to the beta glucuronide and a substantial amount is excreted in the bile. This dual method of excretion may have some advantages in patients with severely impaired renal function.

Table 9.8. Pharmacokinetic values of angiotensin converting enzyme inhibitors

	Captopril	Cilazapril	Enalapril	Fosinopril	Lisinopril	Perindopril	Quinapril	Ramapril
Duration of action	Acute effects 4 hours Long-term effects 12–24 hours	≈24 hours	≈24 hours	12–24 hours	24–36 hours	12–24 hours	12–24 hours	>24 hours
Time to onset of action	20–60 minutes	1–2 hours	<1 hour	≈1 hour	<2 hours	<2 hours	≈30 minutes	1–2 hours
Time to peak	1–1½ hours	≈2 hours	≈4 hours	3–6 hours	5–7 hours	2–4 hours	2–3 hours	3 hours
Plasma half-life	2 hours (free captopril)	9 hours	11 hours	12 hours	13 hours	9 hours	1–2 hours	>13 hours
Metabolism	Mainly unchanged	Converted to cilazaprilat in the liver	Converted to enalaprilat in the liver	Converted to fosinoprilat in the liver. Conjugated to beta glucuronide	No significant metabolism	Converted to perindoprilat in the liver	Converted to quinaprilat and two minor metabolites	Converted to ramaprilat in the liver. Conjugated to two further metabolites
Oral bio-availability (%)	70	60	40	30	30	10	30	40–60
Excretion	Renal as captopril or disulphides	Renal as cilazapril and cilazaprilat	Renal as enalapril and enalaprilat	Eliminated by renal and oral routes	Renal as lisinopril	Renal as perindoprilat	Renal as quinaprilat and quinaprilat	Renal as ramapril, ramaprilat and to conjugated metabolites

All ACE inhibitors are cleared, at least in part by the kidney. This may occur by glomerular filtration alone, e.g. lisinopril or by a combination of glomerular filtration and active tubular secretion (captopril, enalapril). Despite these differences, ACE inhibitors are remarkably similar in their clinical effects, and differ only in terms of the speed of onset and duration of effect. This clearly affects the frequency with which the drugs need to be prescribed. Most ACE inhibitors can be given once daily for the treatment of hypertension – enalapril, lisinopril, cilazapril, fosinopril, perindopril, and ramipril. The duration of action of quinapril is approximately intermediate between that of captopril and enalapril. It is probably effective in most patients when given as a single daily dose, but some patients will require twice dosing to ensure adequate 24-hour control of blood pressure. Captopril should always be administered in divided doses. The majority will show an adequate response to twice daily dosing but in some patients with hypertension doses given three times daily are required.

Pharmacodynamics in hypertensive patients

The antihypertensive efficacy of ACE inhibitors has been documented in numerous comparative studies with placebo and with other antihypertensive drugs. It is worth noting that the antihypertensive doses of captopril have been constantly reduced over the years and are now about one-tenth of those which were used in the early clinical studies. All other ACE inhibitors were introduced at lower dosage partly due to the greater potency determined in pre-clinical studies and partly due to lessons learned from previous experience with the adverse effects of captopril at high dose. For the ACE inhibitors tested so far about 50–70% of patients achieve adequate control. The addition of a diuretic provides adequate blood pressure control in most of the remaining patients.

When ACE inhibitors and diuretics are combined, it is often possible to reduce the doses used as monotherapy. Diuretics stimulate the renin–angiotensin–aldosterone system so that blood pressure control is more dependent on the activation of that system. Inhibitors of ACE tend to be more effective in lowering blood pressure and therefore exert a degree of synergism. Patients with primary hyperaldosteronism respond poorly to ACE inhibitors especially if this is due to an adrenal adenoma. Renal hypertension frequently responds well to this form of therapy provided appropriate precautions are taken beforehand to exclude renovascular disease. ACE inhibitors exert their principal antihypertensive effects by reducing vascular tone in large arteries and resistance vessels. In hypertensive patients, cardiac function remains largely unchanged during chronic therapy. The lack of reflex tachycardia has been attributed to resetting of the baroreceptor reflex without alteration in reflex sensitivity.

Renal effects

The effects of ACE inhibitors in renovascular hypertension have been a matter of great interest both clinically and experimentally. In renal artery stenosis, renal perfusion pressure is reduced to levels of 70–80 mmHg. To compensate, renal autoregulation results in progressive increases in efferent glomerular tone largely due to increased angiotensin II activity. In bilateral renal artery stenosis or stenosis in a solitary kidney, decreases in renal blood flow and elevation in serum creatinine have been observed during ACE inhibitor therapy. These adverse effects are more likely to occur if hypovolaemia is present usually as a result of previous diuretic therapy.

In patients with hypertension and normal renal function the overall effect, however, is to increase renal blood flow despite a decrease in perfusion pressure. Renal vasodilatation has been observed at doses which do not have significant effects on total peripheral resistance. In patients with hypertension and impaired renal function, the effect is more variable. In general, renal function does not deteriorate provided the patient is not volume depleted and there is no evidence of underlying renovascular disease. In other patients, improvements in glomerular filtration and serum creatinine may occur.

CNS effects

The effects of ACE inhibitors on the central nervous system are more difficult to determine. ACE is present in brain tissue and there is evidence from animal work that brain-converting enzyme can be inhibited following acute and chronic systemic treatment. Whether this inhibition contributes to the cardiovascular actions of ACE inhibitors is open to debate. The early changes in fluid and electrolyte balance and the sensitisation of the baroreceptor reflex may be related to inhibition of angiotensin II formation with brain tissue. We do not, as yet, know whether ACE inhibitors penetrate the blood–brain barrier in sufficient amounts to exert their inhibitory actions on the brain. It is possible, however, that effects on brain structures outside the blood–brain barrier could reduce the supply of endogenous angiotensin II for pathways involved in blood pressure control and reduce blood pressure by this mechanism.

Possible clinical advantages for ACE inhibitors

Quality of life

A recent study involving 626 men with mild to moderate hypertension found that, while captopril, propranolol and methyldopa were equally effective in reducing blood pressure, captopril showed the greatest improvements in quality of life. Patients taking captopril, as compared with those taking methyldopa scored significantly higher on measures of well-being, had fewer adverse effects and had better scores of life satisfaction, work performance and visual-motor functioning. When compared with propranolol, patients taking captopril had fewer adverse effects, less sexual dysfunction and greater improvement in measures of general well-being. The choice of comparator drugs in this study is somewhat surprising. When the study was performed, neither propranolol nor methyldopa was considered a drug of first choice and both had previously been shown to have a high incidence of adverse effects. In addition, cough, now known to be the commonest adverse effect of captopril, was not reported as an adverse effect. In a recent comparative study of lower doses of chlorthalidone, acebutolol and enalapril, the diuretic and beta blocker were at least as well tolerated as enalapril in terms of quality of life and incidence of adverse effects. Apart from cough, ACE inhibitors have a low incidence of adverse effects and are generally well tolerated. It is unlikely, however, that they are better tolerated than the currently recommended doses of other widely used antihypertensive agents such as selective alpha blockers, calcium channel antagonists, beta$_1$ selective adrenoceptor antagonists and thiazide diuretics.

Favourable metabolic profile

ACE inhibitors have a neutral effect on plasma lipids, conserve potassium and magnesium and reduce insulin resistance in hypertensive patients. They may also attenuate the hypokalaemia and hyperuricaemia caused by thiazide and loop diuretics. These additional beneficial properties may well represent important advantages over other forms of antihypertensive therapy, but the long-term advantages have not as yet been shown in comparative studies looking at clinical outcome and incidence of adverse effects.

Regression of left ventricular hypertrophy

Left ventricular hypertrophy in patients with hypertension is an important risk factor for morbidity and mortality. Two recent meta analyses concluded that ACE inhibitors were more effective than most other antihypertensive drugs in reducing left ventricular mass. Animal data also suggest that angiotensin II is an important factor in causing hypertrophy in the myocardium and resistance vessels. However, beta adrenoceptors effectively reduce left ventricular mass and the studies with diuretics were either too short, too small or used inappropriately high doses for useful information to be obtained. In addition two recent comparative studies failed to demonstrate any advantage of ACE inhibitors in reducing left ventricular mass compared to other commonly used antihypertensive agents. Left ventricular hypertrophy is an important risk factor for the development of complications in hypertensive patients and reduction of left ventricular hypertrophy is probably beneficial. Whether ACE inhibitors have any advantages over other therapies has still to be demonstrated.

Systolic hypertension

ACE inhibitors are effective in reducing systolic blood pressure. The importance of systolic hypertension as a major risk factor and the favourable outcome of studies in elderly patients with isolated systolic hypertension suggest that the treatment of systolic hypertension should have increasing priority in the years ahead. Diuretics and dihydropyridine calcium antagonists are the first-line agents for this condition, but the addition of ACE inhibitors should be beneficial in the treatment of more resistant cases.

Diabetic patients

ACE inhibitors are not associated with the detrimental metabolic effects on plasma glucose, lipids and electrolytes seen with higher doses of thiazide diuretics or the prolonged hypoglycaemia sometimes seen with non-selective beta adrenoceptor antagonists. They can be safely used in most patients with diabetes. In addition there is growing evidence in insulin dependent diabetics that these agents reduce albuminuria and delay the development of diabetic nephropathy in hypertensive and normotensive patients. This and the observation that ACE inhibitors reduce insulin resistance reinforces the case for their use in diabetic patients. It seems likely that they will become valuable first-line therapy for diabetic patients with hypertension, although recent data demonstrated that captopril and atenolol were equally effective in reducing the renal and eye complications of diabetic patients with hypertension.

Combination therapy

ACE inhibitors can be usefully combined with most other antihypertensive agents with good effect. An additive or possibly synergistic effect has been described with thiazide and loop diuretics. Changes in serum potassium are quite variable on this combination and it is important to check the potassium regularly during chronic therapy. Reducing dietary salt intake can also increase the antihypertensive effect of ACE inhibitors although profound hypotension can result when patients become severely salt-depleted.

Adverse effects

When captopril was first introduced into clinical practice for the treatment of hypertension it was considered to have such serious adverse effects that it could only be used in hypertension resistant to other forms of therapy. Neutropenia, serious renal damage with proteinuria, skin rashes, loss of taste and angio-oedema were identified. Most of these adverse effects were related to the high doses employed when the drug was first used and are rarely, if ever, seen at the currently recommended doses. Angio-oedema, however, remains a truly serious and relatively specific adverse effect.

Class adverse effects

Cough

> The cough usually starts with a tickling sensation in the throat and is persistent, dry and on occasions severe enough to cause vomiting
>
> Yeo and Ramsay (1990)

The most common and irritating adverse effect of ACE inhibitors is cough which occurs in 3–22% of patients receiving the drug depending on the method used to detect the condition. The cough is persistent, non-productive and is often worse when the patient is lying flat. The incidence is greater in women than in men and can be delayed for up to 24 months after starting therapy. It is more commonly reported in non-smokers and is probably dose-related although reducing the dose is rarely successful in preventing cough. It is also unlikely that changing to another ACE inhibitor will reduce the likelihood of cough although post-marketing surveillance data suggest a higher incidence with enalapril than with captopril, or cilazapril. Sulindac and probably other non-steroidal anti-inflammatory drugs appear to reduce the severity and frequency of the cough, but there is a real risk that the antihypertensive activity will be compromised. The angiotensin II receptor antagonists which should have the same advantages as ACE inhibitors, do not cause cough. At present they seem to be the ideal solution in patients who require ACE inhibitors but are unable to tolerate them because of persistent cough.

Hypotension

Although profound hypotension is most commonly seen when ACE inhibitors are used to treat congestive cardiac failure, severe hypotension is also likely to occur in patients with hypertension whose renin angiotensin system is activated as a result of renovascular disease or intensive diuretic therapy. It is most likely to occur after the first dose but can occur after the second and third doses. It is unusual during chronic therapy. The mechanism is not fully understood but seems to involve venodilatation as well as arteriolar dilatation and the absence of reflex tachycardia suggests a parasympathomimetic action similar to vasovagal syncope. The patients with hypertension who are most at risk are those with renin-dependent hypertension, malignant hypertension, renovascular and other causes of secondary hypertension. These patients usually have clinical evidence of renal disease and hypotension is rare in patients with uncomplicated mild to moderate hypertension. There is recent evidence that perindopril is less likely to decrease blood pressure compared with captopril and enalapril after the first dose for the same degree of ACE inhibition in elderly patients with congestive cardiac failure. If the absence of first-dose hypotension is confirmed in larger studies, this agent could become the drug of first choice as initial therapy in "at risk" patients.

Acute renal insufficiency

Acute renal insufficiency has been most commonly described in patients with bilateral renal artery stenosis treated with ACE inhibitors. To maintain glomerular filtration in this condition, marked efferent glomerular arteriolar tone is achieved by high levels of angiotensin II. ACE inhibition removes this tone and decreases the glomerular filtration rate. In the presence of bilateral renal artery stenosis, renal blood flow cannot increase. A similar problem can occur in patients with unilateral renal artery stenosis especially in a single kidney. In patients with severe congestive heart failure in which renal perfusion is decreased bilaterally, due to atheroma, a similar problem can occur when systemic blood pressure decreases. This condition is usually reversible and is less marked if diuretic therapy is reduced before the ACE inhibitor is started.

Hyperkalaemia

ACE inhibitors decrease the release of aldosterone from the adrenal cortex by reducing angiotensin II levels and hence increase serum potassium levels. This is usually mild, but can cause problems in patients with renal impairment receiving potassium supplements or potassium-sparing diuretics and in elderly patients with heart failure.

Angioedema

Although very rare, this is a serious adverse effect. It usually occurs after the first dose or at least within 48 hours of starting therapy. It is characterised by swelling of the tongue, pharynx and vocal cords and is often accompanied by tender swellings in the skin or an urticarial rash. It may be due to subcutaneous effects of kinins, in which case it should not occur with angiotensin II receptor antagonists. Emergency adrenaline may be required to relieve vocal cord oedema.

Adverse effects initially described with high dose captopril therapy

Neutropenia

Neutropenia has only been linked convincingly to high dose captopril therapy and then mostly in patients with connective tissue disease. Neutropenia has been reported following the use of other ACE inhibitors but the incidence is no higher than would normally occur by chance.

Proteinuria

Proteinuria was reported to occur in about 1% of patients receiving captopril, almost all at high dose (more than 150 mg/day) and in patients with pre-existing renal disease.

Impaired taste

Impaired taste also appears to be dose related and was reported to occur with captopril in between 2% and 7% per cent of patients treated with the drug. It is rare at the currently recommended doses. Severe cutaneous reactions also seem to be more common with high dose captopril therapy.

Contraindications

From the renal complications previously described it follows that bilateral renal artery stenosis and unilateral renal artery stenosis in a single kidney are contraindications to the use of ACE inhibitors. ACE inhibitors should also be avoided in patients with severe aortic stenosis due to their effects in reducing afterload. However, they can exert a beneficial effect in patients with milder degrees of aortic stenosis associated with left ventricular failure. Careful observation after starting therapy is clearly required. A few early reports suggested that captopril might have a teratogenic effect so that its use was prohibited in pregnant patients. None of the new ACE inhibitors has been tested in pregnancy, and therefore this is a contraindication or

Table 9.9. Pharmacokinetic values of angiotensin II receptor antagonists

Drugs	Candesartan	Eprosartan	Irbesartan	Losartan	Valsartan
Duration of effect	≤24 hours	≤34 hours	≤36 hours	≤24 hours	≤24 hours
Time to onset of effect	20 minutes	1 hour	1 hour	20 minutes	1 hour
Time to peak action	2–3 hours	3 hours	2 hours	2 hours	4 hours
Plasma half-life	5–11 hours	5–7 hours	1–15 hours	1.5–2.5 hours	5–9 hours
Metabolism	Converted to the active carboxylic acid metabolite	20% metabolised to acyl glucuronide	Acts largely as parent compound	Rapid metabolism to active metabolite	Little metabolism
Oral bioavailability %	19–28	15	60–80	12–67	≈25
Excretion	50% excreted as parent compound and metabolite	10–40% excreted as the parent compound and metabolite	20% of parent compound is excreted in the urine	<5% excreted in the urine	10% of the parent compound and metabolite in the urine

Table 9.10. Principal tissue distribution and function of angiotensin II receptor subtypes

Tissue	Subtype AT_1	Subtype AT_2
Heart	Contractility Hypertrophy	Inhibition of collagenase Antiproliferation
Vasculature	Contraction Hypertrophy Hyperplasia Angiogenesis	Inhibition of angiotenesis Antiproliferation
Brain	Blood pressure elevation Vasopressin release	Thirst Prostaglandin release
Autonomic nervous system	Beta adrenergic stimulation Vagal suppression	— —
Adrenal glands	Aldosterone biosynthesis Catecholamine secretion	— —
Kidneys	Inhibition of renin release Proximal sodium transport Afferent and efferent vasoconstriction	Proximal sodium transport

relative contraindication to their use. Chronic cough but not asthma is also a relative contraindication.

Drug interactions

The most important drug interactions with ACE inhibitors are with potassium-sparing diuretics and potassium supplements, increasing the risk of hyperkalaemia in patients with impaired renal function. Non-steroidal anti-inflammatory drugs blunt the antihypertensive effect of a variety of antihypertensive drugs including ACE inhibitors. Since these drugs can cause deterioration in renal function in patients with poor renal reserve, the combination with ACE inhibitors is likely to be problematical and should be avoided if possible. Other renal interactions of note are the impaired renal clearance of digoxin caused by captopril, increasing steady-state levels by about 30%, and decreased captopril excretion caused by probenecid.

Angiotensin II receptor antagonists

Peptide analogues of angiotensin II have been available for more than 20 years, but were of no clinical benefit due to the extremely low oral

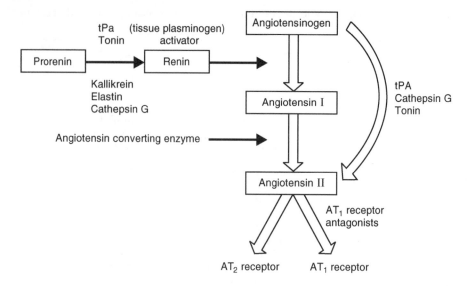

Figure 9.8.   Circulating and tissue enzyme pathways for angiotensin II production and site of action of angiotensin II antagonists.

bioavailability, brief duration of effect and partial agonist activity. Non-peptide, angiotensin II antagonists were developed by innovative chemical modification of the imidazole derivative. This resulted in a number of potent orally active analogues with high specificity and affinity for the angiotensin II receptor. The principal members of the group are listed in Table 9.9.

Mode of action

Angiotensin II produces its effect by stimulating cell membrane subtypes AT1 and AT2. The distribution and proposed mechanisms of these receptors are outlined in Table 9.10. All important cardiovascular effects of angiotensin II receptor antagonists are mediated at the AT1 receptor and all currently available antagonists act principally at this receptor. These agents are also highly specific for the AT1 receptor so that there are no significant effects on pathways outside the renin–angiotensin–aldosterone system such as brady-kinin metabolism (Figure 9.8). Displacement of angiotensin II from the AT1 receptor antagonises angiotensin II induced smooth muscle contraction, aldosterone and catecholamine release, cell growth and proliferation. Blood pressure is reduced in a dose-dependent manner. Angiotensin receptor antagonists demonstrate competitive and non-competitive antagonism at the receptor. Losartan and eprosartan exhibit competitive antagonism, i.e. they cause parallel rightward shifts of the pressor responses to angiotensin II. Candesartan, irbesartan, valsartan and the active metabolite of losartan, EXP 3174, exhibit non-competitive antagonism, i.e. they cause reduced maximal responses and non-parallel rightward shifts of the dose–response relationship.

Pharmacokinetics

Pharmacokinetic values of the principal angiotensin receptor antagonists are listed in Table 9.9. They are all well absorbed following oral administration and undergo hepatic metabolism to active and inactive metabolites which are eliminated in the bile or through the kidney. Losartan, the parent compound, is pharmacologically active but is metabolised to a longer acting and more active compound following hepatic first-pass metabolism. A small number of subjects ($<1\%$) are deficient in the enzyme which converts losartan to EXP 3174. Candesartan cilexetil is an ester pro drug which is converted by the liver to the active carboxylic acid metabolite, candesartan. Plasma concentrations relate to the blood pressure lowering effect up to 15 mg of the drug, but above this dose the effect is less than expected. Irbesartan exhibits linear kinetics over the dose range and alterations in dose are probably not required in renal or liver disease. Dose reductions are required with valsartan and losartan in chronic liver disease.

Pharmacodynamics

Antagonism at the AT_1 receptor results in a dose-related increase in renin and angiotensin II with a variable effect on aldosterone. Blood pressure is progressively reduced over the dose range of most agents secondary to peripheral vasodilatation with no increase in heart rate. All agents which are clinically available are effective over the 24-hour period with trough to peak ratios between 50% and 75%. There is preliminary evidence that 16 mg candesartan cilexetil has greater antihypertensive effect than 50 mg losartan at 24 hours.

Animal studies have shown that angiotensin receptor antagonists have beneficial effects on cardiovascular structure. Reduction in cardiac and vascular hyperplasia, interstitial fibrosis and hypertrophy, similar to those seen with ACE inhibitors has been described. Whether angiotensin II receptor antagonists will prove more effective than other antihypertensives depends on the results of long-term outcome studies. The results of clinical trials in congestive cardiac failure, renal disease and following acute myocardial infarction are also awaited with interest.

Adverse effects and interactions

Angiotensin II receptor antagonists are a very well tolerated group of compounds with an overall incidence of adverse effects and withdrawals due to adverse effects similar to those of placebo. Cough is no more common than placebo and supports the theory that ACE inhibitor cough is mediated by increased levels of bradykinin. Serious adverse effects on blood pressure after the first dose, acute renal failure and hyperkalaemia due to inhibition of the renin angiotensin system are not expected to be different from ACE inhibitors. They are not recommended in pregnancy because of the increased risk of foetal or neonatal malformation and death.

The only important interactions likely to occur are with large doses of loop diuretics predisposing to hypotension and hyperkalaemia caused by co-administration of potassium, potassium-sparing diuretics and non-steroidal anti-inflammatory drugs.

Alpha adrenoceptor antagonists

Alpha adrenoceptors can be divided into two subtypes: alpha$_1$ and alpha$_2$. This subclassification is based on the affinity of selective agonists and antagonists for these two subtypes. Adrenoceptors are also defined in terms of their localisation within the synapse. Pre-synaptic receptors are located on the sympathetic nerve ending and post-synaptic on the target organ, e.g. blood vessel (Figure 9.9). The distribution of these receptors is illustrated in Table 9.10.

Mode of action

Stimulation of the alpha$_1$ adrenoceptors at post-synaptic sites causes vasoconstriction, increases peripheral resistance and hence blood pressure (Table 9.11). Drugs which block the alpha$_1$ adrenoceptors are therefore effective peripheral vasodilators and antihypertensive agents. Non-selective alpha blockers, i.e. those which antagonise the alpha$_1$ and the alpha$_2$ receptor are of little value in the treatment of hypertension because of their propensity to cause tachycardia and blunt the antihypertensive effect due to alpha$_1$ adrenoceptor blockade. Noradrenaline released from the sympathetic nerve ending stimulates the post-synaptic alpha$_1$ receptor to increase blood pressure and the alpha$_2$ pre-synaptic receptor to inhibit the further release of noradrenaline. By antagonising the alpha$_1$ and alpha$_2$ receptors, blood pressure decreases, but the continued release of noradrenaline stimulates the post-synaptic beta$_1$ receptors to increase heart rate (Figure 9.9). On the other hand, drugs such as prazosin and doxazosin selectively block the post-synaptic alpha$_1$ receptor but do not facilitate the

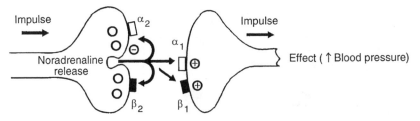

Figure 9.9. Proposed mode of action of alpha antagonists. 1. Non-selective: block alpha₁ and alpha₂ resulting in increased noradrenaline release. 2. Selective: block post-synaptic alpha₁ without preventing the inhibitory effect of the alpha₂ receptor on noradrenaline release.

Table 9.11. Distribution of alpha adrenoceptors and the effect of stimulation

Receptor sub-type	Organ/system	Response to stimulation
Alpha₁ (post-synaptic)	Blood vessels	Contraction
	Heart	Increased force of contraction
	Eye	Mydriasis, increased intraocular pressure
	Central nervous system	Inhibition of afferent inputs to the baroreceptor
Alpha₁ (pre-synaptic)	Gastrointestinal tract	Inhibition of motility
Alpha₂ (post-synaptic)	Central nervous system	Hypotension, bradycardia
	Eye	Increased intraocular pressure
	Pancreas	Inhibition of insulin secretion
Alpha₂ (pre-synaptic)	Sympathetic neurones	Inhibition of noradrenaline release

release of endogenous noradrenaline from the sympathetic nerve endings. As a result they are more effective as antihypertensive agents and do not induce reflex tachycardia. A third group of drugs is much less homogenous in terms of chemistry and pharmacology. This group includes indoramin and ketanserin which combine alpha blockade with blockade of various serotonin receptors (Figure 9.10). Centrally located alpha₁ adrenoceptors may be associated with baroreceptor function. Reduction in this activity may also play a role in the long-term antihypertensive effects of alpha adrenoceptor antagonism.

Pharmacokinetics

The pharmacokinetics of the quinazolines, prazosin, doxazosin and terazosin are outlined in Table 9.12 together with indoramin, a compound structurally related to procainamide with additional antiarrhythmic, antihistamine and antiserotonin activity. Prazosin, the original member of

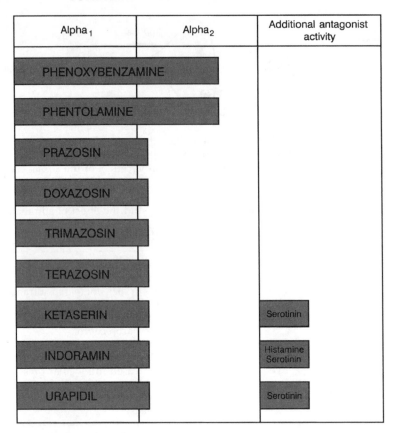

Alpha₁	Alpha₂	Additional antagonist activity
PHENOXYBENZAMINE		
PHENTOLAMINE		
PRAZOSIN		
DOXAZOSIN		
TRIMAZOSIN		
TERAZOSIN		
KETASERIN		Serotinin
INDORAMIN		Histamine Serotinin
URAPIDIL		Serotinin

Figure 9.10. Schematic representation of the range of antagonists of the alpha adrenoceptors and their additional antagonist activities. Modification of table on alpha₁ blockers in Current Cardiovascular Drugs. C. T. Dollery, W. H. Frishman, J. M. Cruickshank. Current Science Ltd, London, 1993. Reproduced with permission.

the group has a short plasma elimination half-life and undergoes rapid hepatic metabolism. Therefore it has to be given two to four times daily. In addition, the time taken to reach peak effect is short and this may explain the higher incidence of "first dose" hypotension with prazosin compared with drugs which have a slower onset of action such as doxazosin. Doxazosin and terazosin have longer elimination half-lives and are extensively metabolised to a number of inactive metabolites. Both drugs can be given once daily although smoother control of blood pressure can be achieved with twice-daily doses of terazosin. Changes in renal function have little impact on the activity of the quinazolines, but accumulation can occur with indoramin in patients with poor renal function.

Table 9.12. Pharmacokinetic values of alpha adrenoceptor antagonists

Drug	Doxazosin	Prazosin	Terazosin	Indoramin
Duration of action	18–36 hours	4–6 hours	18–24 hours	6–8 hours
Time to onset of action	1–2 hours	≈30 minutes	≈30 minutes	Unknown
Time to peak effect	6 hours	1 hour	1–2 hours	≈2 hours
Plasma half life	≈22 hours	≈3 hours	≈12 hours	≈5 hours
Metabolism	Extensive to a variety of inactive metabolites in the liver	Extensive metabolism to several inactive metabolites	Extensive to several inactive metabolites	Metabolism to the 6-hydroxy indoramin and conjugates
% Bioavailability	65	40–80	90	30
Excretion	5–10% excreted unchanged plus metabolites by the kidney	Mainly through the bile and faeces	5–15% renally excreted unchanged plus metabolites	<10% excreted unchanged and metabolites

Pharmacodynamics in hypertensive patients

Selective alpha$_1$ adrenoceptor antagonists, which do not have additional antihypertensive properties, reduce peripheral vascular resistance by dilating peripheral arterioles and increase venous capacitance by reducing venous tone. Cardiac output and heart rate are largely unaltered. Increased activity of the renin angiotensin aldosterone system and sympathetic nervous system has been observed by some investigators. The lack of reflex tachycardia and first-dose syncope has been, in part, related to the venodilator activity.

Efficacy in hypertensive patients

In hypertension, the quinazolines are generally as effective as other antihypertensive agents although there have been some reports to the contrary. Prazosin has been reported to be less effective than calcium channel antagonists in the elderly and a recent large-scale comparative study showed that doxazosin was less effective in reducing systolic blood pressure than chlorthalidone. Overall, however, most comparative studies show similar antihypertensive activity. Follow-up studies with prazosin have demonstrated continued antihypertensive efficacy after 2–5 years of treatment although some studies have suggested reduced antihypertensive effect with long-term use. Prazosin does not have any adverse effects on renal function in hypertensive patients with renal impairment. Doxazosin once daily appears to be as effective an antihypertensive agent as prazosin given twice daily. "First-dose" hypotension seems to occur less frequently than with prazosin but postural hypotension remains a problem. Doxazosin and terazosin are more selective for the alpha$_1$ receptor than prazosin and are now preferred in the treatment of hypertension. In the treatment of hypertension, indoramin and ketanserin are about as effective as other more commonly used agents such as beta blockers and diuretics. Preliminary studies suggest that ketanserin may be beneficial in treating patients with intermittent claudication. Both drugs are ineffective when used once daily and their use is limited because of a high incidence of unpleasant or serious adverse effects. As a result the routine use of indoramin and ketanserin cannot be recommended in the management of hypertension.

Adverse effects

Most adverse effects of alpha adrenoceptor antagonists are due to extension of their pharmacological properties. Hypotension, dizziness, headache, reflex tachycardia, nasal congestion and impaired ejaculation have all been reported especially with non-selective agents. First-dose syncope seems to be related to venodilatation and reduced filling pressure and most commonly occurs when the patient has been receiving large doses of loop diuretics and/or organic nitrates. In most situations, it occurs in patients with predominantly right heart failure. It has been reported more frequently with prazosin than the longer acting drugs doxazosin and terazosin and the phenomenon can often be prevented by careful dose titration. Non-specific adverse effects include drowsiness, lack of energy, depressed mood and positive antinuclear factors without clinical lupus erythematosis in patients receiving long-term prazosin therapy.

Doxazosin and terazosin appear to be better tolerated than prazosin. Most commonly reported adverse effects with these drugs include nasal congestion, headache, vertigo, dizziness, postural hypotension, lethargy and oedema occurring in about 10% of patients treated. The beneficial effects of these drugs on plasma lipids have not been tested in long-term outcome studies.

Indoramin causes significant sedation and depression and ketanserin prolongs the QT intervals especially when combined with diuretics which lower the serum potassium.

Combination with other drugs and adverse interactions

Alpha adrenoceptor drugs combine well with other antihypertensive agents although severe hypotension has been reported when these drugs are combined with calcium channel antagonists and organic nitrates. A diuretic tends to reduce the peripheral oedema which can occur during long-term therapy. Thiazides should not be combined with ketanserin because of the risk of ventricular tachycardia associated with hypokalaemia and a long QT interval.

Contraindications

There are few contraindications to the use of alpha adrenoceptor antagonists in patients with hypertension. First-dose hypotension is more likely to occur in patients with concomitant heart failure or valvular stenosis. There are a few reports of marked hypotension occurring in patients previously receiving beta adrenoceptor antagonists.

Indoramin can worsen the extrapyramidal symptoms of Parkinson's disease, cardiac function in heart failure and increase the risk of epilepsy and depression.

Centrally acting antihypertensive drugs

Centrally acting inhibitors of the sympathetic nervous system have been available for the treatment of hypertension for almost 40 years. However, due to their central sedative and depressive properties and the development of several non-sedating antihypertensive agents, their use has declined over the last 20 years. They are, however, as effective as other antihypertensive drugs and can be usefully combined with other agents in the management of resistant hypertension.

Mode of action

Clonidine and methyldopa act by similar mechanisms. They stimulate the alpha$_2$ adrenoceptors in the vasomotor centre of the medulla oblongata reducing sympathetic outflow from the brain. Clonidine produces its effect directly but methyldopa requires metabolism within the brain to alpha methyl noradrenaline (Figure 9.11). Stimulation of the pre-synaptic alpha$_2$ receptors by clonidine and alpha methyl noradrena-

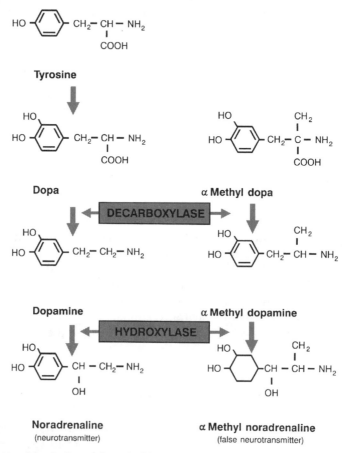

Figure 9.11. Metabolism of methyldopa showing the relationship with the bio synthetic pathway for noradrenaline.

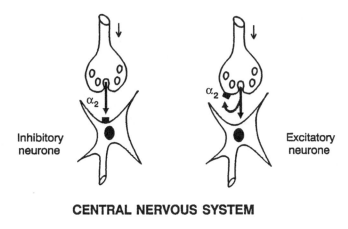

CENTRAL NERVOUS SYSTEM

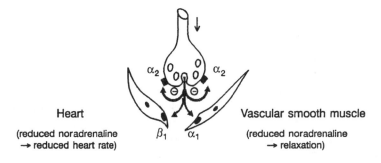

PERIPHERAL NERVOUS SYSTEM

Figure 9.12. Possible sites of action of centrally acting alpha$_2$ agonist antihypertensive drugs.

line in the peripheral nervous system probably makes a contribution to their antihypertensive activity (Figure 9.12). Following acute intravenous administration, clonidine causes a transient elevation in blood pressure probably due to stimulation of the post-synaptic alpha adrenoceptors on peripheral blood vessels. Blood pressure subsequently falls due to central alpha$_2$ stimulation.

Moxonidine is a centrally acting antihypertensive drug with a high affinity for I$_1$-imidazole receptor in the rostral–ventrolateral medulla. Through this mechanism moxonidine lowers blood pressure by reducing excessive sympathetic vasomotor activity without impairing normal reflex control within the cardiovascular system. Central agonist activity at the alpha$_2$ adrenoceptor is minimal. Antiarrhythmic and natriuretic activity has also been described.

Pharmacokinetics

The pharmacokinetics of clonidine, alpha methyldopa and moxonidine are illustrated in Table 9.13. Methyldopa has a relatively short elimination half-life of 1–2 hours while clonidine has a long and rather variable half-life of 12–16 hours. Methyldopa and clonidine are usually given in divided doses although a sustained release preparation of clonidine is available which is effective once daily. A sustained antihypertensive effect can be achieved with clonidine lasting several days by using transdermal preparations. Moxonidine produces a sustained antihypertensive effect over a 24-hour period when given once or twice daily. Renal impairment decreases the clearance of methyldopa, moxonidine and clonidine so that reductions in dosage are necessary in patients with chronic renal impairment. Biotransformation of methyldopa and clonidine is also impaired in patients with hepatic disease and reductions in dosage may be necessary. Adjustment of the dose of moxonidine is unnecessary in patients with renal impairment.

Clinical indications

The centrally acting antihypertensive agents are highly effective as monotherapy and when combined with other agents. They reduce blood pressure in the elderly, and in the young, and are equally effective in blacks and whites. They have a very good track record in patients with diabetes and renal disease. Their main limitation, however, relates to their unwanted adverse effects which can produce poor quality of life in a significant number of patients. These drugs combine well with diuretics and can be usefully used with beta adrenoceptor antagonists provided care is taken to avoid sudden withdrawal of clonidine during long-term treatment. Centrally acting drugs now have a limited role in the management of essential hypertension; however, methyldopa continues to be used in patients with renal insufficiency and in the hypertension of pregnancy. Moxonidine may have a role in patients with resistant hypertension unresponsive to or intolerant of first-line agents.

Adverse effects

The commonest adverse effects of methyldopa and clonidine relate to their central mode of action on the $alpha_2$ adrenoceptors. These include sedation, dry mouth and a variety of other central nervous system effects such as fatigue, headache, unpleasant dreams, confusion and depression. Tolerance develops to the sedative effects during continuous therapy without a reduction in the antihypertensive activity. Impotence and vertigo have also been reported. Dry mouth, sedation and fatigue occur with moxonidine but at a lower incidence than clonidine and methyldopa.

285

Table 9.13. Pharmacokinetic values of centrally acting antihypertensive drugs

	Clonidine	Moxonidine	Alpha methyldopa
Duration of action	Up to 8 hours	≈24 hours	Up to 24 hours
Time to onset of action	30–60 minutes	30 minutes	Unknown
Time to peak action	2–4 hours	1–2 hours	4–6 hours (single dose) 2–3 days (multiple dose)
Plasma half-life	12–16 hours	2–3 hours	1–2 hours
Metabolism	50% metabolised to five inactive metabolites	5–10% metabolised to dihydromoxonidine and guanidine derivative	Initially converted to alpha methyl noradrenaline in the brain. Conjugated to sulphate in the liver
Oral bioavailability %	90	50–60	Unknown
Excretion	30% as parent compound in the kidney. 20% excreted in the bile. Remainder excreted through the kidney as metabolites	Almost 100% of parent compound and metabolites excreted in the urine	Most excreted by the kidney unchanged. Remainder as the sulphate conjugate

Table 9.14.   Interactions with clonidine and methyldopa

Drug	Interaction
Centrally acting sedative drugs, e.g. benzodiazepines, phenothiazines, alcohol	Additional sedative effect
Beta adrenoceptor antagonists	Rebound hypertension is more likely to occur
Anaesthetics	Severe hypotension
Levodopa	Methyldopa may potentiate the response to levodopa
Lithium	Increased risk of toxicity
Monoamine oxidase inhibitors	Antihypertensive effect of methyldopa may be decreased
Non-steroidal anti-inflammatory drugs	Reduced antihypertensive efficacy
Tricyclic antidepressants	Antihypertensive effect may be reduced
Sympathomimetics	Increase the effect of clonidine and reduce the effects of methyldopa

Sudden cessation of drug therapy can result in rebound hypertension. This was first described following withdrawal of clonidine, but was later documented in association with other centrally acting antihypertensive agents. The condition is characterised by symptoms and signs associated with sympathetic overactivity. As well as increases in blood pressure and heart rate, behavioural changes such as anxiety, insomnia and tremor have been described. Increased excretion of urinary catecholamines also occurs. The condition usually presents within 24 hours of the last dose, lasts for 1–5 days and is more commonly associated with higher doses of the drug.

Methyldopa causes severe hypersensitivity reactions in a small number of patients which are not seen with other centrally acting drugs and presumably related to the methyldopa molecule. A positive direct Coombs antiglobulin_test has been reported in 20–30% of patients after 6–12 months of therapy although only a very small number develop haemolytic anaemia. Other rare hypersensitivity reactions include pancreatitis, allergic rashes, myocarditis, a lupus-like syndrome and hepatocellular necrosis. Deaths from hepatic necrosis have been described. Parkinson's disease has occasionally been reported, probably related to reduced dopamine activity within the brain.

Interactions and contraindications

The main interactions with clonidine and methyldopa are listed in Table 9.14. Patients who are likely to be poorly compliant with drug therapy should not receive centrally acting drugs because of the risk of rebound hypertension.

These drugs are also best avoided in patients who operate machinery or who drive regularly as part of their occupation. Clonidine, moxonidine and methyldopa are best avoided in patients with depression, particularly if they are already receiving antidepressant medication. Caution should also be exercised in patients with Raynaud's disease, other occlusive peripheral vascular disease, cerebrovascular or coronary artery disease because of reported sudden decreases in tissue perfusion pressure. Moxonidine also increases the sedative effects of anxiolytics and hypnotics. It is contraindicated in sick sinus syndrome, heart block, severe angina and is best avoided in Parkinson's disease and epilepsy.

Direct-acting vasodilator drugs

The direct-acting vasodilator antihypertensive drugs represent a hetero-geneous group of compounds which relax vascular smooth muscle by a variety of mechanisms. Within this group we generally include two orally active agents, minoxidil and hydralazine, and two parenteral vasodilators, nitroprusside and diazoxide. All four drugs relax arteriolar smooth muscle and so reduce systemic vascular resistance. Decreased arteriolar resistance and decreased blood pressure, elicit compensatory responses mediated by baroreceptors, sympathetic and renin–angiotensin–aldosterone systems. These effects on heart rate, blood volume and inotropic activity oppose the antihypertensive effects of vasodilators (Figure 9.13), but can be largely prevented by co-administration of diuretics and beta adrenoceptor antagonists.

Mode of action

Hydralazine appears to produce its vasodilator effect by interfering with the cellular calcium movements responsible for initiating or maintaining muscle contraction. Minoxidil prevents the uptake of calcium by the cell membrane of vascular smooth muscle cells and may enhance the opening of the potassium channels. The observation that endogenously formed nitric oxide from the vascular endothelium is a potent vasodilator suggests that organic nitrates may mimic this action in vascular smooth muscle. Diazoxide acts directly on smooth muscle by opening potassium channels and exerts its effect on all circulatory beds. Direct-acting vasodilators differ substantially in their effects on small and large arteries and their differential vasodilatory action on arterial and venous vessels. Overall, however, diazoxide, hydralazine and minoxidil act principally on the resistance arterioles while sodium nitroprusside has combined arteriolar and venodilator activity.

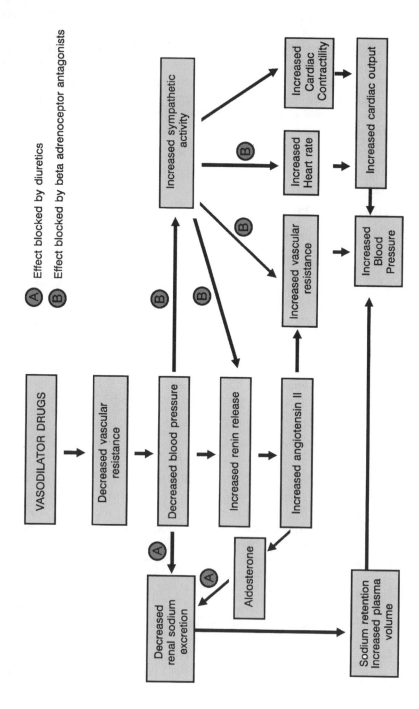

Figure 9.13. Effects of direct acting vasodilator drugs on heart rate, blood volume and inotropic activity.

Pharmacokinetics

The pharmacokinetic values of diazoxide, hydralazine, minoxidil and sodium nitroprusside are listed in Table 9.15. Diazoxide is chemically related to the thiazide diuretics but has no diuretic activity. It is extensively protein bound to vascular tissue and serum albumin. About 50% of the drug is metabolised and the remainder is excreted unchanged in the urine. It has a plasma elimination half-life of about 24 hours but there is a poor relationship between plasma concentration and effect. Although the drug rapidly lowers blood pressure when administered as an intravenous bolus, it is better to administer it as a continuous infusion to achieve smoother control of blood pressure. Hydralazine is well absorbed from the gastrointestinal tract, and is rapidly metabolised by the liver during "first-pass" metabolism. The oral bioavailability is consequently low. Hydralazine is metabolised partly by acetylation with a distribution which shows a bimodal pattern (see Figure 3.2). Patients consequently divide into fast and slow acetylators. Rapid acetylators have greater first-pass metabolism, lower bioavailability and less antihypertensive activity for a given dose than those who acetylate the drug slowly. Toxic effects are consequently more common in slow acetylators. The elimination half-life of hydralazine is short, but the antihypertensive effects last longer than would be predicted from the plasma concentrations, probably due to avid binding to vascular tissue. Minoxidil is also well absorbed from the gut and is extensively metabolised by conjugation within the liver. Minoxidil is not protein bound, but like hydralazine the antihypertensive effects persist even when plasma concentrations are unrecordable. This may be due to the persistence of an active metabolite, minoxidil sulphate. Nitroprusside is a complex of iron, cyanide groups and a nitroso moiety. It is rapidly metabolised by uptake into erythrocytes with the formation and liberation of cyanide. This in turn is metabolised to thiocyanate by the mitochondrial enzyme rhodanase in the presence of a sulphur donor. Thiocyanate is distributed in extracellular fluid and slowly eliminated by the kidney. Nitroprusside rapidly lowers blood pressure and its effects disappear within 1–10 minutes of stopping a continuous intravenous infusion. In aqueous solution, sodium nitroprusside is sensitive to light and has to be covered with opaque foil. It should also be made up fresh before each administration and changed after every few hours if possible.

Clinical indications

Owing to the presence of severe unpleasant adverse effects with hydralazine and minoxidil, they are now considered to be fourth-line drugs as adjunctive therapy in patients with uraemia and severe resistant hypertension. Diazoxide

Table 9.15. Pharmacokinetic values of direct acting vasodilator drugs

	Diazoxide	Hydralazine	Minoxidil	Sodium nitroprusside
Duration of action	<8 hours	3–8 hours	Up to 75 hours	1–10 minutes after stopping infusion
Time of onset of action	≈1 hour	45 minutes	30 minutes	Intermediate (iv)
Time to peak action	≈2 hours	≈1 hour	2–3 hours	1–2 minutes
Plasma half-life	28 hours	2–3 hours	2–4 hours	2 minutes / 3 days (thiocyanate)
Metabolism	Hepatic	Extensive to active and inactive metabolites	Extensive to active and inactive metabolites	Rapid to cyanide and thiocyanate
Oral bioavailability %	Unknown	30 and 50 (slow and fast acetylators)	Low	100 (iv)
Excretion	50% renal unchanged	Renal 10% unchanged	Renal <50% unchanged	Renal largely as the thiocyanate

and nitroprusside are powerful, fast-acting, antihypertensive drugs which are used principally for rapid reduction of blood pressure in hypertensive crises and to maintain hypotensive anaesthesia. Nitroprusside is particularly beneficial in patients with cardiac failure due to hypertension. In general, sodium nitroprusside is preferred to diazoxide in hypertensive crises although in most situations oral therapy with other antihypertensive drugs is preferred. It acts on peripheral arteriolar and venous capacitance vessels. The effects are dose related and depend on the pre-existing haemodynamic state of the patient. In hypertensive and normotensive subjects, a slight increase in heart rate is observed accompanied by a slight fall in cardiac output. In those with heart failure, substantial improvements in left ventricular function are seen with a slight decrease in heart rate. As the drug is metabolised rapidly to the cyanide radical, cyanogen, and then to thiocyanate in the liver, care must be taken to ensure that the rate of infusion does not exceed the patient's capacity to remove the cyanide radical. As a general rule the period of administration should not exceed 24 hours.

Adverse effects

Diazoxide

The most important adverse effect of diazoxide has been excessive hypotension resulting in stroke and myocardial infarction. This has usually occurred following rapid intravenous injections of 300 mg. The reflex sympathetic response can also provoke angina, cardiac failure and evidence of myocardial ischaemia on the electrocardiograph. Diazoxide inhibits insulin release from the pancreas probably due to opening potassium channels in the beta cell membrane and is used to treat hypoglycaemia secondary to insulinaemia. Occasionally, hyperglycaemia can occur especially in patients with renal insufficiency. Unlike the thiazide diuretics, to which it is related, diazoxide causes salt and water retention. For these reasons intravenous diazoxide is almost never used.

Sodium nitroprusside

The most serious adverse effect of sodium nitroprusside is due to the accumulation of cyanide. This can result in metabolic acidosis, arrhythmias, excessive hypotension and death. Thiocyanate may also accumulate during prolonged administration, especially in patients with renal insufficiency. This presents with weakness, disorientation, psychosis, muscle spasms and convulsions and the diagnosis is confirmed by finding serum concentrations > 10 mg/dl. Sodium thiosulphate to increase cyanide metabolism and to reduce affinity for the red cell, and hydroxycobalamine to form relatively non-toxic cyancobalamine have been advocated for prophylaxis and treatment of cyanide poisoning due to long-term nitroprusside administration. Rarely hypothyroidism occurs due to the inhibition of iodide uptake by the thyroid by thiocyanate. Methaemoglobinaemia has occasionally been reported during infusion. There is no justification for the long-term administration of this compound.

Hydralazine

The most common adverse effects of hydralazine relate to the drug's potent vasodilator activity. Headache, palpitations, sweating and flushing as well as nausea and anorexia are widely reported. In patients with ischaemic heart disease, reflex tachycardia and sympathetic nerve stimulation can result in angina and cardiac arrhythmias. With high dose therapy, especially in patients who acetylate the drug slowly, a syndrome resembling lupus erythematosis has been described. Features include arthralgia, myalgia, skin rashes and fever. Unlike systemic lupus erythematosis renal damage is not a feature and the condition settles when the drug is discontinued. Peripheral neuropathy has also been described.

Minoxidil

Because of the drug's potent vasodilator activity, minoxidil commonly causes palpitations, headache, sweating, flushing and peripheral oedema. As a result the drug is always combined with beta adrenoceptor antagonists and diuretics which further enhance the antihypertensive effect. Sweating and hypertrichosis, particularly unpleasant for females, are relatively common and severely limit the use of the drug.

Interactions and contraindications

A variety of drugs interact with the direct acting vasodilator agents. Alcohol and calcium channel antagonists enhance the vasodilator activity while it is reduced by non-steroidal anti-inflammatory drugs, sympathomimetics and oestrogens. Diazoxide has been reported to potentiate the anticoagulant effects of warfarin. Contraindications and special precautions are listed in Table 9.16.

Treatment of severe hypertension

In view of the graded nature of the risk associated with hypertension there is no clear dividing line between those who require treatment and those

Table 9.16. Contraindications and special precautions in the use of direct-acting vasodilators

Condition	Reason
Valvular stenosis especially aortic stenosis. Hypertrophic obstructive cardiomyopathy	Increased gradient across the obstruction and reduced cardiac output
Glaucoma	Condition may get worse
Hypothyroidism	Sodium nitroprusside can make the condition worse
Severe obstructive coronary artery disease	Steal phenomenon and aggravation of angina
Conditions associated with salt and water retention – heart failure, cirrhosis, nephrotic syndrome	Increased salt and water retention if diuretics are not given concurrently
Diabetes	Diazoxide can increase plasma glucose concentrations

who do not. Medical treatment, however, has greatly improved the prognosis of patients with marked increases in blood pressure and advanced retinopathy. Despite the high levels of blood pressure in these patients there is no justification for rapid lowering of blood pressure unless additional factors are present such as encephalopathy, pulmonary oedema or a dissecting aneurysm. In the absence of these factors oral regimens should be used which are similar to those recommended for non-malignant hypertension although these should be initiated with the patient in hospital.

For urgent therapy of acute severe hypertension sublingual nifedipine is now a relatively standard therapy in this country. It consistently reduces systolic and diastolic blood pressure by about 20% within 20–30 minutes and seems to be relatively safe even in the presence of cerebral symptoms. It has also been shown to be of value in heart failure due to hypertension.

Nitroprusside is extensively used especially in the United States but has no clear advantages over sublingual nifedipine. Rebound hypertension is more common and nitroprusside is less effective in lowering blood pressure. Oral labetalol is also effective and produces a smooth reduction in blood pressure without an associated tachycardia (Table 9.17). Diazoxide is best avoided and there is no place for other direct acting vasodilator drugs.

The non-selective alpha adrenoceptor antagonists have a limited role in the management of hypertensive emergencies. In theory they should be effective when increased blood pressure is due to excess of circulating concentrations of alpha agonists. This may occur in patients with phaeochromocytoma, an overdose of sympathomimetic drugs, interactions with monoamino oxidase inhibitors and following clonidine withdrawal. Phentolamine given

Table 9.17. Precautions and adverse effects of the three principal drugs used to treat severe hypertension

Drug	Precautions	Adverse effects
Nifedipine (bite and swallow every 4–6 hours)	Caution in patients with papilloedema and hypertensive encephalopathy	Ischaemia. 'Overshoot' is rare
Labetalol (oral or intravenous)	Avoid in patients with heart failure	May aggravate heart failure
Nitroprusside (infusion)	Avoid except in patients with encephalopathy and hypertensive heart failure	Hypotension

intravenously can be used in these situations. However, other antihypertensive drugs are generally preferred since considerable experience is necessary to use phentolamine safely in these settings.

New antihypertensive drugs

Renin inhibitors

Compounds which inhibit renin to prevent the formation of angiotensin I from angiotensinogen (Figure 9.14) have been developed. These include intravenous peptides and orally active non-peptide compounds. They have the advantage of preventing the rise in renin which accompanies the use of ACE inhibitors and angiotensin receptor antagonists. The results of early clinical trials have proved disappointing.

Atrial natriuretic peptidase inhibitors

Atrial natriuretic peptide is a substance produced by the atria in response to volume expansion which produces vasodilatation and natriuresis. To prolong these physiological effects, a variety of inhibitors have been developed. They clearly could be potentially valuable in heart failure and hypertension and orally active inhibitors are now available. Some of these drugs also inhibit ACE which could increase their efficacy and extend their role.

Potassium channel activators

Nicorandil is a new vasodilator drug which produces its vasodilator effect by activating the potassium channels and facilitating potassium efflux. It

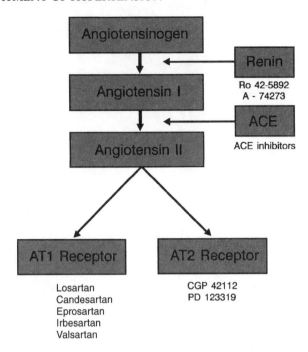

Figure 9.14. New antihypertensive drugs which inhibit the renin–angiotensin system.

has recently been introduced as an antianginal agent and could have a role in the management of hypertension in the future.

Endothelin receptor antagonists

Endothelin I is a small peptide which produces an extremely potent and long-lasting vasoconstrictor effect. The vasoconstrictor effect is largely mediated via the ET_A receptor while stimulation of the ET_B receptor mediates endothelium dependent vasodilatation. Ro 16–2005 (Bosentan) is a small non-peptide antagonist of the ET_A receptor. Evidence to date has confirmed that the compound is orally active and reverses vasospasm in a variety of animal models. The compound may have potential as an antihypertensive agent and the results of early clinical studies are awaited.

10 Drug Treatment of Thromboembolic Disease

Introduction

Blood coagulates when soluble fibrinogen is converted to insoluble fibrin. A number of circulating proteins interact in a cascade of limited proteolytic reactions. At each stage a clotting factor zymogen, for example factor IX becomes an active protease, factor IXa, as a result of limited proteolysis. This in turn activates the next clotting factor (X) until a solid clot is formed. Fibrinogen (factor I), the soluble precursor of fibrin is the substrate for the enzyme, thrombin (factor IIa). This protease is found during coagulation by activation of prothrombin (factor II). Prothrombin is bound by calcium to the phospholipid surface of the platelet where factors Va and Xa convert it to circulating thrombin (see Figure 5.2).

Coagulation is initiated *in vivo* when factor VII is activated by its product, factor Xa. Tissue factor accelerates the activation of factor X by VIIa, phospholipids and calcium ions and it is likely that the release of this substance at the site of injury plays an important role in the initiation of haemostasis. VIIa can also activate factor IX in the presence of tissue factor. Tissue factor pathway inhibitor helps to regulate the production of tissue factor and hence the clotting cascade. The oral anticoagulant drug warfarin inhibits the hepatic synthesis of several vitamin K-dependent clotting factors. Heparin also inhibits the action of a number of activated clotting factors. Other naturally occurring anticoagulants such as protein C and protein S down-regulate the clotting pathways involving the proteolysis of factors Va, VIIIa and XIa.

Heparin

In 1916, a medical student called Jay McClean discovered a phospholipid anticoagulant while investigating ether soluble pro-coagulants. Six years later Howell discovered a water-soluble mucopolysaccharide in the same laboratory. His work was published in the *American Journal of Physiology*, and in that publication Howell referred to the substance as heparin since it was found to be abundant in the liver.

Chemistry and mode of action

Heparin is a heterogeneous mixture of sulphated mucopolysaccharides which bind to the surface of endothelial cells. Its pharmacological activity is largely dependent on its interaction with the plasma protease inhibitor antithrombin III. This inhibitor forms stable complexes with a variety of clotting factor proteases. Heparin binds tightly to the antithrombin, alters the shape of the molecule and greatly increases its antithrombin activity. Heparin catalyses the antithrombin–protease reaction and is then released intact for renewed binding to more antithrombin. The region of antithrombin binding consists of repeated sulphated disaccharide units composed of D-glucosamine–D-glucuronic acid (Figure 10.1).

Heparin has a variety of pharmacological actions. By maintaining electronegativity of the surface of blood vessels, heparin may reduce platelet adhesiveness to endothelial cells and so reduce platelet-derived growth factor and the development of atherosclerotic plaques involving smooth muscle cell proliferation. Although heparin is a potent anti-coagulant it has no effect on the synthesis of blood-clotting factors. One-stage tests of coagulation such as whole-blood clotting time or activated partial thromboplastin generation time are prolonged by heparin in proportion to the plasma heparin and antithrombin III concentrations. Heparin also has anticomplement and antihistamine activity.

Pharmacokinetics and dosage

The principal pharmacokinetic values of heparin are listed in Table 10.1. Heparin is not absorbed through the intestinal mucosa when given orally and is administered parenterally. The drug is therefore given by continuous intravenous infusion, intermittent intravenous injection or subcutaneously. When given intravenously the onset of action is immediate, but following subcutaneous administration the action can be delayed for up to 1 hour. The elimination half-life increases with increasing dose and is prolonged in patients with severe renal and hepatic failure. The half-life may be reduced in patients with thromboembolic disease.

Until recently most heparin was administered by continuous intravenous infusion often preceded by a bolus injection. Commonly used doses are 5000 U as an intravenous injection followed by 1000–1500 U per hour delivered by an infusion pump. Monitoring of the anticoagulant effect is

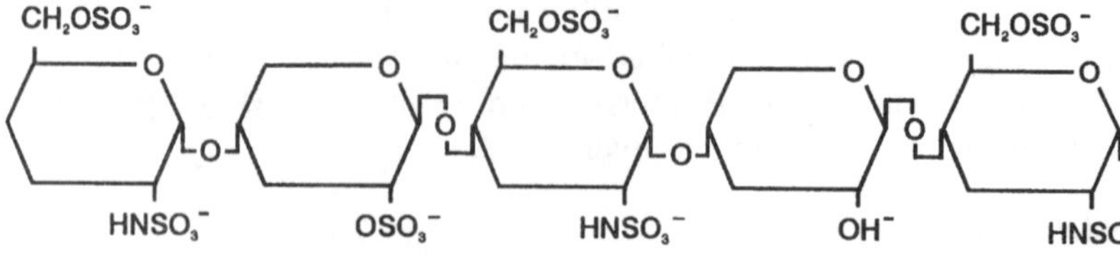

Figure 10.1.   A section of the heparin polymer illustrating the sequence of disaccharide units, most of which are sulphated.

Table 10.1. Pharmacokinetic values of the three most commonly used anticoagulants

	Heparin	Warfarin	Phenindione
Time to onset of action	Immediate (iv) 20–60 minutes (sc)	12 hours–3 days	1½–2 days
Time to peak action	Few minutes (iv)	3–6 days	1½–2 days
Plasma half-life	½–2½ hours	12 hours–3 days	Not known
Metabolism	Hepatic and uptake by reticuloendothelial system	Hepatic hydroxylation to inactive metabolites	Hepatic hydroxylation
Oral bioavailability %	100 (iv)	Very variable	Very variable
Excretion	Renal as metabolites and unchanged drug	Inactive metabolites in bile and urine	Inactive metabolites in bile and urine
Protein binding	>90%	97%	>97%

achieved by measuring the partial thromboplastin time (PTT) and maintaining it 1.5–2.5 times the normal value (usually 50–80 seconds). The risk of recurrence of thromboembolism is reduced if these values are achieved compared with values <1.5 times normal. It has been conventional clinical practice to continue heparin for up to 10 days starting warfarin on the fifth to tenth day. Recent randomised clinical trials in patients with proximal vein thrombosis indicate that this period can be shortened to 5 days without loss of efficacy. With these regimens, oral anticoagulants are started on the first or second day of treatment. Intermittent intravenous heparin is associated with a greater risk of bleeding than continuous intravenous infusion. A common regimen is 5000 units every 4 hours.

Subcutaneous heparin can be used in place of warfarin for chronic therapy when oral anticoagulants are contraindicated, for example, during pregnancy. A total daily dose similar to that given intravenously is usually administered every 8–12 hours to achieve a PTT of 1.5 times the control value, midway between doses. Low-dose subcutaneous heparin is also used prophylactically to reduce the risk of thromboembolic disease in susceptible patients. A commonly employed regimen is 5000 units administered subcutaneously twice daily. In this situation monitoring of the PTT is unnecessary.

Low molecular weight heparins

Low molecular weight heparins have a mean molecular weight between 4000 and 5000 and exert their anticoagulant activity primarily through

Table 10.2. Comparison of the modes of action, bioavailability and dose–response relationships of unfractionated heparin, low molecular weight heparin and hirudin. Modified table Schussheim, A. E., "Fuster Valentin Thrombosis, antithrombin agents and the antithrombin approach in cardiac disease", *Prog. Cardiovasc. Disease*, 1997; 40 3: 205–238 (Copyright © 1997 by W. B. Saunders Company).

Unfractionated heparin	Low molecular weight heparin	Hirudin
Inhibits thrombin, factor VII more than IXa and XIa	Mainly affects factor Xa. Thrombin to some degree	Specific and potent inhibitor of thrombin
Antithrombin III dependent	Antithrombin III dependent	Non-antithrombin III activity
No effect on clot-bound thrombin and factor VII	No effect on clot-bound thrombin and factor VII	Inactivates clot-bound thrombin
Thrombocytopaenia relatively common	Thrombocytopaenia rarely occurs	No thrombocytopaenia
Subcutaneous bioavailability 30%	Subcutaneous bioavailability >90%	Subcutaneous bioavailability ≈85%
Poor dose response relationship	Satisfactory dose response relationship	Satisfactory dose response relationship
Not immunogenic	Not immunogenic	Rarely immunogenic

antithrombin III-dependent inhibition of factor Xa (Figure 10.2). Unfractionated heparin has an antifactor Xa to antithrombin ratio of 1:1. Low molecular weight heparins have a ratio between 4:1 and 2:1. This is because an additional 15 saccharides (molecular weight >5400) are needed for the antithrombin activity (Figure 10.2). Table 10.2 illustrates some of the advantages of low molecular weight heparins over fractionated heparin. Low molecular weight heparins bind less to plasma proteins and endothelial cells making their bioavailability and dose–response relationships more predictable. The prolonged clearance allows for less frequent drug administration. Interactions with platelets and the von Willebrand factor are less than with unfractionated heparin, which may account for the lower bleeding rates and reduced incidence of thrombocytopaenia observed in clinical trials. The more predictable response permits administration without clinical monitoring.

Low molecular weight heparins given subcutaneously have been compared with unfractionated heparin given by intravenous infusion in a variety of clinical situations. Overall they are as effective as conventional heparin in preventing venous thromboembolism (certoparin, dalteparin, enoxaparin and tinzaparin) and treating deep venous thrombosis (dalteparin, enoxaparin and tinzaparin) unstable angina (dalteparin) and for the prevention of clotting in extracorporeal circuits (dalteparin, enoxaparin, tinzaparin).

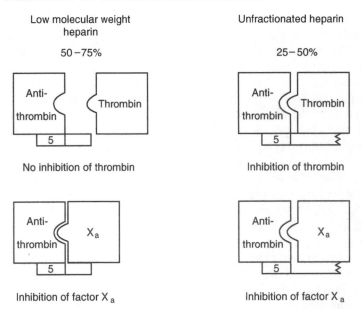

Figure 10.2. A comparison of low molecular weight heparin and unfractionated heparin on thrombin and factor X_a activity. Reproduced from Schussheim, A. E., "Fuster Valentin Thrombosis, antithrombin agents and the antithrombin approach in cardiac disease", *Prog. Cardiovasc. Disease*, 1997: 40; 3; 205–238. (Copyright © 1997 by W. B. Saunders Company).

Heparin resistance

The amount of heparin required to produce a desired anticoagulant effect in patients is variable due largely to differences in the concentrations of heparin-binding proteins in the plasma. Occasionally a PTT cannot be prolonged more than 1.5 times the mean control value with doses greater than 50 000 units. Some patients have very short pre-treatment values and are not truly resistant, others eliminate the drug very rapidly while those with chronic liver disease, nephrotic syndrome and disseminated intravascular coagulation have severe acquired antithrombin deficiency.

Clinical indications

Heparin is the treatment of choice for most acute venous thromboembolism. The development of accurate objective tests to detect thromboembolic disorders, together with improved methods of anticoagulant control, has allowed heparin therapy to be evaluated effectively in a number of clinical situations. Information now available confirms that 4–5 days of heparin therapy as initial treatment is as effective as longer periods of therapy and patients with PTT values lower than 1.5 have a higher risk of recurrent venous thromboembolism than those with values between 1.5 and 2.5. In patients, however, with a very high risk of bleeding it may be preferable to delay starting oral therapy for a longer period of time since the anticoagulant effect of heparin is easier to reverse than that of warfarin. Low dose subcutaneous heparin is also widely used in patients undergoing general and orthopaedic surgical procedures to prevent post-operative deep venous thrombosis and pulmonary embolism in high risk patients. "At risk" patients include those with a previous history of thromboembolic disease, those who are obese, have malignant disease, are elderly and/or immobile and those undergoing complicated and prolonged surgery. Low molecular weight heparins may have some advantages in these situations.

There remains considerable controversy about the role of heparin as adjunctive therapy to thrombolysis in patients following an acute myocardial infarction. When used as the single adjunctive therapy with thrombolytic agents no trials show clear benefit over thrombolysis alone and in patency studies no trial has shown a benefit over aspirin. Beneficial effects of adjunctive therapy with aspirin and heparin are probably due to the antiplatelet effects of aspirin.

Low dose heparin has also been shown to have a number of anti-inflammatory effects involving adhesion, activation and movement of leucocytes. There are preliminary reports of beneficial effects in asthma and ulcerative colitis, but good clinical evidence is lacking.

Adverse effects

Bleeding is by far the most common and important adverse effect of heparin. The incidence of bleeding varies with the type of patient studied but values varying from 1% to 33% for serious bleeding have been reported. There is a clear positive relationship between the number of bleeding episodes, the dose of heparin and the duration of the aPTT. Recent evidence suggests that low molecular weight heparin is associated with a lower incidence of bleeding complications.

Thrombocytopaenia (a platelet count $<100\,000/\mu l$) occurs in 1–5% of patients after 7–14 days of initiating treatment. Occasionally it may occur earlier in patients previously exposed to heparin. In a small number of patients, thrombocytopaenia is associated with thrombotic complications including arterial thrombosis with platelet-fibrin "white" clots. Thrombocytopaenia is less common with porcine than bovine heparin and is reversible after discontinuation of the drug.

Mild elevations of hepatic transaminases have been reported but are generally of little clinical significance. Osteoporosis resulting in sponta-neous vertebral fractures occurs infrequently in patients who have received full therapeutic doses for several months. Heparin, unlike oral anti-coagulants, does not cross the placenta and has not been associated with foetal abnormalities, prematurity or increased foetal mortality.

Interactions and contraindications

Drugs which inhibit platelet aggregation or cause platelet dysfunction, e.g. aspirin, non-steroidal anti-inflammatory drugs, dipyridamole, etc. are associated with increased risk of bleeding when heparin is co-administered. Severe thrombocytopaenia is usually a contraindication.

Heparin is best avoided in patients with past or present gastrointestinal ulcerative conditions, severe hypertension, recent surgery involving the eye, brain or spinal cord, and those with active or occult bleeding. Adverse reactions to heparin are particularly common in elderly patients. Oral anticoagulants and heparin have synergistic effects on blood coagulation.

Antagonists to heparin

The anticoagulant effect of heparin decreases rapidly after discontinuing a continuous infusion of heparin. Mild bleeding can therefore be controlled by stopping the drug. If life-threatening haemorrhage occurs, however, the anticoagulant effect can be rapidly reversed by a slow intravenous infusion of protamine sulphate. The protamines are low molecular weight basic proteins isolated from fish sperm which neutralise the anticoagulant effect of heparin. Protamine needs to be given at the lowest dose required to reverse the anticoagulant effect since protamine interacts with platelets, fibrinogen and other plasma proteins to exert its own anticoagulant effect. This amount is approximately 1 mg of protamine for every 100 units of heparin. Anaphylactic reactions sometimes occur as well as a very rare hypersensitivity reaction consisting of pulmonary vasoconstriction, right ventricular dysfunction, systemic hypertension and transient neutropenia.

Hirudin

Hirudin, initially isolated as a leech peptide, is now synthesised as recombinant hirudin with a molecular sequence similar to the catalytic site of the thrombin receptor on platelets and smooth muscle cells. It does not require endogenous co-factors such as antithrombin III for its activity and can inhibit thrombin-induced platelet aggregation (Table 10.2). Preliminary evidence suggests an efficacy similar to heparin but a higher incidence of bleeding complications.

Oral anticoagulants

Introduction

The discovery of orally active anticoagulants resulted from investigations into an unusual cattle disease in North Dakota and Alberta in the early 1920s. In 1922, a veterinary surgeon, F. W. Schofield in Alberta, demonstrated that haemorrhagic septicaemia in cattle was caused by eating hay containing spoiled sweet clover. In 1931, another veterinary surgeon, L. M. Roderick of North Dakota, discovered that the haemorrhagic factor reduced the activity of prothrombin. It took another 8 years before H. A. Campbell isolated crystals of the anticoagulant. Two members of his group, Mark Strahmann and Charles Huebner, spent the next 9 months improving the efficacy of the isolation procedure and on the 1 April 1940 they confirmed that the active substance was 3,3'-methylene-bis-(4-hydroxycoumarin), a chemical which had already been synthesised in 1903.

In 1942, the first oral anticoagulant, dicoumarol, was marketed and since then hundreds of coumarins and analogues have been developed with significant anticoagulant activity. Warfarin was finally chosen as the anticoagulant of first choice, being longer acting and 5–10 times more potent than dicoumarol. It quickly achieved popularity as a rat poison and later in the treatment of thromboembolic diseases. The name was derived from the Wisconsin Alumini Research Foundation which obtained substantial royalties from the product.

Mechanism of action

Oral anticoagulants produce their effects by antagonising the action of vitamin K. Vitamin K is required for the synthesis of factor II prothrombin, factor VII, factor IX and factor X by the liver. These factors and the anticoagulant proteins C and S are biologically inactive unless 9–12 of their amino-terminal glutamic acid residues are carboxylated. The γ-carboxy-glutamate residues provide calcium ion binding properties which are essential in the formation of effective catalytic complexes. This reaction requires vitamin K, carbon dioxide, molecular oxygen and a precursor of the target protein containing a pro-peptide recognition site (Figure 10.3). Carboxylation is directly coupled to the oxidation of vitamin K to the epoxide. Reduction in the amount of vitamin K has to be regenerated from the epoxide for the sustained carboxylation and synthesis of biologically active proteins. Oral anticoagulants block this recycling process. At therapeutic concentrations the process is reversible and administration of vitamin K can reduce the anticoagulant effect.

305

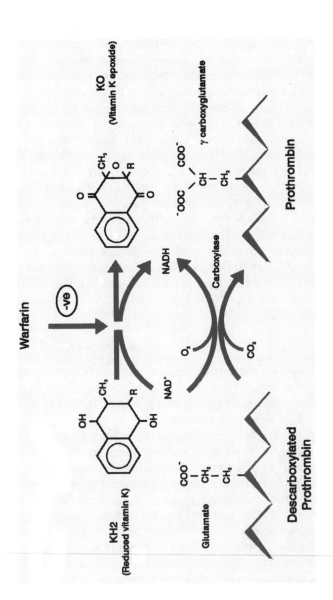

Figure 10.3. Proposed actions of warfarin on vitamin K and prothrombin synthesis.

Pharmacokinetics and dosage

Warfarin is well absorbed from the gastrointestinal tract with detectable levels occurring after 1 hour and peak levels between 2–8 hours. The amount of drug absorbed is reduced by the presence of food in the gut. Warfarin is almost completely bound to plasma proteins (97%), mainly albumin, and distributes rapidly into a volume equal to the albumin space. It rapidly crosses the placenta and achieves plasma concentrations in the foetus comparable to those in the mother. Intra-uterine bleeding is therefore more common and serious birth defects affecting bone formation have been described. Active warfarin is not secreted into breast milk. Warfarin is metabolised by hydroxylation in the liver to inactive metabolites which are then excreted in the bile and urine (Table 10.1). The elimination half-life ranges from 12 to 72 hours with a mean value of about 40 hours.

Regimens for the administration of warfarin vary widely, but in general most involve a loading dose between 10 and 20 mg followed by a maintenance dose to achieve an international normalised ratio (INR) between 2 and 3.5. Alternatively, especially in an outpatient setting, the loading dose can be omitted. Therapeutic doses of warfarin decrease the total amount of each vitamin K-dependent coagulation factor synthesised in the liver by up to 50%. For some coagulation factors, notably factor II, the full antithrombotic effect following initiation of warfarin therapy may not be achieved for several days even though the INR is increased within 1 to 2 days due to activity on factor VII.

Clinical indications

The main indications for oral anticoagulation are deep venous thrombosis, pulmonary embolism, atrial fibrillation and in the treatment of patients with prosthetic heart valves. Warfarin is sometimes indicated in patients with transient cerebral ischaemic episodes.

Oral anticoagulants are effective in the primary and secondary prevention of venous thromboembolism. Warfarin should be given to those patients with proximal or distal vein thrombosis for a period of 3–6 months although the optimal duration of therapy remains uncertain. Several studies have confirmed over the last 25 years that patients with venous thromboembolic disease have a high risk of recurrence if untreated or if treated with subtherapeutic doses of anticoagulants. Recurrences would be reduced if therapy were continued indefinitely in all patients, but overall most patients would be exposed to unnecessary inconvenience and risk. Oral anticoagulation should be given during the first week of treatment with heparin and may be started as early as the first day of heparin treatment.

Patients who develop recurrent venous thrombosis without additional risk factors following a 3-month course of adequate anticoagulant therapy have a high risk of recurrence. The duration of further anticoagulation should, however, be tailored to the individual patient. Those with slowly resolving risk factors, such as prolonged immobilisation, would probably benefit from a further three months of treatment while those with underlying malignancy, antithrombin III protein C or S deficiency, homocysteinuria, lupus anticoagulant or recurrent thromboembolism, should receive therapy indefinitely. Attempts to reduce oral anticoagulant therapy to 4 weeks following diagnosis have been unsuccessful.

Oral anticoagulant therapy is approximately 50% more effective than aspirin in preventing ischaemic stroke in patients with atrial fibrillation. The benefit, however, depends on the presence of associated risk factors. These include mitral valve disease, prosthetic valves, diabetes, hypertension, a previous stroke or transient ischaemic episode and increasing age. Patients with ischaemic heart disease and heart failure also benefit more from oral anticoagulation than those without additional risk factors.

Individuals less than 60 years of age without clinical risk factors (lone atrial fibrillation) do not require warfarin therapy to prevent stroke. In patients greater than 75 years with atrial fibrillation, oral anticoagulation requires more careful monitoring due to the increased risk of intracerebral bleeding.

Thromboembolism is a major complication of prosthetic heart valves. Long-term oral anticoagulation is essential and even with satisfactory control, an incidence of transient weakness, dysphasia and visual disturbances of 1–2% per annum has been reported. In this small group of patients the addition of an antiplatelet drug may be appropriate.

Oral anticoagulation should not be used in the treatment of peripheral arterial disease or acute cerebral thrombosis, but may be of value in patients with transient ischaemic attacks if aspirin is contraindicated.

Adverse effects

Like heparin, the major adverse effect of oral anticoagulants is bleeding. The most important sites include those where the bleeding will cause compression of vital structures such as the brain, spinal cord or heart, or from massive internal haemorrhage from the gastrointestinal tract, behind or within the peritoneal cavity. The risk of intracerebral or subdural haematoma is greatest in patients more than 50 years of age. In view of these significant risks, patients must be informed and well supervised with arrangements made to treat any serious bleeding episodes should they arise. If mild bleeding occurs the dose of anticoagulant should be omitted and the INR measured. A reduction in drug dosage is then required.

For continued and serious bleeding vitamin K_1 is the effective antidote, although it takes several hours to reduce the anticoagulant effect since the coagulation proteins have to be fully carboxylated before the clotting activity can be restored. If an immediate effect is required, this can be achieved by fresh frozen plasma, although vitamin K_1 is still required since the clotting factors, especially factor VII, are cleared from the circulation more quickly than the remaining anticoagulant. Usually 5–10 mg is sufficient given orally, subcutaneously or intravenously, but some patients require larger doses. Repeated administration is occasionally necessary in deliberate overdose situations or if the oral anticoagulant is one with an excessively long half-life. Vitamin K administration tends to make subsequent anticoagulant control difficult and short-term heparin therapy may be required before full anticoagulant effect can be achieved with oral therapy.

Warfarin administration during pregnancy can cause intra-uterine bleeding, birth defects and abortions. During the first trimester, exposure can result in nasal hypoplasia and stippled epiphyseal calcification. Central nervous system abnormalities have been reported during the second trimester while bleeding is the most common problem in the third trimester and in the newborn. Cutaneous necrosis with reduced activity of protein C occasionally occurs during the first weeks of treatment. In severe cases, infarction of the breasts, fatty tissues, intestine and extremities can occur.

Drug interactions

Interactions with warfarin are among the most common and important in clinical practice (Tables 10.3, 10.4). A variety of drugs have been implicated as well as changes in dietary vitamin K and alcohol intake.

Interactions with warfarin can be broadly classified into pharmacokinetic and pharmacodynamic effects. The most important pharmacokinetic

Table 10.3. Drugs which decrease the anticoagulant effect of warfarin

Drug	Possible cause of the interaction
Antiepileptic drugs	Reduced effect probably due to enzyme induction occurs with phenobarbitone, primidone and carbamazepine. Reduced and enhanced anticoagulant effects have been described with phenytoin
Antifungal agents	Griseofulvin reduces the anticoagulant effect
Hormone antagonists	Reduced anticoagulant effect by aminoglutethimide
Hormones	Oestrogen and progestogens in the oral contraceptive reduce anticoagulant activity
Retinoids	Acitretin decreases effect
Vitamin K	High intake of vitamin K reduces the anticoagulant effect

Table 10.4. Drugs which increase the anticoagulant effect of warfarin

Drug	Possible cause of the interaction
Alcohol	Large amounts tend to increase the anticoagulant effect, but responses are variable
Anti-inflammatory drugs	Aspirin and all non-steroidal anti-inflammatory drugs increase the risk of gastrointestinal bleeding. Antiplatelet effect of aspirin and anticoagulant effect of azopropazone, phenylbutazone, diclofenac, diflunisal, flurbiprofen, mefenamic acid, piroxicam and other anti-inflammatory drugs increase the risk of bleeding
Antiarrhythmic drugs	Amiodarone, propafenone and quinidine increase anticoagulant activity
Antibacterial agents	Chloramphenicol, ciprofloxacin, co-trimoxazole, erythromycin, metronidazole, ofloxacin and sulphonamides enhance the anticoagulant activity. Experience from anticoagulant clinics suggest that any broad spectrum antibiotic, especially ampicillin, can increase the INR
Antifungal agents	Imidazole antifungal agents fluconazole, itraconazole, ketoconazole and miconazole increase anticoagulant activities
Hormone antagonists	Danazol, flutamide, tamoxifen and possibly bicalutamide, enhance the anticoagulant effect
Lipid lowering drugs	Fibrates and simvastatin enhance anticoagulant activity
Ulcer healing drugs	Cimetidine and omeprazole increase anticoagulant effect, probably by enzyme inhibition
Uricosuric agents	Sulphinpyrazone enhances anticoagulant activity

mechanisms are enzyme induction and inhibition and decreased plasma protein binding. Important enzyme inducers include barbiturates, carbamazepine and rifampicin and these drugs decrease the effective plasma concentrations of warfarin. Cimetidine, co-trimoxazole and metronidazole inhibit cytochrome P450 oxidative enzyme systems and increase drug concentrations. Protein binding displacement is one of the mechanisms involved in the increased anticoagulant effect of warfarin observed with phenylbutazone. Pharmacodynamic mechanisms include synergism in which the synthesis of clotting factors is further impaired, competitive antagonism (vitamin K) and additional factors such as reduced platelet adhesiveness and increased risk of gastric erosion, which make bleeding more likely. Phenylbutazone and sulphinpyrazone not only increase hypoprothrombinaemia but inhibit platelet function and increase the risk of peptic ulceration and erosion. Broad spectrum antibiotics reduce the intestinal bacteria which produce vitamin K and third-generation cephalosporins have been shown to inhibit vitamin K epoxide reductase. Heparin directly prolongs the prothrombin time by inhibiting the activity of several clotting factors. Cholestyramine binds warfarin in the intestine and reduces its absorption and overall bioavailability.

Contraindications

There are several clinical conditions for which warfarin is contraindicated. These include active bleeding from any site but in particular the gastrointestinal, respiratory or genito-urinary tracts. Warfarin is also best avoided in bleeding disorders such as thrombocytopaenia and pregnancy, and in patients who have had recent surgery to the central nervous system or eye, or who have a space-occupying lesion within the brain. Relative contraindications are severe, uncontrolled hypertension, patients with proliferative retinopathy, recurrent falls, poor compliance and alcoholism.

Appendix 1: Some Important Cardiovascular Drug Interactions

Appendix 1. Some Important Cardiovascular Drug Interactions

Drug group	Interacts with	Result of interaction	Possible mechanism
Positive inotropic drugs *Digoxin*	1. Non-steroidal anti-inflammatory drugs	Increased plasma concentrations. Reduced digoxin effect in heart failure	Reduced glomerular filtration Salt and water retention
	2. Antiarrhythmic drugs: amiodarone, propafenone, quinidine	Increased digoxin levels	Reduced renal elimination Reduced apparent volume of distribution?
	3. Beta adrenoceptor antagonists	Increased bradycardia and atrioventricular block	Additive pharmacodynamic effects
	4. Calcium channel antagonists	Increased digoxin levels: diltiazem, verapamil, nicardipine. Bradycardia and atrioventricular block	Reduced digoxin elimination Additive pharmacodynamic effects
	5. Diuretics (thiazides and loop diuretics)	Hypokalaemia increases digoxin toxicity	Enhanced inhibition of $Na^+K^+ATPase$
Diuretics	1. ACE inhibitors	Hyperkalaemia (with potassium-sparing diuretics) Hypotension	Additive pharmacodynamic effect, especially with renal impairment. Volume depletion
	2. Non-steroidal anti-inflammatory drugs	Impaired renal function and reduced diuretic activity Hyperkalaemia	Renal prostaglandin inhibition
	3. Antiarrhythmic drugs: amiodarone, disopyramide, flecainide, quinine	Increased toxicity of antiarrhythmic drugs	Hypokalaemia increases toxicity
	4. Antibacterials: Aminoglycosides	Increased toxicity of aminoglycosides	Additive renal tubular effects
	5. Antidiabetic agents: with loop diuretics, thiazides	Reduced hypoglycaemic effect	Probable effects on insulin release
	6. Antihypertensives: alpha blockers, ACE inhibitors	Hypotension	Volume depletion and hyponatraemia
	7. Lithium with loop and thiazide diuretics	Lithium toxicity	Impaired renal excretion of lithium

Drug	Interacting drug	Effect	Mechanism
	8. Potassium salts with potassium-sparing diuretics	Hyperkalaemia	Additive pharmacodynamic effect on the kidney
Antiarrhythmic drugs			
Adenosine	1. Dipyridamole	Increased toxicity	Effects on adenosine metabolism
	2. Theophylline	Reduced effect	
Amiodarone	1. Other antiarrhythmic drugs: disopyramide, flecainide, procainamide, quinidine	Increased toxicity	Additive proarrhythmic and negative inotropic effects
	2. Warfarin	Increased anticoagulant effect	Reduced metabolism
	3. Antiepileptic drugs: phenytoin	Increased phenytoin toxicity	Impaired metabolism
	4. Beta adrenoceptor antagonists	Increased bradycardia and myocardial depression	Additive pharmacodynamic effects
	5. Calcium antagonists, especially verapamil and diltiazem	Increased bradycardia and myocardial depression	Additive pharmacodynamic effects
	6. Digoxin	Increased digoxin concentrations	Impaired elimination
	7. Cimetidine	Increased plasma concentrations of amiodarone	Enzyme inhibition
Disopyramide	1. Amiodarone	Increased risk of arrhythmias	Pharmacodynamic interaction
	2. Other antiarrhythmic drugs (especially class 1a)	Depressed myocardial contractility	Additive pharmacodynamic effect
	3. Enzyme-inducing drugs – phenobarbitone, phenytoin and rifampicin	Reduced plasma concentrations	Enzyme induction
	4. Anticholinergic drugs	Enhanced anticholinergic effects	Additive pharmacological effects
	5. Beta adrenoceptor antagonists and verapamil	Depressed myocardial function	Additive pharmacodynamic effects
	6. Diuretics	Increased cardiotoxicity	Reduced potassium due to diuretics
Flecainide	1. Amiodarone	Increases the risk of ventricular arrhythmias	Additive pharmacodynamic effects
	2. Other antiarrhythmic drugs (especially class 1a)	Depressed myocardial contractility	Additive pharmacodynamic effects

Continued

Appendix 1. *Continued*

Drug group	Interacts with	Result of interaction	Possible mechanism
Flecainide (continued)	3. Quinine	Increased risk of arrhythmias	Increased plasma flecainide concentrations
	4. Beta adrenoceptor antagonists and verapamil	Depressed myocardial function	Additive pharmacodynamic effect
	5. Cimetidine	Increased toxicity	Enzyme inhibition
	6. Diuretics	Increased cardiotoxicity	Reduced potassium due to diuretics
Procainamide	1. Captopril	Increased toxicity	Impaired renal elimination
	2. Amiodarone	Increased toxicity	Pharmacokinetic interaction
	3. Other antiarrhythmic drugs (especially class 1a)	Depressed myocardial contractility	Additive pharmacodynamic effects
	4. Tricyclic antidepressants	Increased risk of arrhythmias	Pharmacodynamic interaction
	5. Beta adrenoceptor antagonists and verapamil	Depressed myocardial function	Additive pharmacodynamic effects
	6. Antihistamines and phenothiazines	Increased risk of arrhythmias	Additive pharmacodynamic effects
	7. Cimetidine	Increased toxicity due to elevated plasma concentrations	Enzyme inhibition
Propafenone	1. Quinidine	Increased toxicity of propafenone	Reduced clearance of propafenone
	2. Other antiarrhythmic drugs (especially class 1a)	Depressed myocardial contractility	Additive pharmacodynamic effects
	3. Rifampicin and other enzyme inducing drugs	Reduced antiarrhythmic activity	Enzyme induction
	4. Warfarin	Increased risk of bleeding	Increased plasma concentrations of warfarin
	5. Tricyclic antidepressants	Increased risk of arrhythmias	Additive pharmacodynamic effects
	6. Antihistamines	Increased risk of arrhythmias	Additive pharmacodynamic effects
	7. Beta adrenoceptor antagonists	Increased beta blocking effects	Increased plasma levels of propranolol and metoprolol
	8. Digoxin	Increased digoxin concentrations	Reduced clearance of digoxin
	9. Cyclosporin	Increased cyclosporin concentrations	Reduced cyclosporin clearance

Drug	Interacting drug	Effect	Mechanism
	10. Theophylline	Increased plasma theophylline concentrations	Reduced theophylline clearance
	11. Cimetidine	Increased propafenone concentrations	Enzyme inhibition
Quinidine	1. Amiodarone	Increased quinidine plasma concentrations	Reduced clearance of quinidine
	2. Antiarrhythmic drugs (especially class 1b)	Impaired myocardial contractility	Additive pharmacodynamic effects
	3. Rifampicin and other enzyme-inducing drugs	Reduced quinidine effect	Enzyme induction
	4. Warfarin	Increased bleeding tendency	Reduced warfarin clearance
	5. Tricyclic antidepressants	Increased risk of ventricular arrhythmias	Additive pharmacodynamic effects
	6. Antihistamines	Increased risk of ventricular arrhythmias	Additive pharmacodynamic effects
	7. Beta adrenoceptor antagonists	Increased risk of ventricular arrhythmias	Additive pharmacodynamic effects
	8. Calcium channel antagonists Nifedipine Verpamil	Reduces quinidine effects Increased quinidine toxicity	Increases clearance of quinidine Increased plasma concentrations and additive pharmacodynamic effects
	9. Cimetidine	Increased quinidine toxicity	Enzyme inhibition
Bretylium	1. Other antiarrhythmic drugs (especially class 1b)	Increased risk of ventricular arrhythmias	Additive pharmacodynamic effects
	2. Tricyclic antidepressants (higher doses)	Increased risk of ventricular arrhythmias	Additive pharmacodynamic effects
	3. Antihypertensive drugs	Increased risk of hypotension	Additive pharmacodynamic effects
	4. Levodopa, alcohol, phenothiazines	Increased hypotension	Additive hypotensive effect
Lignocaine	1. Other antiarrhythmic drugs (especially class 1a)	Depressed myocardial function	Additive pharmacodynamic effect
	2. Beta adrenoceptor antagonists	Depressed myocardial function	Additive pharmacodynamic effect
	3. Diuretics	Reduced antiarrhythmic effect	Hypokalaemia

Continued

Appendix 1. *Continued*

Drug Group	Interacts with	Result of interaction	Possible mechanism
Lignocaine (continued)	4. Cimetidine	Increased lignocaine toxicity	Enzyme inhibition
Mexiletine	1. Other antiarrhythmic drugs (especially class 1a)	Depressed myocardial function	Additive pharmacodynamic effects
	2. Rifampicin and other enzyme-inducing agents	Reduced antiarrhythmic effect	Enzyme induction
	3. Diuretics	Reduced antiarrhythmic activity	Hypokalaemia
	4. Theophylline	Increased risk of theophylline toxicity	Impaired theophylline clearance
Moracizine	1. Other antiarrhythmic drugs (especially class 1a)	Depressed myocardial function	Additive pharmacodynamic effects
	2. Theophylline	Reduced theophylline effect	Increased theophylline clearance
	3. Cimetidine	Increased toxicity with moracizine	Enzyme inhibition
Tocainide	1. Other antiarrhythmic drugs (especially class 1a)	Reduced myocardial contractility	Additive pharmacodynamic effects
	2. Beta adrenoceptor antagonists, and verapamil	Bradycardia and reduced myocardial contractility	Additive pharmacodynamic effects
	3. Diuretics	Reduced antiarrhythmic effects	Hypokalaemia
Beta adrenoceptor antagonists	Rifampicin and other enzyme-inducing drugs	Reduced effectiveness of propranolol and bisoprolol	Enzyme induction
	Hypoglycaemic agents	Prolonged hypoglycaemia and masking of the signs of hyperglycaemia	Reduced sympathetic responses to hypoglycaemia
	Clonidine	Increased risk of rebound hypertension on drug withdrawal	Increased sympathetic activity
	Calcium channel antagonists	Increased risk of bradycardia and heart block (diltiazem and verapamil) and heart failure (verapamil and nifedipine)	Additive pharmacodynamic effects

Drug class	Interacting drug	Effect	Mechanism
	Digoxin	Increased risk of bradycardia and heart block	Additive pharmacodynamic effects
	Cimetidine	Increased effect of latetalol and propranolol	Enzyme inhibition
	Diuretics	Increased risk of arrhythmias with sotalol	Hypokalaemia
Alpha adrenoceptor antagonists	Antidepressants, alcohol, anaesthetics and antipsychotics	Hypotension	Additive pharmacodynamic effects
	Beta blockers	Increased risk of first dose hypotension	Additive pharmacodynamic effects
	Calcium channel blockers	Increased risk of first dose and long-term hypotension	Additive pharmacodynamic effects
	Diuretics	Increased risk of first dose hypotension	Additive pharmacodynamic effects
ACE inhibitors. Angiotensin II receptor antagonists	Alcohol and other anaesthetic agents	Increased risk of hypotension	Additive pharmacodynamic effects
	Non-steroidal anti-inflammatory drugs	Attenuation of the antihypertensive and beneficial effects in heart failure	Sodium and water retention related to prostaglandin inhibition
	Other antihypertensive agents, especially diuretics	Increased risk of hypotension	Additive pharmacodynamic effects
	Cyclosporin	Increased risk of hyperkalaemia	Additive renal effects
	Potassium-sparing diuretics and potassium supplements	Increased risk of hyperkalaemia	Additive renal effects
	Lithium	Increased risk of lithium toxicity	Reduced renal excretion of lithium
	Grapefruit juice	? Increased drug effect	Enhanced absorption
Calcium channel blockers	Other antihypertensive drugs	Enhanced hypotensive effects	Additive antihypertensive effects
	Antiarrhythmic drugs, especially with verapamil and diltiazem	Increased risk of bradycardia and heart block	Additive pharmacodynamic effects. Increased plasma concentrations of quinidine

Continued

Appendix 1. *Continued*

Drug Group	Interacts with	Result of interaction	Possible mechanism
Calcium channel blockers (continued)	Rifampicin and other enzyme-inducing agents	Reduced clinical effects	Enzyme induction
	Cyclosporin	Increased risk of cyclosporin toxicity with diltiazem, verapamil and nicardipine	Reduced clearance of cyclosporin
	Lithium	Increased risk of lithium toxicity with diltiazem and verapamil	Reduced lithium clearance
	Theophylline	Enhanced theophylline effect with diltiazem and verapamil	Reduced theophylline clearance
	Cimetidine	Increased risk of toxicity	Enzyme inhibition
Direct-acting vasodilators Antihypertensive arteriolar dilators (diazoxide, minoxidil and hydralazine)	Other vasodilator drugs – ACE inhibitors, alcohol, anaesthetics, calcium channel antagonists and nitrates	Hypotension	Additive pharmacodynamic effect
	Other drugs which reduce blood pressure – beta blockers, neuroleptics and diuretics	Hypotension	Additive pharmacodynamic effect
	Non-steroidal antiinflammatory drugs	Impaired antihypertensive effect	Antiprostaglandin effects with sodium retention
Centrally acting vasodilator drugs (clonidine and methyldopa)	Other antihypertensive drugs, notably beta blockers, calcium channel antagonists and diuretics	Hypotension	Additive pharmacodynamic effect
	Other drugs which reduce blood pressure – alcohol, anaesthetics antidepressants, neuroleptics	Hypotension	Additive pharmacodynamic effect
	Non-steroidal anti-inflammatory drugs	Impaired antihypertensive effect	Antiprostaglandin effects with sodium retention

Drug class	Interacting drug	Effect	Mechanism
	Antidopaminergic agents	Reduced effectiveness of L-dopa in Parkinson's disease (methyldopa)	Central pharmacodynamic interaction
Lipid lowering drugs Cholestyramine Colestipol	Paracetamol Sodium valproate Digoxin Thiazide diuretics Thyroxine	Reduced drug effect	Reduced gastrointestinal absorption
	Warfarin		Reduced absorption Reduced vitamin K absorption?
Fibrates	Acarbose	Decreased blood glucose	Unknown
	Warfarin	Increased anticoagulant effect	Additive effects
	Warfarin	Increased anticoagulant effect	
	Statins	Increased risk of myopathy	
Statins	Rifampicin	Reduced lipid lowering effect (fluvastatin)	Enzyme induction
	Warfarin	Increased anticoagulant effect (simvastatin)	Unknown
	Digoxin	Increased risk of digoxin toxicity with atorvastatin	Unknown
	Itraconazole Cyclosporin Nicotinic acid	Increased risk of myopathy	Additive effects

Appendix 2: Glossary of Some Common Terms Used in Cardiovascular Pharmacology

ACE	Angiotensin converting enzyme.
Acetylcholine	A neurotransmitter, the effects of which can be divided into nicotinic and muscarinic responses.
Nicotinic effects	Actions of acetylcholine (resembling those of nicotine) at cholinoreceptors on the post-synaptic membrane of autonomic ganglion cells, skeletal muscle and adrenal medulla.
Muscarinic effects	Actions of acetylcholine (mimicked by muscarine) at cholino-receptors on structures receiving post-ganglionic cholinergic innervation. Important cardiovascular effects include bradycardia and negative inotropic activity which can be blocked by atropine.
Adenylyl cyclase	Enzyme responsible for producing cyclic AMP from ATP. Synonyms include adenylate cyclase and adenyl cyclase, both of which are chemically inaccurate.
ADP	Adenosine diphosphate.
Adrenaline	Transmitter/hormone produced by the adrenal medulla.
Adrenergic	Working through adrenaline. Since noradrenaline is now known to be the neurotransmitter, noradrenergic is more appropriate for describing activity of the sympathetic nervous system.
Adrenoceptor	A receptor responsible for mediating the physiological and pharmacological actions of adrenaline and noradrenaline. They are classically divided into alpha$_1$ and alpha$_2$, and beta$_1$, beta$_2$ and beta$_3$ sub-types.
Adrenoceptor antagonist	A substance which selectively inhibits responses to adrenergic nerve stimulation and injected catecholamines by combining with the adrenoceptor on the effector organs.
Agonist	A drug, hormone or neurotransmitter which when combined with a receptor induces a change in the receptor which in turn results in a biological or pharmacological response.
Angiotensin converting enzyme (ACE)	The enzyme responsible for the conversion of angiotensin I (inactive) to angiotensin II, a potent vasoconstrictor and stimulator of aldosterone release from the adrenal medulla.
Antiarrhythmic	A drug which is used to prevent, control or terminate a cardiac dysrhythmia. Most antiarrhythmic drugs can, under certain circumstances, increase the risk of developing arrhythmias, i.e. proarrhythmic.
Antiplatelet drugs	Drugs which modify platelet function by altering their adhesive properties and/or thromboxane production and so reduce the number of thrombo-embolic episodes. Examples include aspirin, sulphinpyrazone and dipyridamole.

Arachidonic acid	A 20-carbon unsaturated fatty acid with four double bonds which is the starting material for the synthesis of prostaglandins, endoperoxides and leukotrienes.
ATP	Adenosine triphosphate. The principal energy source in cell metabolism.
Automaticity	The tendency of excitable cardiac tissue to initiate spontaneous impulses and give rise to arrhythmias.
Autoreceptor	Presynaptic receptor involved in the regulation of transmitter release. It usually mediates negative feedback such as the presynaptic alpha$_2$ receptor on noradrenergic neurones.
Beta adrenoceptor antagonists	Drugs which prevent the activation of beta adrenoreceptors. Widely used to reduce heart rate and blood pressure in patients with angina pectoris, cardiac dysrhythmias, hypertension, thyrotoxicosis and anxiety.
Bradykinin	A non-peptide autacoid produced from a plasma protein precursor. Increased levels are thought to be associated with ACE inhibitor cough.
Buccal administration	A form of administration for organic nitrates in angina pectoris. The tablet is placed between the cheek and the jaw and allowed to dissolve, producing similar absorption to sublingual administration.
Calcium channel blocker	A drug which prevents the entry of calcium ions through the calcium channels in the cell membrane.
Cardiac glycoside	A glycoside having important effects on the heart. The majority are derived from the foxglove leaf and chemically are sugars in which the hydroxyl group has been replaced by another chemical group.
Catecholamine	An ethylamine derivative of catechol (1,3-dihydroxyphenol). Important catecholamines in cardiovascular pharmacology include adrenaline, noradrenaline and dopamine.
Cyclic AMP	Cyclic adenosine 3'5'-monophosphate. A substance present in most cells which is produced from ATP (adenosine-5'-triphosphate) by the membrane-bound enzyme, adenylyl cyclase. Cyclic AMP acts as a second messenger by which a variety of hormones and drugs produce their intracellular effects. cAMP regulates the activity of a protein kinase which phosphorylates other enzymes resulting in a variety of physiological responses.
Cyclic GMP	Cyclic guanosine monophosphate. Another intracellular second messenger.
Cyclooxygenase	The enzyme responsible for generating the endoperoxides and prostaglandins from arachidonic acid. It is the principal site of action for non-steroidal antiinflammatory drugs and the antiplatelet action of aspirin.
Cytochrome P450	A mixed function oxidase enzyme system present in the rough endoplasmic reticulum and in the microsomal fraction of liver extract. It consists of about 100 isoenzymes which are involved in oxidation reactions involving drugs and a variety of other chemicals. The system is inducible by barbiturates, rifampicin and carbamazepine.
Desensitisation	A change in which the receptor becomes less sensitive to the agonist and high concentrations are required to produce the original effect. A slow decrease in responsiveness is often referred to as tolerance while a more rapid effect is known as tachyphylaxis. However, these latter two terms do not

specifically refer to receptors and can occur by a variety of mechanisms.

Discontinuation syndrome A clinical condition experienced when a drug is withdrawn. Most commonly this results in recurrence of the original condition, but rebound in which the original condition is transiently more intense can also occur (chest pain and tachycardia following withdrawal of beta adrenoceptor antagonists).

Enantiomer Optical isomer.

Endothelins A family of vasoconstrictor isopeptides consisting of 21 amino acids in a sequence almost identical to the sarafotoxins produced by *Atractaspis engaddensis*, the burrowing asp. Endothelin I produced by the vascular endothelium is presently the most powerful vaoconstrictor known.

Endothelin derived relaxing factor (EDRF) A substance produced by the vascular endothelium in response to a variety of mechanical factors, hormones and neurotransmitters, notably sheer stress, acetylcholine and serotonin. It is responsible for the relaxation of smooth muscle and is now known to be nitric oxide produced from L-arginine in the endothelium.

Enzyme induction/inhibition

Induction An increase in microsomal activity usually by increased enzyme synthesis caused by a drug or other substance which acts as a substrate. This results in increased metabolism of the original drug (autoinduction) or of other drugs and physiological substances.

Inhibition Reduced or absent microsomal enzyme activity usually due to reversible or irreversible inactivation of the enzyme.

First-dose effect The rapid and excessive action of a drug following its first dose which is not repeated with subsequent doses. ACE inhibitors and short-acting alpha blockers produce greater reduction in blood pressure after the first dose than with chronic therapy in a significant percentage of patients.

Free radical An atom or molecule which has a short-lived independent existence with an unpaired electron. It is consequently very reactive and plays an important role in many biological functions and in causing cell damage.

Free radical scavenger A chemical that inactivates free radicals preventing their adverse effects on the body. Common examples include vitamin C, vitamin E, superoxide dismutase and nitric oxide.

G proteins Family of GTP-dependent trimeric proteins associated with the cell membrane. G proteins link receptors on the membrane to an enzyme which then catalyses the production of the second messenger or ion channel.

GTP Guanosine-5'-triphosphate. A high-energy phosphate enzyme synthesised from guanine, ribose and phosphate groups. Its main function is as a high-energy phosphate transfer medium, but it also acts as a second messenger in signal transduction.

Inotrope A drug which influences myocardial contractility. Positive inotropic action increases contractility and negative inotropic action reduces contractility.

Ion channel A protein structure which spans the cell membrane providing a hydrophilic pathway that permits small ions to cross the membrane. Ion channels can respond to changes in electrical potential (voltage-gated), the presence of a neurotransmitter (receptor-gated) and the level of intracellular calcium (calcium gated).

Ion channel blocker An antagonist which produces its pharmacological effect by plugging the ion channel and preventing electrical current flow through the channel.

Natriuretic A substance which increases sodium excretion by the kidney.

Nitric oxide (NO) A potent vasodilator and neurotransmitter. It carries an unpaired electron and is therefore highly reactive and after synthesis from L-arginine lasts only a few seconds. Nitric oxide is synonymous with EDRF and acts by stimulating guanylcyclase to produce the second messenger, cyclic GMP.

Partial agonist A drug which combines with specific receptors, but does not produce a response equal to the maximum that can be produced by the full agonist acting on the same receptors, even when all the receptors are occupied.

Phases of metabolism

Phase 1 reactions Reactions in which a polar group (–OH, COOH, –SH, –NH$_2$) is produced or introduced into a molecule by oxidation, reduction or hydrolysis. These metabolites usually retain a high degree of biological activity and many are sufficiently polar to be eliminated in the urine without further metabolism.

Phase II reactions Conjugation reactions in which an endogenous substrate (glucuronic acid, sulphate or glutathione) combines with a reactive group in the drug molecule or metabolite from a phase I reaction. These metabolites are rarely active and are very polar so that they are easily eliminated in the bile or urine.

Phosphodiesterase inhibitors Drugs which act by inhibiting phosphodiesterase such as milrinone, enoximone and theophylline. They have a variety of effects on the heart, bronchi and central nervous system.

Pro drug A biologically inert chemical which is metabolised (usually in the liver or gut wall) to a biologically active substance. Enalapril and most longer acting ACE inhibitors are converted to their active diacid metabolite.

Prostaglandin Twenty carbon atom fatty acids formed in tissues from phospholipids via arachidonic acid in response to a wide variety of chemical stimuli. They have important roles in inflammation, the control of smooth muscle activity, platelet function and temperature control.

Sublingual drug administration Administering a drug below the tongue to permit rapid absorption and to avoid "first-pass" metabolism, e.g. glyceryl trinitrate in angina pectoris.

Surrogate endpoint If a drug effect can be related reliably to a long-term therapeutic benefit (reduction in stroke due to lowering blood pressure) then the regulatory authorities can approve a therapeutic claim without long-term outcome data. While not ideal, the abandoning of surrogate endpoints would severely diminish the incentive to develop new drugs.

Trimeric proteins Proteins composed of three identical (homotrimeric) or different (heterotrimeric) subunits. Important examples are the G proteins.

Appendix 3: Key References for Further Reading

General reading

Brody, S. L., Larner, J. M. and Minneman, K.P. *Human Pharmacology: Molecule to Clinical* (Third Edition). Mosby Year Book Inc., St Louis, 1998.

Dollery, C. T., Frishman, W. H. and Cruickshank, J. M. *Current Cardiovascular Drugs*. Current Science Lt, London, 1993.

Goodman and Gilman. Drugs affecting renal and cardiovascular function. In *The Pharmacological Basis of Therapeutics* (Ninth Edition), Hardman, J. G. and Limbird, L. E. (Eds), New York: McGraw-Hill, Health Professions Division, 1996, pp. 683–897.

Katzung, B. G. (Ed.) *Basic and Clinical Pharmacology* (Sixth Edition). Prentice Hall International Inc. Cardiovascular-Renal Drugs, Appleton and Lang, East Norwalk Connecticut, 1995, pp. 147–249.

Melmon, K. L., Morrelli, H. F., Hoffman, B. B. and Nurenberg, D. W. (Eds). *Clinical Pharmacology: Basic Principles in Therapeutics* (Third Edition). New York: McGraw-Hill, 1992, pp. 52–185.

Rowland, M. and Tozer, T. N. In *Clinical Pharmacokinetics – Concepts and Applications* (Third Edition). Philadelphia: Lea and Febiger, 1995.

Yocobi, A., Skelly, J. P., Shah, V. P. and Benet, L. Z. (Eds) *Integration of Pharmacokinetics, pharmacodynamics and Toxicokinetics in Rational Drug Development*. New York: Plenum, 1993.

Chapter 1—Principles of Cardiovascular Function

Calver, A. J., Collier, J. and Vallance, P. Nitric oxide and cardiovascular control. *Experimental Physiology* 78 (1993): 303–326.

Chien, S., Usami, D. S. and Skalak, R. Blood flow in small tubes. In *Handbook of Physiology* (Second Edition). Section 2, Volume 4, E. M. Rankin and C. C. Michel (Eds). American Physiological Society, Bethesda, 1984, pp. 217–250.

Cowley, A. W. Long term control of arterial blood pressure. *Physiological Review* 72 (1992): 231–300.

Johnson, P. C. Autoregulation of blood flow. *Circulation Research* 59 (1986): 483–495.

Katz, A. M. *Physiology of the Heart* (Second Edition). New York: Raven Press, 1992.

Rowell, L. B. The venous system. In *Human Circulation: Regulation during Physical Stress*. New York: Oxford University Press, 1986, pp. 44–47.

Zipes, D. P. and Jalife, J. *Cardiac Electrophysiology. From Cell to Bedside*. Philadelphia: Saunders, 1990.

Chapter 2—Cellular Mechanisms of Cardiovascular Drug Action

Bristow, M. R., Kantrowitz, N. E., Ginsberg, R. and Fowler, M. B. Beta adrenergic function in heart muscle disease and heart failure. *Journal of Molecular Cell Cardiology* 17 (Suppl. 2) (1985): 41–52.

Broddie, O. E. The functional importance of beta$_1$ and beta$_2$ adrenoceptors in the human heart. *American Journal of Cardiology* 62 (1988): 24C–29C.

Catterall, W. A. Structure and function of voltage-gated ion channels. *Annual Review of Biochemistry* 64 (1995): 495–531.

Clapham, D. E. Mutations in G protein-linked receptors: novel insights on disease. *Cell* 75 (1993): 1237–1239.

Davey, M. Mechanism of alpha blockade for blood pressure control. *American Journal of Cardiology* 59 (1987): 18G–28G.

Kenakin, T. P., Bond, R. A and Bonner T. I. Definition of pharmacological receptors. *Pharmacological Reviews* 44 (1992): 351–362.

Kobilka, B. Adrenergic receptors as models for G protein-coupled receptors. *Annual Review of Neuroscience* 15 (1992): 87–114.

Kuntz, I. D. Structure based strategies for drug design and discovery. *Science* 257 (1992): 1078–1082.

Neer, E. J. Heterotrimeric G proteins: organisers of transmembrane signals. *Cell* 80 (1905): 249–257.

Perkins, J. P, Hansdorff, W. P. and Lefkowitz, R. J. Mechanisms of ligand-induced desensitization of β-adrenergic receptors. In *β-adrenergic Receptors*, J. P. Perkins (Ed.). New York: The Human Press, 1991: pp. 73–124.

Wickman, K. and Clapham, D. E. Ion channel regulation by G-proteins. *Physiological Reviews* 75 (1995): 865–885.

Chapter 3—Cardiovascular clinical pharmacology: Rational dose selection and the time course of drug action

Holford, N. H. G. and Sheiner, L. B. Understanding the dose–effect relationship. *Clinical Pharmacokinetics* 6 (1981): 429–453.

Rowland, M. and Tozer, T. N. *Clinical Pharmacokinetics* (Third Edition). Philadelphia: Lea and Febiger, 1995.

Chapter 4—Drug Treatment of Angina Pectoris

Hampton, J. R. Choosing the right β-blocker: a guide to selection. *Drugs* 48 (1994): 544–568.

Kar, S., Warkada, J. and Norlander, R. The high risk unstable angina patient. An approach to treatment. *Drugs* 43 (1992): 837–848.

Kerins, D. M. and Fitzgerald, G. A. The current role of platelet-active drugs in ischaemic heart disease. *Drugs* 41 (1991): 665–671.

Lowenstein, C. J., Dinerman, J. L. and Snyder, S. H. Nitric oxide: a physiologic messenger. *Annual of Intern Medicine* 120 (1994): 227–237.

Parker, J. D. and Parker, J. O. Nitrate therapy for stable angina pectoris. *New England Journal of Medicine* 338 (1998): 520–531.

Parratt, J. R. Nitroglycerin—the first one hundred years: new facts about an old drug. *Journal of Pharmaceutical Pharmacology* 31 (1979): 801–809.

Purcell, H., Patel, D. J. and Mulcahy, D. Nicorandil. In *Cardiovascular Drug Therapy* (Second Edition), F. H. Messerli (Ed.). Philadelphia: Saunders, 1996, 178: 1638–1645.

Rutherford, J. D. Pharmacologic management of angina and acute myocardial infarction. *American Journal of Cardiology* 72 (1993): 16C–20C.

Thandani, U. Role of nitrates in angina pectoris. *American Journal of Cardiology* 70 (1992): 43B–53B.

Tiara, N. Differences in cardiovascular profile among calcium antagonists. *American Journal of Cardiology* 59 (1987): 24B–29B.

Turpie, A. G. G. New frontiers in the management of unstable coronary artery disease. *American Journal of Cardiology* 80(5A) (1997): 21E–24E.

Van Zwieten, P. A. and Pfaffendorf, M. Similarities and differences between calcium antagonists: pharmacological aspects. *Journal of Hypertension* 11 (Suppl. 1) (1993): S3–S11.

Weiner, D. A. Calcium antagonists in the treatment of ischaemic heart disease: angina pectoris. *Coronary Artery Disease* 5 (1994): 14–19.

Chapter 5—Drug Treatment of Acute Myocardial Infarction

Anderson, H. V. and Willerson, J. T. Thrombolysis in acute myocardial infarction. *New England Journal of Medicine* 329 (1993): 703–709.

Antiplatelet Trialists' Collaboration. Collaborative overview of randomised trials of antiplatelet therapy I: prevention of death, myocardial infarction, and stroke by prolonged antiplatelet therapy in various categories of patients. *British Medical Journal* 308 (1994): 81–106.

Antman, E. M., Lau, J., Kupelnick, B. *et al.* A comparison of results of meta-analyses of randomised control trials and recommendations of clinical experts. Treatments for myocardial infarction. *Journal of the American Medical Association* 268 (1992): 240–248.

Collen, D. Towards improved thrombolytic therapy. *Lancet* 342 (1993): 34–36.

Dalen, J. E. and Hirsh, J. Third ACCP consensus conference on antithrombin therapy. *Chest* 102 (1992): 303S.

Ertl, G. Angiotensin converting enzyme inhibitors in angina and myocardial infarction. What role will they play in the 1990s? *Drugs* 46(2) (1993): 209–218.

Gershlick, A. H. and More, R. S. Treatment of myocardial infarction. *British Medical Journal* 316 (1998): 280–284.

Greenbaum, A. B. and Ohman, E. M. An update on acute myocardial infarction from recent clinical trials. *Current Opinion in Cardiology* 12 (4) (1997): 418–426.

ISIS-2 (Second International Study of Infarct Survival) Collaborative Group. Randomisation of intravenous streptokinase, oral aspirin, both or neither among 17,187 cases of suspected acute myocardial infarction. *Lancet* 2 (1988): 349–360.

Johnston, G. D. Digoxin after myocardial infarction: Does it have a role? *Drugs* 37 (1989): 577–582.

Jugdutt, B. I. Nitrates in myocardial infarction. *Cardiovascular Drugs Therapy* 8 (1994): 635–646.

Radford, M. J, Krumholz, H. M. Beta-blockers after myocardial infarction—for few patients, or many? *New England Journal of Medicine* 339 (1998): 551–552.

Verstraete, M. Thrombolytic treatment. *British Medical Journal* 311 (1995): 582–583.

Yusuf, S., Held, P. and Furberg, C. Update of effects of calcium antagonists in myocardial infarction or angina in light of the second Danish Verapamil Infarction Trial (DAVIT-II) and other recent studies. *American Journal of Cardiology* 67 (1991): 1295–1297.

Chapter 6—Drug Treatment of Heart Failure

Armstrong, P. W. and Moe, G. W. Medical advances in the treatment of congestive heart failure. *Circulation* 88 (1994): 2941–2952.

Arnold, J. M. The role of phosphodiesterase inhibitors in heart failure. *Pharmacology and Therapeutics* 57 (1993): 161–170.

Bigger, J. T., Eleiss, J. L., Roinitzky, L. M., et al. Effect of digitalis treatment on survival after acute myocardial infarction. Ameican Journal of Cardiology 55 (1985): 623–630.

Blatt, C. M., Marsh, J. D. and Smith, T. W. Extracardiac effects of digitalis. In Digitalis Glycosides, T. W. Smith (Ed.). Orlando Fla: Grune and Stratton, 1986, pp. 209–216.

Brater, D. Clinical pharmacology of loop diuretics. Drugs 41 (1991): 14–22.

Braunwald, E. ACE inhibitors—a cornerstone of the treatment of heart failure. New England Journal of Medicine 325 (1991): 351–353.

Captopril. Digoxin Multicentre Research Group. Comparative effects of therapy with captopril and digoxin in patients with mild to moderate heart failure. Journal of the American Medical Association 259 (1988): 539–544.

Cohn, J. N. The management of chronic heart failure. New England Journal of Medicine 335 (1996): 490–498.

Conti, C. R. Use of calcium antagonists to treat heart failure. Clinical Cardiology 17 (1994): 101–102.

Dormans, T. P. J., Gerlag, P. G. G., Russel, F. G. M. and Smits, P. Combination diuretics therapy in severe congestive heart failure. Drugs 55(2) (1998): 165–172.

Doughty, R. N., MacMahon, S. and Sharpe, N. Beta blockers in heart failure: promising or proved? Journal of the American College of Cardiology 23 (1994): 814–821.

Fleg, J. L., Gottlieb, S. H., Lakatta, E. G. Is digoxin really important in the treatment of compensated heart failure? A placebo controlled cross over study in patients with sinus rhythm. American Journal of Medicine 73 (1982): 244–250.

German and Austrian Xamoterol Study Group. A double blind placebo-controlled comparison of digoxin and xamoterol in chronic heart failure. Lancet 1 (1988): 489–493.

Guyatt, G. H., Sullivan, M. J. J., Fallen, E. L., et al. A controlled trial of digoxin in congestive heart failure. American Journal of Cardiology 61 (1988): 371–375.

Johnston, G. D. Adverse reactions profile: Digoxin. Prescribers Journal 1 (1993): 29–35.

Lee, D. C., Johnston, R. A., Bingham, J. B., et al. Heart failure in outpatients: a randomised trial of digoxin versus placebo. New England Journal of Medicine 306 (1982): 699–705.

Madsen, E. B., Gilpin, E., Henning, H., et al. Prognostic importance of digitalis after acute myocardial infarction. Journal of the American College of Cardiology 3 (1984): 681–689.

Milrinone Multicentre Trial Group. A comparison of oral milrinone, digoxin and their combination in the treatment of patients with chronic heart failure. New England Journal of Medicine 320 (1989): 677–683.

Muller, J. E., Turi, Z. G., Stone, R. H., et al. Digoxin therapy and mortality after myocardial infarction: experience in the MILIS study. New England Journal of Medicine 314 (1986): 265–271.

Packer, M. The development of positive inotropic agents for chronic heart failure: how have we gone astray? Journal of the American College of Cardiology 22 (1993): 119A–126A.

Packer, M., Bristow, M. R., Cohn, J. N. et al. The effects of carvedilol on morbidity and mortality in patients with chronic heart failure. New England Journal of Medicine 334 (1996): 1349–1355.

Pugh, S. E., White, N. J., Aronson, J. K., et al. Clinical, haemodynamic and pharmacological effects of withdrawal and re-introduction of digoxin in patients with heart failure in sinus rhythm after long term treatment. British Heart Journal 61 (1989): 529–539.

Ryan, T. J., Bailey, K. R., McCabe, C. H., et al. The effects of digitalis on survival in high risk patients with coronary artery disease: the Coronary Artery Surgery Study (CASS). Circulation 67 (1983): 735–742.
Singh, S. N. Congestive heart failure and arrhythmias: therapeutic modalities. Journal of Cardiovascular Electrophysiology 8 (1997): 89–97.
Smith, T. W. Digoxin in heart failure. New England Journal of Medicine 329 (1993): 51–53.
Steeds, R. P. and Charnier, K. S. Drug treatment in heart failure: lowering heart rate may reduce mortality. British Medical Journal 316 (1998): 567–568.
Taggart, A. J., Johnston, G. D., McDevitt, D. G. Digoxin withdrawal after cardiac failure in patients with sinus rhythm. Journal of Cardiovascular Pharmacology 5 (1983): 229–234.
The Digitalis Investigation Group: the effect of digoxin on mortality and morbidity in patients with heart failure. New England Journal of Medicine 336 (1997): 525–583.

Chapter 7—Drug Treatment of Hyperlipidaemia

Coro, J., Klittich, W., McGuire, A., et al. The West of Scotland Coronary Prevention Study: economic benefit analysis of primary prevention with pravastatin. British Medical Journal 315 (1997): 1577–1582.
Criqui, M. H. The emerging role of statins in the prevention of coronary heart disease. British Medical Journal 315 (1997): 1554–1555.
Drugs and Therapeutics Bulletin (1996). Management of hyperlipidaemia 34: 89–93.
Grundy, S. M. and Vega, G. L. Fibric acids: effects on lipids and lipoprotein metabolism. American Journal of Medicine 83 (1987): 9–20.
Law, M. R., Wald, N. J. and Thompson, S. G. By how much and how quickly does reduction in serum cholesterol concentration lower risk of ischaemic heart disease? British Medical Journal 308 (1994): 367–373.
Levine, G. N., Kearney, J.F. and Vita, J. A. Cholesterol reduction in cardiovascular disease: clinical benefits and possible mechanism. New England Journal of Medicine 332 (1995): 512–521.
Lipid Research Clinics Program. The Lipid Research Clinics Coronary Primary Prevention Trials Results II. The relationship of reduction in incidence of coronary heart disease to cholesterol lowering. Journal of the American Medical Association 251 (1984): 365–374.
McMurray, J. V. Reductions in mortality post-myocardial infarction: recent clinical trial data. British Journal of Cardiology 2 (Suppl 2) (1995): S15–S17.
Poole-Watson P. Recent atherosclerosis prevention studies: the message for cardiologists. British Journal of Cardiology 2 (Suppl 2) (1995): S2–S4.
Sacks, F. M., Pfeffer, M.A., Moye, L. A. et al. for the Cholesterol and Recurrent Events Trial Investigators. The effect of pravastatin on coronary events and myocardial infarction in patients with average cholesterol levels. New England Journal of Medicine 335 (1996): 1001–1009.
Scandinavian Simvastatin Survival Study Group. Randomised trial of cholesterol lowering in 4444 patients with coronary heart disease: the Scandinavian Simvastatin Survival Study. Lancet 344 (1994): 1383–1389.
Shepherd, J., Cobbe, S. M., Ford, I. et al. for the West of Scotland Coronary Prevention Study Group. Prevention of coronary heart disease with pravastatin in men with hypercholesterolaemia. New England Journal of Medicine 333 (1995): 1301–1307.
Wilztum, J. P. The oxidation hypothesis of atherosclerosis. Lancet 344 (1994): 793–795.

Chapter 8—Drug Treatment of Cardiac Dysrhythmias

Akhtar, M., Tchou, P. and Jazayeri, M. Use of calcium entry blockers in the treatment of cardiac arrhythmias. *Circulation* 80 (Suppl. IV) (1989): 31–39.

Anon. Drugs for cardiac arrhythmias. *Medical Letter on Drugs and Therapeutics* 38 (982) (1996): 75–82.

McAlister, F. A. and Teo, K. K. Antiarrhythmic therapies for the prevention of sudden cardiac death. *Drugs* S4(2) (1997): 235–252.

Nair, L. A. and Grant, A. O. Emerging class III antiarrhythmic agents: mechanisms of action and proarrhythmic potential. *Cardiovascular Drugs and Therapy* 11 (1997): 149–167.

Roden, D. M. Risks and benefits of antiarrhythmic drug therapy. *New England Journal of Medicine* 331 (1994): 785–791.

Roden, D. M, Echt, D. S, Lee, J. T. *et al.* Clinical pharmacology of antiarrhythmic agents. In *Sudden Cardiac Death*, M. E. Josephson (Ed.). Blackwell Scientific, Blackwell Science Ltd, Oxford, 1993, pp. 182–185.

Singh, B. N. Advantages of beta blockers versus antiarrhythmic agents and calcium antagonists in secondary prevention after myocardial infarction. *Journal of the American College of Cardiology* 66 (1990): 9C–20C.

Van Gelder, I. C., Brügemann, J. and Crijns, H. J. G. M. Current treatment recommendations in antiarrhythmic therapy. *Drugs* 55(3) (1998): 331–346.

Vaughan Williams, F. M. Classifying antiarrhythmic actions: by facts or speculation. *Journal of Clinical Pharmacology* 32 (1992): 964–977.

Chapter 9—Drug Treatment of Hypertension

Collins, R., Peto, R., MacMahon, S. *et al.* Blood pressure, stroke and coronary heart disease, Part 2. Short term reductions in blood pressure: overview of randomised drug trials in their epidemiological context. *Lancet* 335 (1990): 827–838.

Freis, E. D. and Papademetriou, V. Current drug treatment and treatment patterns with antihypertensive drugs. *Drugs* 52 (1996): 1–16.

Johnston, G. D. Dose response relationships with antihypertensive drugs. *Pharmacology and Therapeutics* 55 (1992): 53–93.

Johnston, G. D., Wilson, R., McDermott, B. J. *et al.* Low dose cyclopenthiazide in the treatment of hypertension: a one year community-based study. *Quarterly Journal of Clinical Pharmacology* 78 (1991): 135–141.

Joint National Committee on Detection, Evaluation and Treatment of High Blood Pressure: the sixth report of the Joint National Committee on Detection, Evaluation and Treatment of High blood Pressure (JCN V). *Archives of Internal Medicine* 157 (1997): 2413–2416.

Materson, B. J., Reda, D. J., Cushman, W. C. *et al.* Single drug therapy for hypertension in men: a comparison of six antihypertensive agents with placebo. *New England Journal of Medicine* 328 (1993): 914–921.

Messerli, F. H., Weber, M. A. and Brunner, H. R. Angiotensin II receptor inhibition. A new therapeutic principle. *Archives of Internal Medicine* 156 (1995): 1957–1965.

Neaton, J. D., Grimm, R. H. Jr, Prineas, R. J. *et al.* Treatment of Mild Hypertension Study: final results. *Journal of the American Medical Association* 270 (1993): 713–724.

Reid, J. L. New therapeutic agents for hypertension. *British Journal of Clinical Pharmacology* 43 (1996): 37–41.

SHEP Co-operative Research Group. Prevention of stroke by antihypertensive drug treatment in older patients with isolated systolic hypertension. *Journal of the American Medical Association* 265 (1991): 3255–3264.

Siscovik, D. S., Raghinathan, T. E., Psaty, B. M. *et al.* Diuretic therapy for hypertension and the risk of primary cardiac arrest. *New England Journal of Medicine* 330 (1994): 1852–1857.

van Zwieten, P. A. Different types of centrally acting antihypertensive drugs. *European Heart Journal* 13 (Suppl A) (1992): 18–21.

van Zwieten, P. A. and Pfaffendorf, M. Similarities and differences between calcium antagonists: pharmacological aspects. *Journal of Hypertension* 11 (Suppl 1) (1993): S3–S11.

Yeo, W. W. and Ramsay, L. E. Persistent dry cough with enalapril: incidence depends on method used. *J. Human Hypertens.* 1990; 4: 517–520.

Chapter 10—Drug Treatment of Thromboembolic Disease

American College of Chest Physicians Consensus Conference on Antithrombin Therapy. *Chest* 102 (1992): 305S–349S.

Baker, W. F. Thrombosis and haemostasis in cardiology: review of pathophysiology and clinical practice. *Thrombosis and Haemostasis* 4(1) (1998): 51–75.

Collen, D. and Lynon, H. R. Fibrinolysis and the control of haemostasis. In *Molecular Basis of Blood Diseases* (Second Edition), G. Stamatoyannopoulos, A. W. Nienhuis, P. W. Majerus and H. Varmur (Eds). Philadelphia: Saunders, 1992, pp. 725–752.

Collins, R., Peto, R., Baigent, C. and Sleight, P. Drug therapy: aspirin, heparin and fibrinolytic therapy in suspected acute myocardial infarction. *New England Journal of Medicine* 336 (1997): 847–860.

Griffin, J. P., D'Arcy, P. F. and Spiers, C. J. Anticoagulants. In *A Manual of Adverse Drug Reactions* (Fourth Edition). London: John Wright, 1988, pp. 137–158.

Hirsh, J. and Levine, M. N. Low molecular weight heparin. *Blood* 79 (1992): 1–17.

Hull, R. D., Raskob, G. E. and Hirsh, J. Prophylaxis of venous thrombosis: an overview. *Chest* 89 (1986): 374S–383S.

Kearon, C. Drug trials that have influenced our practice in the treatment of venous thromboembolism. *Thrombosis and Haemostasis* 78(1) (1997): 553–557.

Schussheim, A. E. and Fuster, V. Thrombosis, antithrombotic agents, and the antithrombotic approach in cardiac disease. *Progress in Cardiovascular Diseases* 40(3) (1997): 205–238.

Thomson, R., McElroy, H. and Sudlow, M. Guidelines on anticoagulant treatment in atrial fibrillation in Great Britain: variation in content and implications for treatment. *British Medical Journal* 316 (1998): 509–513.

Index